W0043310

Recent Advances in Burns and Plastic Surgery – The Chinese Experience

Recent Advances in Burns and Plastic Surgery – The Chinese Experience

Editors-in-chief:
Chang Tisheng, M.D.
Shi Jixiang, M.D.
Yang Zhijun, M.D.

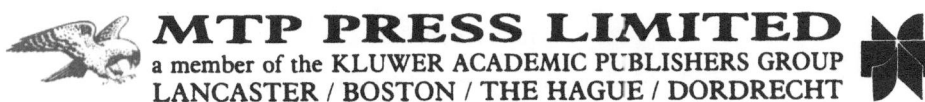

MTP PRESS LIMITED
a member of the KLUWER ACADEMIC PUBLISHERS GROUP
LANCASTER / BOSTON / THE HAGUE / DORDRECHT

Published in the UK and Europe by
MTP Press Limited
Falcon House
Lancaster, England

British Library Cataloguing in Publication Data

Recent advances in burns and plastic surgery — The Chinese Experience.
1. Burns and scalds
I. Chang, Ti-sheng   II. Shi, Ji-xiang
III. Yang, Chih-chun
617'.1106   RD96.4
ISBN-13: 978-94-010-8670-7   e-ISBN-13: 978-94-009-4900-3
DOI: 10.1007/978-94-009-4900-3

Published in the USA by
MTP Press
A division of Kluwer Boston Inc
190 Old Derby Street
Hingham, MA 02043, USA

Library of Congress Cataloging in Publication Data

Recent advances in burns and plastic surgery

Selected papers from a congress held May 16-24, 1982, in
Shanghai.
Includes bibliographies and index.
1. Burns and scalds—Treatment—Congresses. 2. Surgery,
Plastic—China—Congresses. I. Chang, Ti-sheng. II. Shi, Ji-
xiang. III. Yang, Chih-chun, 1930-   . [DNLM: 1. Burns—
surgery—congresses. 2. Surgery, Plastic—China—congresses.
W0 704 R295 1982]
RD96.4.R38 1985   617'.11059   85-19787

Copyright©1985 MTP Press Limited
Softcover reprint of the hardcover 1st edition 1985

All rights reserved. No part of this publication
may be reproduced, stored in a retrieval
system, or transmitted in any form or by any
means, electronic, mechanical, photocopying,
recording or otherwise, without prior permission
from the publishers.

Typesetting by Georgia Origination, Liverpool.

Contents

CONTENTS

Part II
Recent Advance in Burns Surgery in China

CONTENTS

Introduction

In 1958, a severely burned steel worker, the extent of whose burns was 89% of the body surface, with 20% of third degree burns, was saved by the Kwangts'e hospital (now the Rui Jin hospital) of Shanghai Second Medical College. It was the first report in the world of such a critically injured patient recovering, and seemed like a miracle at that time. During the 24 following years, a great number of papers reporting the development and advances in burn therapy in clinics and in research showed that Chinese medical investigations in the field of burns have ranked among the most advanced in the world. Plastic surgery, as an independent branch of general surgery, has been established gradually since Liberation. Recently, new techniques, including microsurgical techniques, in plastic surgery have emerged and developed, permitting rapid progress in clinical work and attracting attention and appreciation in other parts of the world.

The first national congress of Burns and Plastic Surgery was held from May 16–24 1982 in Shanghai. Over 800 papers were presented and showed how advances have been made in recent years in these two specialities. Here we present selected articles as a symposium. It is hoped that this symposium will be of value to its readers.

About the Editors

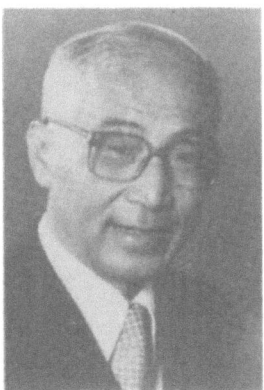

Chang Ti-sheng (Zhang Di-sheng), who was born 12 June 1916, is Professor of Surgery, Shanghai Second Medical College, Shanghai, Chief of the Department of Plastic and Reconstructive Surgery, and Director of Shanghai Ninth People's Hospital, Shanghai. Graduating from China National Central University Medical School in 1941, he studied at the Graduate School of Medicine, University of Pennsylvania, Philadelphia, USA, 1946–1948. He was Professor of Surgery, Tung Chi University Medical School, Shanghai, 1949–1955, and Professor of Surgery, Shanghai Second Medical College, Kwangts'e Hospital, Shanghai, 1956–1966, becoming Professor of Surgery, Shanghai Second Medical College, The People's Ninth Hospital, in 1966.

His publications include:

Plastic and Reconstructive Surgery (Shanghai Science and Technologic Publishing Co., 1979);

Microsurgery (edited with Dr C. W. Chen *et al.*) (Shanghai Science and Technologic Publishing Co., 1979);

Micro-Reconstructive Surgery (Beijing People's Health Publishing Co. (in press); and

over 80 articles on plastic surgery and microsurgery published in Chinese and foreign medical journals and books.

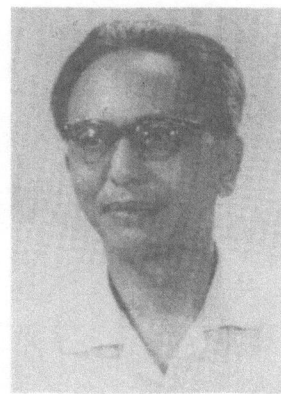

Professor Shi Jixiang (Shih Tsi-siang) born in December 1921 in Shanghai, China, graduated from the Medical Faculty of Aurora University in Shanghai. He is Chief, Burn Center of Rui-jin Hospital, Shanghai and Professor of Surgery, Shanghai Second Medical College. Author and editor of five books and numerous publications on shock, infection and burn care. Dr Shi has more than 20 years of experience in all phases of burn patient management, clinical research and teaching.

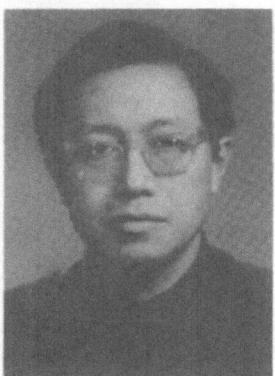

Professor Yang Zhijun (Yang Chih-chun) was educated at the School of Science (Premedical), St John's University, Shanghai (1947–1950), the School of Medicine, St John's University, Shanghai (1950–1952), graduating BS, and Shanghai Second Medical College (1952–1954), graduating MD. He was Resident Surgeon, Surgical Department, Rui-jin Hospital (1954–1960), Visiting Surgeon, Surgical Department, Rui-jin Hospital (1960–1966), and Chief of the Burn Unit, Rui-jin Hospital (1966–1978). Since 1978 he has been Professor of Surgery, Rui-jin Hospital, and Chief of the Burn Unit again since 1979.

Part I

Recent Advances in Plastic Surgery in China

1 Corrections of Contractures in Patients Surviving Very Extensive Deep Burns

CHEN WENYUAN, ZHU ZHAOMING, GUO ZHENRONG and YIN SHAOJIE

Trauma Center, Postgraduate Medical College and 304 Hospital of the PLA

In recent years, along with significant advances in the management of burns, more and more patients have survived the ravages of very extensive deep burns. As a result, an increasing number of people are in urgent need of plastic and reconstructive surgery because of their multiple scar contractures, which either seriously hamper their daily activities or cause disfigurements so grotesque that they are afraid of going outdoors. On the other hand, these patients usually lack virgin donor sites to donate entirely normal skin for repair purposes. In addition, it is often very hard to establish peripheral venous lines because of the deep burns which have destroyed many superficial veins, rendering the replacement of fluid and blood lost during operations quite difficult. Another frequently encountered problem is the difficulty in inserting an endotracheal tube for anesthesia due to chin–neck or even chin–chest adhesions. All the four patients who came into our hands for the correction of their scar contractures had the above features. A retrospective study was made on them, in the hope that some useful lessons could be derived from it.

CLINICAL MATERIALS

The extent of the original burns, early treatment, contracture sites and conditions of contractures of the four patients are summarized in Table 1.1.

Determination of operative priority for different sites of contractures depends upon the extent and depth of the burn and the selection of anesthetic technique. The techniques we used to correct various contractures included Z-plasties, Z-plasties with free skin grafting, severance of the scar to release its contraction plus free grafting, and excision of the scar followed by free skin grafting (Table 1.2).

Due to the inadequacy of donor areas, the scalp which had been repeatedly used in the treatment of acute burn, and areas of healed superficial burn were again used to donate skin (Table 1.3).

3

Table 1.1 Extent of original burn and early treatment

Patient/sex/age	1/M/8 y	2/F/21 y	3/M/23 y	4/F/22 y
Burn area total/III°	90/70	90/85	96/76	95/75
Early management for III°	Natural separation (NS) & auto-graft	Excision, chest, abd., limbs; NS remaining	Excision, chest, abd., limbs; NS remaining	Excision, chest, abd., limbs, NS remaining
Sites and conditions of contractures	1. Chin–chest, eversion of lip, scoliosis of spine.	1. Chin–chest, eversion of lip.	1. Both axillas, no abduction.	1. Chin–neck, lip eversion.
	2. Both axillas, abduction impossible.	2. Both axillas, abduction less than 30°.	2. Ectropion eyelids, corneal opacity.	2. Axillary webs.
	3. Perineal web.	3. Both knees, 110–170°.	3. Perineal web, false passage outside anus.	3. Perineal web.
	4. Both popliteal with cracks.	4. Both elbows, extension 160°.	4. Chin–neck, lip eversion.	4. Both elbows, extension 160°.
	5. Equina deformity, bil.	5. Perineal web, no abduction of thighs.	5. Both knees extension 170°, flexion 100°.	5. Unstable scars.
	6. Both elbows with cracks.	6. Multiple ulcers in scars.	6. Gluteal flexion of hips 60°.	
	7. Clawhand, left.		7. Multiple ulcerations.	
Normal skin (% TBSA)	Lower abd. (2%) Scalp (2%)	Scalp (2%)	Scalp (2%)	Scalp (3%)

Table 1.2 Various procedures used and number of operations in the four cases

Patient	Z-plasties	Z-plasties & grafts	Severance & grafts	Excision & grafts
1	1	2	9	5
2	5	1	—	4
3	—	4	6	2
4	11	1	3	2

After multiple plastic operations, patients 1, 2 and 4 are able to carry out simple work, while patient 3 is also able to take care of his daily life by himself.

Table 1.3 Number of donations from various donor areas and their healing time

Patient	Number of donations		Average healing time (days)		Secondary grafting in BSS* after donating
	Scalp	BSS*	Scalp	BSS*	
1	9	5	7	24	—
2	2	6	7	40	1
3	9	4	10	32	2
4	1	5	7	33	—

* Burn-scarred skin

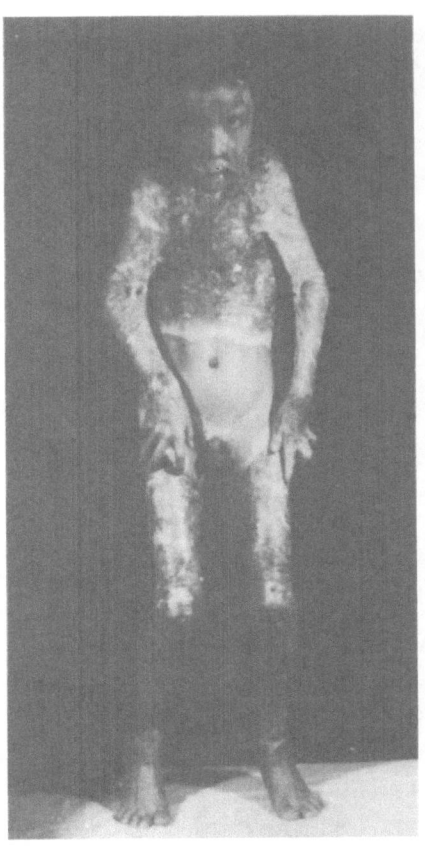 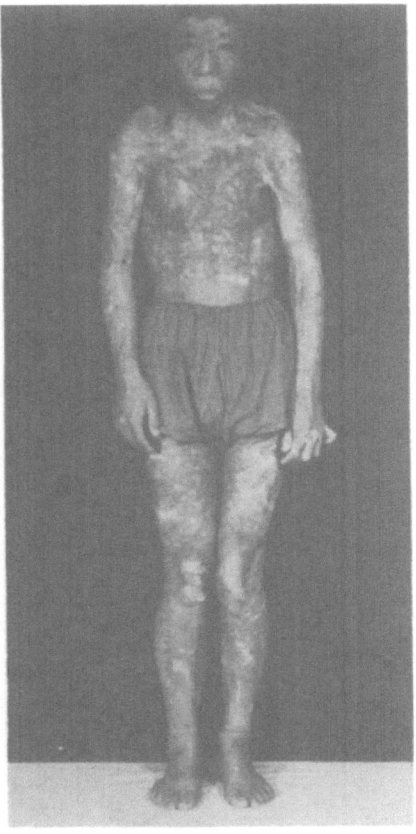

a   b

Figure 1.1 **a,** Before correction (8 years old) **b,** After correction (16 years old)

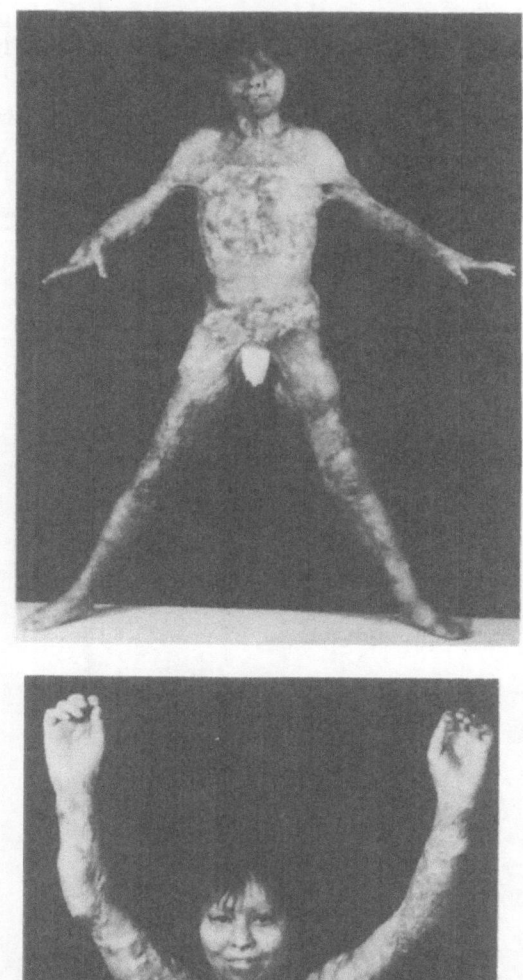

Figure 1.2   Case 4. **a,** Before correction. **b,** After correction

DISCUSSION

There are invariably multiple disabling cicatricial contractures all over the body in the survivors of very extensive deep burns, demanding a number of plastic operations before they become self-dependent or esthetically acceptable to society, not to say able to return to their previous work. To achieve this goal, our experiences gained from the management of these four patients make us realize that the following problems should be seriously considered prior to the beginning of a series of operations.

Operative priority and anesthetic technique

Which contracture should be given the priority for operation, and what anesthetic technique should be chosen?

Generally speaking, the operative sites of priority are the ones with the worst deformity, those contractures whose correction facilitates subsequent operations, those which are most crippling, or those the patient has the strongest desire to have corrected. For example, patient 3 was unable to abduct either of his arms, preventing him from taking care of himself. Therefore, we decided that the axillary contractures should be tackled first. After Z-plasties and free skin grafting in the right axilla had been performed, the patient regained a good range of movements of his right hand, enabling him to take meals by himself. In addition, he was able to lie prone so that his back could be used as a donor site. Because multiple operations were necessary in all the patients, we preferred to use local infiltrating anesthesia or nerve blocks (e.g. brachial plexus block). However, many patients tolerated pain less and less during operations with elapse of time, and we were compelled to resort to general anesthesia in some extensive plastic operations. In case of a cervical contracture, transnasal introduction of an endotracheal tube was the only feasible way to give general anesthesia. If there was difficulty in introducing the endotracheal tube, it would be mandatory that the contracture be released under local anesthesia before operations in any other sites can be attempted. Therefore, it is wise to give the neck contracture priority if it is serious enough to prevent easy introduction of an endotracheal cannula. In all of the four patients we have handled, the chin–chest adhesion was released before any operation for which general anesthesia was indicated.

Owing to the fact that all these patients had had their extremity eschar excised, the peripheral veins eligible for venepuncture were lacking over such areas as the elbow, forearm and ankles. Sometimes, some veins were left over the dorsum of the foot or hand, and they were accessible for infusions of small amounts of fluids and medication. Although they were not good enough for rapid infusions of fluids and blood, they were good enough to meet the needs of anesthesia. However, if blood loss is expected to be great during the operation, a jugular venous line should be established before the operation. If this jugular line is not feasible, either because it might interfere with the surgical procedure or it is inaccessible, a subclavian or femoral line should be made available before the operation begins. In our series, a subclavian venous line was employed during the perineal repair in patient 3 and inguinal repair in patient 4.

Extent of operations, and intervals between

What should be the appropriate extent of each operation, and how long should be the interval between two operations?

Although it is the general opinion that operations should begin after the hypertrophic scars become softened and all remaining wounds are healed, serious ectropion of eyelids or contractures of the hand should be corrected as early as possible. Patient 3 was admitted for plastic and reconstructive surgery 2 years after the development of ectropion of his left eyelids, and there was already corneal opacity. The ectropion was corrected successfully, but his vision never recovered.

As there was always difficulty in establishing an adequate venous line for blood transfusion, it is preferable to limit the extent of each operation. It is advisable to allow the patient to recover from each operation, and to schedule the next operation for when the hemoglobin value returns to within normal range. After several operative procedures, it is also advisable that the patient be discharged from the hospital to recuperate further at home, and then readmitted for repair of other contractures. Sometimes, operations are postponed because of episodes of acute cellulitis or erysipeloid infections arising from some minor cracks in the scar. For the parts where repeated attacks of such infections occur, it is advisable to remove the infection foci followed by immediate skin grafting under the cover of appropriate antibiotics.

Selection of operative procedures

The most frequently used reconstructive techniques consist of Z-plasty and its various modifications, Z-plasty supplemented by free skin grafting, severance of scar tissue plus free skin grafting, and excision of scar tissues followed by grafting. We believe the procedures of choice should be Z-plasty and its modifications. Although the presence of extensive scars in the vicinity of the Z-plasty necessarily limits its gain in length, it still has the advantage of sparing skin grafting and less contraction in the long run. The latter is especially important in children. In patient 1, Z-plasties were done in the perineal region at the age of 8 years, and contraction has not recurred 10 years later. On the other hand, in the correction of his bilateral popliteal contractures, the scars were severed and the defects were grafted with split thickness grafts. At the time of operation, the result seemed to be quite satisfactory, but with the growth of the child, chaps developed frequently and contracture finally recurred, and it took three more operations to overcome the contraction. Nevertheless, the contraction was partially due to the thinness of skin grafts harvested from the scalp.

Sometimes, Z-plasty alone is not sufficient to gain the desired length of skin in correcting the contracture; then, transposition of local skin flaps supplemented by free skin grafting can be used to good avail. Contraction of free skin grafts will be prevented by the interposed skin flaps, albeit they themselves are scarred. The bilateral arm–chest adhesions and marked perineal web with buried anal opening in patient 3 were all repaired by this technique with satisfactory results.

When the tissues surrounding the contracting scar are unyielding and taut, it is desirable to sever the scar, correct the contracture, and cover the expanding raw surface with ample skin grafts, instead of doing Z-plasty. Or the scar is excised, especially if there are chaps and ulcers, and then the resulting open wound is covered with skin grafts. As the donor sites are usually inadequate, excision should be limited to the unstable scars only.

Selection of donor sites

In a case of very extensive deep burn such as the four patients presented here, even the tiny areas of unburned skin have been used as donor sites more than once in an effort to cover all the deep burn wounds in the acute stage. Therefore, the donor sites which are going to donate skin grafts are themselves scarred. Although the scalp has been repeatedly used as a donor site, only a small amount of scar tissues have been formed, so that they can again be used in later reconstructive work.

The scalp is a very good donor site, because it heals rapidly, and new crops of split thickness skin can usually be harvested at 1 week intervals, provided only thin split thickness grafts are taken. The disadvantage of using scalp as a donor site is that the grafts are narrow and thin, so that they have a stronger tendency to contract and they do not tolerate friction well.

The areas of healed superficial burn or previously used donor sites have sometimes been used to obtain continuous strips of skin grafts with the aid of a drumtype dermatome. The results have been quite satisfactory. Unfortunately, such a donor site is so difficult to re-epithelialize by itself without a secondary grafting. In patient 3, the donor site on the back showed no sign of epithelialization until grafted with skin taken from the scalp.

It is our experience that the scalp can be used as a donor site in repairing contractures situated on the extremities and trunk. But for the face and hands we prefer skin grafts obtained from areas of healed superficial burn to give better functional and cosmetic results.

SUMMARY

Four patients who had suffered from very extensive burns previously (total burn area exceeded 90% and third degree burn over 70%) were admitted for correction of contractures. Experience gained from management of these patients is summarized as follows.

(1) A plan should be drawn up as regards the sequence of operations for various sites of contractures and disfigurements. It is preferable to give the neck contracture priority for surgery, in order to facilitate the administration of general anesthesia in subsequent operations.

(2) Lack of peripheral veins in such patients hinders rapid replacement of fluids and blood. Therefore, it is advisable that the extent of each operation be limited and intervals between operations prolonged.

(3) Z-plasties supplemented by skin grafts from the scalp are the procedures of first choice.

(4) For the extremities and trunk, the scalp is used as the major donor site, while for the hands and face, the healed superficially burned areas may be used as donor sites to obtain better functional and cosmetic results.

2 Experiences in Treatment of 713 Patients with Postburn Scar Contracture (1966–1980)

CHANG TI-SHENG, WANG TEH-CHAO, GUAN WEN-XIANG, WEI LIAN-CHUN, WANG WEN-I, WANG WEI and TING CHO-SHEN
Department of Plastic and Reconstructive Surgery, Shanghai Second Medical College

From 1966 to 1980, there were 713 patients admitted to our hospital for the treatment of scar contracture over various parts of the body, of whom 468 were males and 245 females, a ratio of about 2:1. More than half (461 patients, 64.7%) of the patients were within the age range 21–50 years. The hand, the face and the neck are the three commonest sites of burn, in that order of frequency[1,2]. The commonest cause of burn is flame (65%).

TREATMENT OF THE DESTRUCTIVE FACIAL SCAR

Generally speaking, the result of treatment of destructive facial scar is still far from satisfactory. The relevant factors are hyperpigmentation of the grafted area and the mask-like appearance of the grafted face due to lack of expression.

However, skin grafting in the area around the mouth was always gratifying in our experience, because the scar contracture over this area was usually the most striking and functional interference the severest. For instance, eversion of the lips usually resulted in exposure of gingiva which later became chronically infected and bled easily. Incisors were often seen protruding from the mouth owing to lack of constant pressure exerted by the lips. The patient would also experience difficulty in opening his mouth and this to some degree interfered with speech and feeding. Drooling was also noted in some patients as a result of inability to close their lips. Underdeveloped chin was occasionally observed in those who sustained burn in childhood. In fact, many of our patients requested operation in this region even after they had been informed of or had seen the shortcomings of the skin graft.

Our experience has shown that the skin taken from the upper chest, the inner aspect of the upper arm or lower chest wall usually has less color change after transplantation than that from any other regions of the body, though this does not necessarily mean the final solution of the problem. Therefore, these three regions have become the first choice of donor site in our hospital unless they have already been destroyed by the burn.

Full thickness graft versus split thickness graft is still a subject of controversy. In our hands they have not so far shown any significant difference in color change, but we prefer thick split thickness skin graft because the management of its donor site is much simpler and easier than that of the full thickness graft. Figure 2.1 shows our favored way of skin grafting around the mouth. The lateral margin of the graft should either lie along or preferably a little bit lateral to the nasolabial fold and should be in a curved shape. It is advisable to make the new mouth slightly larger than the normal purposely to compensate the contraction of the skin graft which usually occurs at a later date. Avoidance of a conspicuous straight line at the upper margin of the graft is another important measure to improve the appearance. This can be accomplished by inserting a small triangular piece of skin in the region between the nasolabial fold and the alar and another piece into the nostril floor on both sides. Care should also be taken to build the new upper lip with its longitudinal length not longer than 2 cm, otherwise the vermilion will be inverted and looks too thin.

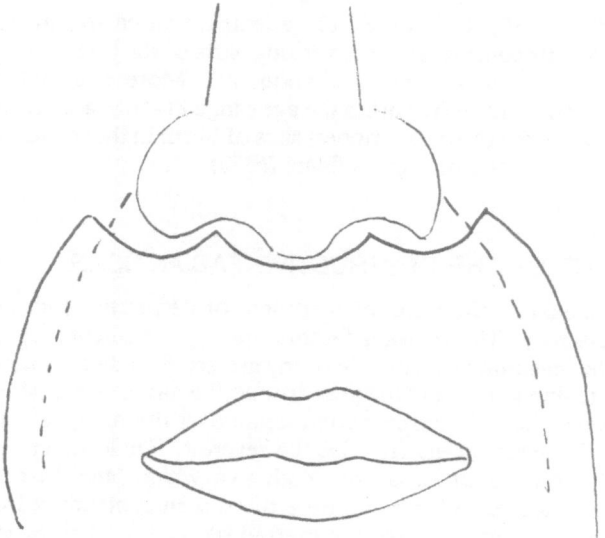

Figure 2.1   Sketch showing favored way of skin grafting around the mouth. Dotted lines represent the nasolabial fold

Everted lower lip in a longstanding case usually becomes hypertrophied and necessitates excision of excessive tissue before a normal-looking appearance of the lower lip can be expected. Transverse excision or sagittal wedge shaped excision of the lower lip can be done depending on the need of the individual case (Figure 2.2).

Though color change is less striking with the flap or tube, they are still usually too bulky for a good appearance. For this reason, a flap or tube procedure is

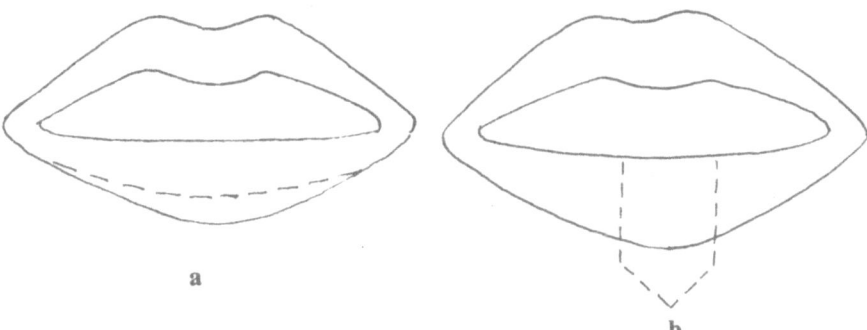

Figure 2.2 a, Sagittal wedge shaped excision of the hypertrophied lower lip. **b,** Transverse excision of the hypertrophied lower lip

only indicated for cases whose facial muscles have already been severely damaged or for cases who have an underdeveloped chin, for in either case a skin graft is no longer a benefit to the patient. In recent years a free forearm flap has been introduced in our patients with underdeveloped chin in order to shorten hospitalization and operative stages.

TREATMENT OF SCAR CONTRACTURE OF THE NECK

In our present series, 192 patients had scar contracture over the neck which required treatment, constituting 26.9% of the series.

In our opinion, almost all scar contractures of the neck can be satisfactorily corrected with a free skin graft. In order to achieve a complete release of scar contracture, it has been our routine to excise the scar together with the platysma which always shows signs of fibrosis. On rare occasions the excision should include the prethyroid muscles if they are also involved in the contracture.

The mandibulocervical angle is a precious gem for the cosmetic appearance of the neck. Therefore, every effort should be made to dissect and remold it out. We used to carry out the dissection in the groove between the hyoid bone and the thyroid cartilage. It is important to leave as little areolar tissue as possible in the groove if a conspicuous angle is expected.

The lateral margin of the wound should be made in a zigzag fashion in order to avoid linear scar contraction of the wound edge postoperatively. Not infrequently, we found that a straight line wound edge lying along or even posterior to the midlateral line of the neck had a tendency to move forward postoperatively because of the contraction of the skin graft later. This lineal junctional scar would to some extent restrict the movement of the neck.

The continuous wearing of a splint for 6 months or more will help prevent postoperative contraction of the grafted skin. Poor surgical result or even recurrence of contracture was often seen in patients who did not follow this advice strictly, especially in children. In recent years we have devised a foam rubber collar which has been proved effective and comfortable for this purpose.

It is inexpensive and also so simple that it can easily be made by the patient himself or members of his family.

An equally good result can also be obtained by local flap transfer if one takes good care to see that the flap is not improperly brought up to a level higher than that of the mandibulocervical angle, otherwise the cosmetic result will be un-satisfactory.

TREATMENT OF POSTBURN DEFORMITIES OF THE HAND

In our series, there were 701 postburn hands, of which 114 had developed into 'clawhand' deformity, constituting 6.2% of this series.

Our experience showed that clawhand was a considerable disaster to the patient, especially to those who were crippled by involvement of both hands. The deformed hand lost most of its vital functions, so that the patient was not only unable to resume his former work but in some cases such patients even had difficulty in taking care of themselves in their daily life.

Prevention is imperative, because once clawhand deformity is established surgery can only restore a part of the lost function. The development of the deformity depends largely on the depth of the burn, but the interval between the burn and the appropriate reconstructive operation also plays an important role in its development. Some of our cases had only sustained a superficial burn on their hands as evidenced by clinical signs, but the deformity was as severe as that of a deep burn, only because of lack of early treatment.

In our opinion, a hand with deep second degree burn or even third degree burn will retain most of its vital function if it is treated appropriately with a skin graft during the early postburn period. Even the established clawhand will benefit greatly if it is treated early. Therefore, we suggest that reconstructive surgery should be carried out within 3–6 months after the healing of the hands and the interval should not exceed 6 months. In the early case, there is no or little secondary changes in the joint and its surrounding soft tissue, therefore a free skin graft is all that is needed. As for a longstanding clawhand, severe secondary changes are usually present and a complete reduction of the joints is often associated with exposure of deep structures. Hence, a flap or tube is necessary for the reconstruction and this requires several stages to complete. Recently, we have used an island forearm flap, a free forearm flap, or a free scalp fascia with superimposed skin graft in some carefully selected cases, thus reducing the operative stages to one. The result is much the same as the conventional flap or tube graft procedure.

In this series, we also tried Krukenberg's operation on both heavily scarred forearm stumps of a girl, and obtained an excellent result (Figure 2.3).

TREATMENT OF SCAR CONTRACTURE OF THE AXILLARY REGION

There were 60 cases with scar contracture of the axillary region, constituting 8.4% of the series.

For a web scar in which there is enough surrounding normal skin, a single Z-

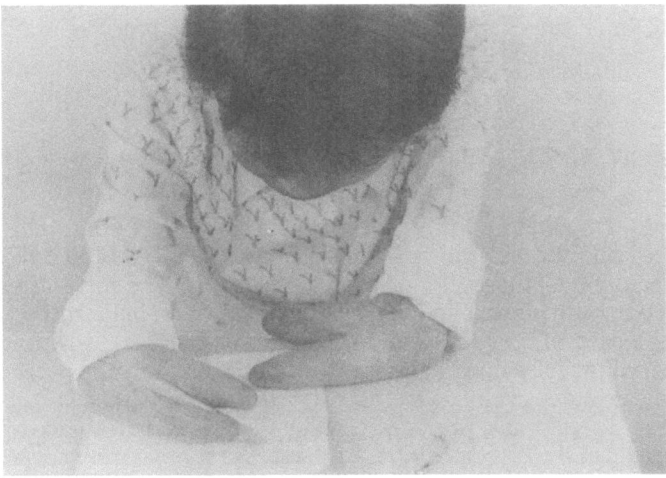

Figure 2.3 Functional restoration of the amputated hands after Krukenberg's operation

plasty or multiple Z-plasties are recommended, while in a severe case where considerable deficiency of skin is present, additional tissue is often needed.

Our past experience convinced us that a mere skin graft usually did not serve well because of its late postoperative contraction. Local flap or flaps were always associated with a better result even when they were designed on a matured scar.

Many patients with scar contracture in the axillary region had a small piece of normal skin hidden at the apex of the axilla. This piece of skin had escaped the burn because of its location, and was usually the source of repeated infection and the cause of sinus formation. Excision of the scar should always include this piece of skin before a radical cure can be expected.

In longstanding cases the brachial plexus usually became shortened with the passing of time. Care should be taken not to injure it after the contracture is released. This complication occurred once in a child in this series. Fortunately paralysis of the brachial plexus was only temporary and recovery took place a few months after the operation.

TREATMENT OF TALIPES EQUINUS AND TALIPES EQUINOVARUS DUE TO SCAR CONTRACTION AND SHORTENING OF TENDON CALCANEUS

Extensive and severe scar contracture over the posterior aspect of the leg, especially over the region overlying the calcaneal tendon, occasionally caused talipes equinus or talipes equinovarus in our patients. Solution of this problem often required excision of the responsible scar and lengthening of the calcaneal tendon. Formerly we used to replace the scar tissue with a flap or a tube before proceeding to lengthen the calcaneal tendon. This always took time and gave much discomfort to the patient because of the cross-leg immobilization required. In recent years we have begun to solve the problem in different ways without the preliminary flap replacement of scar tissue.

Lengthening of scar tissue together with calcaneal tendon as a whole by Z-plasty

This type of operation was indicated for a less severe case, and it has been performed on four legs with good result. A Z incision was placed directly over the lower third of the posterior aspect of the leg. The incision went directly through the overlying scar and the underlying calcaneal tendon. Two rectangular flaps composed of scar tissue and calcaneal tendon were thus formed. When these two rectangular flaps were interpositioned, not only the overlying scar but also the calcaneal tendon were lengthened and the ankle joint was thereby reduced to a right angle position. Usually there were two small triangular raw areas created at the two extremities of the Z. These areas were covered with skin graft which usually took well because no denuded tendon was present in the wound.

Correction of talipes equinovarus by triple or quadruple arthrodesis

Two female patients had extensive burn scar over their bodies with severe talipes equinovarus of both legs. In one patient, triple arthrodesis was performed on both legs through incisions which went through the scar and bone tissue. A wedge block consisting of scar tissue and bone was removed from each foot so as to correct the equinovarus deformity. The ankle was maintained in a right angle position by a plaster of Paris cast after the operation. The scar wound healed uneventfully and bone union was also noted in due time. The patient is now able to walk with her heels touching the ground.

In the other patient, as her deformity was too severe for a triple arthrodesis, a quadruple arthrodesis was performed first on one of her legs. Wound healing and bone union were good and the operative result was satisfactory. Therefore, a second similar operation was scheduled on the other leg. During operation, separation of the scar from the underlying bone was done for a short distance in order to gain better access to the joint space. It was this portion of scar that necrosed after the operation. As a result, the bone surface was exposed, and it was complicated by chronic osteomyelitis. After intensive care, the wound took several months to heal and bone union was also effected. However, equinovarus deformity still persisted, although with less severity.

SUMMARY

A total of 713 patients with postburn scar contracture are analysed in this chapter and treatment of scar contractures on the face, neck, axilla, hand and leg is discussed. A good result was obtained in all regions except the face, the problems in this region being due to hyperpigmentation and mask-like appearance.

REFERENCES

1. Chang Ti-sheng (1979). *Plastic and Reconstructive Surgery*. (Shanghai: Shanghai Scientific and Technologic Publishing Co.)
2. Chang Ti-sheng *et al*. (1978). Treatment and prevention of scar contraction on the face, neck and hand after extensive burn. *Chinese J. Surg.*, **16**, 76

3 Surgical Treatment of Postburn Contracture Deformities – An Analysis of 686 Cases

PENG FU-REN

Department of Surgery, Guangxi Medical College, Nanning, Guangxi

A series of 686 cases (928 sites) of postburn contracture deformities were surgically treated in our department from 1971 to 1981. Good–excellent results of 91.6% were obtained, according to a long-term follow-up study.

CLINICAL DATA

Of the 686 patients, 419 were male and 267 female (364 adults and 322 children). Their ages ranged from 1 to 55 years. Topographic distribution of deformities is shown in Table 3.1.

Table 3.1 Topographic distribution of deformities

Location	Patients (n)	%
Face and neck	171	18.5
Trunk	13	1.4
Axilla	40	4.3
Elbow	46	5.0
Hand	415	44.9
Knee	82	8.9
Foot	139	15.0
Perineum	19	2.0

SURGICAL TECHNIQUE

Scar excision and contracture release

Thorough scar resection and complete contracture release are essential, taking constant care not to injure the underlying nerves and blood vessels. A general consideration of the scar contracture should be made before surgical intervention and any deep incision and hasty wide scar excision be avoided.

Generally, the incision has to be started at the critical point of the scar and contracture released gradually under the scar. In cases of excessive tension of the deep fascia or tendons, multiple transverse incisions on the deep fascia and cutting or lengthening of the tendons are useful. The nerves and vessels should not be under tension after contracture release. In the case of secondary bone and joint deformities, violent traction should be avoided; otherwise, bone fracture and joint capsular tearing are very probable. Contracture releasing followed by skin grafting to the maximum is a sine qua non of a good postoperative result. Staged operations are often necessary in longstanding contracture of the neurovascular bundle.

Skin defect cover

The wound after scar excision can be covered in the following ways:

(1) Split thickness or full thickness skin grafts (647 sites, 70%): this method is used in large skin defects. Thorough scar excision, complete hemostasis, even pressure dressing and local immobilization are the key points to success in skin grafts. This technique was successful in all of our 647 skin grafts (Figures 3.1, 3.2).

(2) Local skin flap (103 sites, 11.1%): this is used to repair small areas of skin loss. Satisfactory results were obtained in our 103 local flap repairs.

(3) Free skin graft combined with local skin flap (125 sites, 13.5%): this is used to cover the large skin defect in dynamic regions (joint with exposed

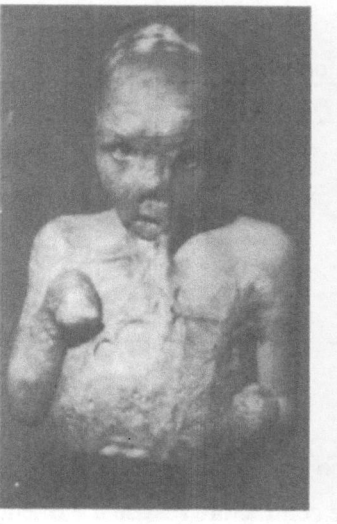 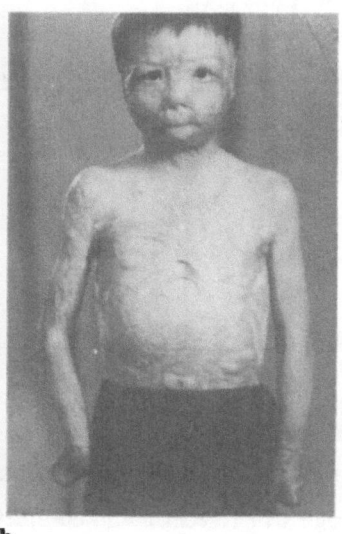

a   b

Figure 3.1 a, Before surgical correction. b, One year after surgical correction by free skin graft

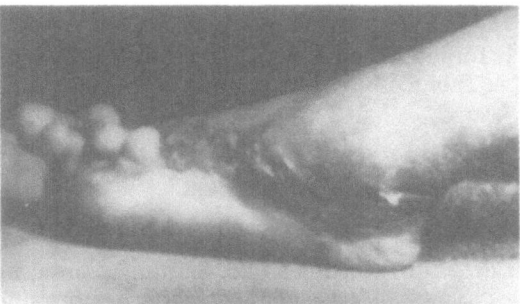

a

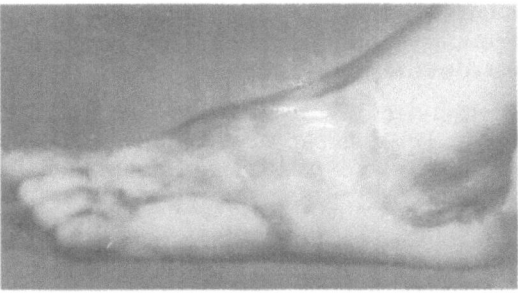

b

Figure 3.2 **a,** Before surgical correction. **b,** After surgical correction by free skin graft

tendons and neurovascular bundle). Postoperative retraction of the skin flap is insignificant and functional recovery has been quite good in our series.

(4) Distant skin flap or tubular flap (50 sites, 5.4%): this is used to cover the wound where the tendons, bones, nerves or vessels are exposed and split skin grafts are difficult to take.

Table 3.2 Operative results in 405 patients

Grades	Clinical criteria	Case (n) (%)
Excellent	Deformity corrected & complete or nearly complete functional recovery	237 (67.4)
Good	Deformity nearly corrected with functional improvement	98 (24.2)
Poor	No apparent esthetic & functional recovery	34 (8.4)

RESULT

A follow-up study for more than 2 years was carried out on 405 patients and the results are listed in Table 3.2.

DISCUSSION

The deciding factors of the operative results are as follows:

(1) Duration of deformity: the longer the deformity duration, the poorer the postoperative results. In longstanding postburn deformity, the underlying tendons, nerves and blood vessels are shortened and the joints deformed and surgical correction will be very difficult if not impossible, and very poor postoperative results will ensue. All of our 34 cases of longstanding postburn deformity (more than 7 years) had poor postoperative results. Early surgical correction is reasonable[1].

(2) Extent of deformity: the deeper the scar involvement, the poorer the postoperative results. For example, electric burns, which always involve the deep structures, had poorer postoperative results than the thermal ones.

(3) Thickness of the skin grafts: the thicker the skin graft, the less the postoperative graft contraction. Full thickness skin grafts are advisable in the reconstructive surgery of the head, neck and hand regions.

(4) Survival rate of skin grafts: complete take of skin grafts is essential to good postoperative results[2].

REFERENCES

1. Chang Ti-sheng *et al*. (1978). Prevention and treatment of scar contracture after extensive burns in the face, neck and hands. *Chinese J. Surg.*, **16**, 76
2. Huang, T. T. *et al*. (1978). Ten years of experience in managing patients with burn contractures of the axilla, wrist, elbow and knee joints. *Plast. Reconstr. Surg.*, **61**, 70

4 Severe Local Radiation Injury of the Skin – a Report of 22 Cases

GAO XUE-SU
Department of Plastic and Reconstructive Surgery, Second Army Medical College
CHANG TI-SHENG
Department of Plastic and Reconstructive Surgery, Shanghai Second Medical College

Since 1956, 22 cases of severe local radiation injury of the skin have been admitted to our two colleges. This chapter is devoted to a brief account of our experiences in the diagnosis, treatment and prevention of such injuries.

CLINICAL DATA

Fifteen cases in this series sustained radiation injuries from overexposure to X-ray during screening; 12 of the 15 were injured during fracture reduction or removing of foreign bodies. Eight of these were members of staff – orthopedic surgeons or X-ray technicians – and the other four were patients being screened. Both hands were involved in five staff members and the left hand alone in the remaining three. The dorsal aspects of the second, third, fourth and fifth fingers together with their tips were commonly seen and the injury tended to be more severe in the distal parts of these digits than the proximal. Fortunately the thumb was always spared. The ulcers, though shallow, usually involved full thickness of the skin. As the surgeon would hold the patient's limb with his left hand, which was then motionless and nearest to the tube, the left hand was more often injured than the right, and the dorsal aspect more often than the volar. In the four patients being screened the radiation injury occurred at the fracture line or around the site of a foreign body and the injury they sustained tended to be deeper than the surgeons'. Two of the injuries were so deep that they destroyed the structures down to the bone. The remaining three patients were injured in the back and waist regions during barium meal examination of the gastrointestinal tract; the ulcers were oval and 10 cm deep, penetrating into their spines and spinal muscles.

23

LESSONS AND DISCUSSION

Problems related to diagnosis

The clinical signs of radiation injury of the skin are similar to those of thermal burn. However, as the biological response induced by ionizing radiation does not manifest itself as immediately as that induced by thermal burn, and the incidence of injury is relatively low when compared with the other injuries, the definite diagnosis of radiation injury may be delayed. For example, in six of our series the condition was diagnosed only after a search of several months to 1 year for causes of a stubborn ulcer not responding to any treatment. In one patient with erythema and swelling in the fingertip, the condition was misdiagnosed as paronychia and the site was mistakenly incised and drained. Another case, where the patient was injured during exploratory surgery under screening and had erythema and swelling in the involved area, was mistaken for infection and accordingly the patient was treated with a 50% alcohol wet dressing. As a result, abrupt breakdown of the local skin occurred the next day. Dermatitis was diagnosed in another three cases, and the subjects continued working under direct exposure to the X-ray beams until unbearable pain intervened as a result of severe injury. Such a mistake should never occur.

Early diagnosis of acute radiation injury is often difficult but a timely diagnosis is by no means impossible because a positive exposure history combined with specific clinical signs can still provide valuable clues if one is on the alert. Most patients in this series experienced in the early stage an abnormal feeling of numbness or pain and showed signs of erythema and swelling in the irradiated area similar to that of allergic reaction or acute infection. Therefore, the possibility of radiation injury must be considered first if those signs manifested themselves after radiation. Blisters that soon break down to become radiation ulcers are often encountered in severe cases during the basic reactive stage. The typical ulcer has a sharp edge and irregular base with dirty yellowish thick discharge. Granulation is scarce because the healing process is retarded. The skin around the ulcer always shows signs of involvement; the nearer it is to the ulcer, the more severe the damage will be. The skin immediately adjacent to the ulcer is pale, dry and glistening, encircled by another zone of brown (hyperpigmentation), thin and atrophic skin. Beyond that zone is normal skin. All these prominent features are helpful clues for the establishment of a definite diagnosis. In addition, pain not only is a common and suggestive symptom but tends to intensify with the passage of time. Sometimes the pain may be of intolerable severity. In one case of radiation injury of the hand, the pain was so terrible that it could only be relieved by 6-hourly intramuscular administration of Dolantine 100 mg. Nevertheless, most pains subside or become less severe after the ulcer is grafted. Therefore, intractable pain at the irradiated site is also a reliable diagnostic clue.

Treatment

For a local radiation injury of the skin, treatment must also include improving the patient's general condition in order to enforce tissue regenerative capability and its resistance against infection. Local treatment is often ineffective because the pathologic changes in the irradiated tissue are of degenerative nature. The intima of the capillary vessels becomes inflamed, resulting in narrowness or thrombosis of the vascular lumen. The ulcer persists as a result of the low regenerative capability of the tissue and poor nutrition. All these unfavorable factors combined together pose a great problem in treatment. Surgical excision of the ulcer followed by skin grafting has been reported in the literature to be effective.

Some authors have stressed that skin grafting should be postponed for 6 months after initial injury until new tissues and vascular networks appear in the ulcer. In the present authors' experience, skin grafting can be successfully carried out as early as the reparative phase, provided that polymorphonuclear and macrophage cells can be detected by cytologic smear examination. This phenomenon indicates that the wound has reached the reparative phase and will respond well to skin grafting. This has been proved by one of our cases in which the ulcer did heal satisfactorily after skin grafting at this stage.

The extent of excision of the ulcer must, if possible, encompass all the surrounding zone of the skin involved. Failure to do this means running a great risk of recurrence or leads to some other unexpected adverse outcomes. Generally, the depth of excision must accord with the surgical principles to include all the necrotic tissues, thus leaving a base covered with a layer of living tissue. However, if there are important structures such as internal organs, major nerve trunks and vessels, pleura or pericardium, right underneath the ulcer, a more conservative excision is advised so as to avoid exposure of these structures. In such a case, excision should be limited to a plane where the residual scar at the

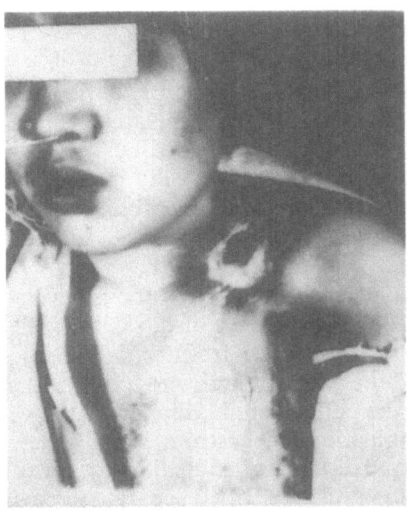
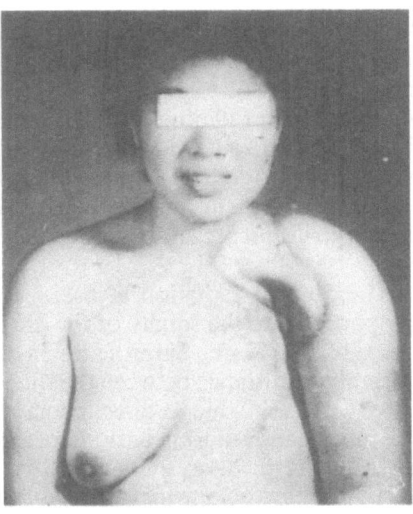

Figure 4.1 a, Preoperative view.   **b,** Postoperative view

base just begins to show signs of bleeding points, because such a recipient bed would be adequate to support a thin skin graft.

One patient in this series had undergone mastectomy for breast cancer but was highly suspected of lymph node metastasis in the supraclavicular fossa. After operation, she received radiation therapy for the region but an unfortunate overdose led to the occurrence of a local ulcer penetrating into the subclavicular tissue resulting in exposure of the clavicle. Moreover, involvement of sub-clavicular vessels was also suspected. Therefore, excision of the ulcer together with the clavicle did not go beyond such level as would expose the subclavicular vessels. On the contrary, a thin layer of necrotic tissue was intentionally left to overlie the vessels and the wound covered with a pedicled flap. Eventually the flap took well on such a bed and the wound subsequently healed (Figure 4.1). The mechanism of healing in such a wound with a thin layer of dead tissue covered by a flap is probably due to the effect of the biologic debridement, as stated by Marino.

The type of skin graft to be chosen depends on the nature and depth of the ulcer. For a superficial ulcer with fresh and pink granulation, a thin medium-thickness skin graft is selected to insure good functional restoration. But for an ulcer with poor blood supply and lack of healthy granulation, it is best to cover it with a very thin or Thiersch skin graft as a preliminary step. Should the necessity for further reconstruction arise later, that piece of thin skin graft could be replaced by a more convenient flap to meet the requirements of a definitive operation. Ten cases in this series required a flap reconstruction and the longest follow-up time was more than 15 years. All attained a good surgical result.

CAUSES OF RADIATION INJURY AND PROTECTIVE MEASURES AGAINST IT

Direct causes of radiation injury include technical errors and neglect of protection. All 22 cases in this series suffered from radiation injury during either fluoroscopy or radiotherapy. The output from an X-ray tube is closely related to its voltage, current, filter, distance, size of field and other factors. Too high a voltage or current, inadequate filter, too short a distance, faulty indication of voltage and current ampere meters are common causes of overdose. And both the surgeon and patient might receive overdoses when a large field of radiation is used.

The dose of radiation at a certain point from the X-ray tube is inversely proportional to the square of the distance. The shorter the distance, the greater the radiation dose. Seven cases in this series suffered from radiation injury because the distance between the tube and the patient's limb was too short, and three cases were due to direct contact of the patient's lumbodorsal region with the tube window during barium meal examination of a gastrointestinal series. A large diagnostic X-ray unit usually has a fixed distance of 35 cm between the tube focus and the table, while a portable unit is equipped with a separate screening plate because there is no tube attached. Therefore, carelessness in placing the plate too close to the tube might result in overdose and this deserves special attention during operation of the machine.

The absorbed radiation is proportional to exposure time. Eleven cases suffered from radiation injury because of prolonged exposure in addition to short distance and neglect of protective measures. One surgeon suffered radiation injury because of a 30–40 min overexposure during fracture reduction in four patients consecutively within a short period. In another instance, both surgeon and patient were injured during the surgical removal of a foreign body under fluoroscopy. Reduction of fracture and removal of a foreign body under fluoroscopy are therefore likely to induce overexposure and these procedures require special attention.

Violation of the precaution regulations and failure to check the status of the X-ray before use may also result in radiation injury. Two cases sustained radiation injury because of failure to check the machine before use. As a result, a current of 15 mA was mistakenly used during screening (this amount had been set the day before for taking a film and the machine had not been readjusted before screening – which requires only 3 mA).

Generally, the window of the tube is masked with an aluminum filter plate 0.5 mm thick to absorb the useless soft rays in order to reduce the total amount of the emitting ray and improve the quality of the X-ray beam. Failure to replace the filter plate during installation or fixing of the machine will result in an increased X-ray dose. Two of our cases sustained radiation injury in this way.

In the literature, medical workers who sustained radiation injury were mostly not trained in this specialty. Although they had comparatively less chance of coming into contact with X-rays, they were injured more often. This higher incidence closely relates to their habitual neglect of protective measures and reluctance to observe the precaution regulations strictly. For example, the eight medical workers who were injured in this series were either general surgeons or orthopedic specialists – none were radiologists.

In conclusion, we should like to suggest the following precautions to avoid improper operation of the machine.

(1) Those who use X-ray apparatus must have competent basic knowledge of the generator and its functions. They must observe strictly the operational regulations including protective measures. Full cooperation of the radiologists is advised during operation of the machine.

(2) Unprotected hands should not be placed directly under the X-ray beam during reduction of a fracture or removal of a foreign body. Use of the X-ray should be restricted to checking and correcting the position of the reduced fracture and dislocation, or just localizing a foreign body.

(3) In a medium or small sized X-ray unit, the distance between the tube and the limb must always be adjusted to shorter than 30 cm.

(4) The amount of radiation must not exceed 10 rad/min in a diagnostic X-ray unit; if it is found to be higher the machine should be checked and the malfunction identified.

(5) The accuracy of the machine meters should be regularly checked.

5 Musculus Frontalis Rotation Flap in the Treatment of Blepharoptosis Gravis

SONG YE-GUANG and ZHAO MIN
Plastic Surgery Hospital, Chinese Academy of Medical Sciences, Beijing

Unilateral or bilateral, congenital or acquired blepharoptosis is a clinical entity in which the musculus levator palpebrae superioris, paralyzed by agenesis or traumatic injury of the oculomotor nerve, is unable to lift the upper lid. The surgical treatment of ptosis of the upper eyelid is both cosmetic and functional. The various surgical procedures may be classified into three groups: (1) advancement of the elevator, (2) suspension of the elevator and (3) substitution

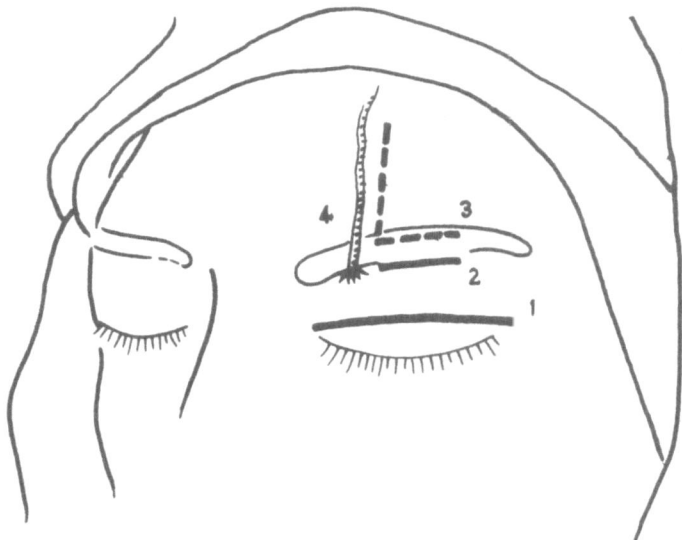

Figure 5.1 Design of skin incisions. (1) Lid fold incision; (2) infrabrow incision; (3) an angular incision at lower part of musculus frontalis and (4) supraorbital neurovascular bundle

29

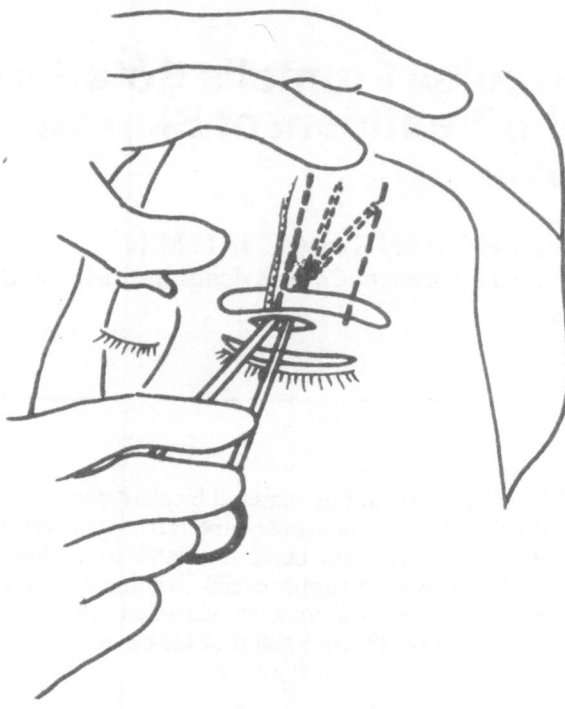

Figure 5.2   Two wide underminings are made, one between the skin and the musculus frontalis, the other between the undersurface of the musculus frontalis and the periosteum of the frontal bone

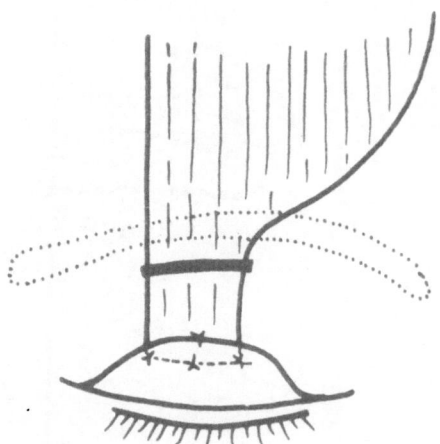

Figure 5.3   The musculus frontalis flap is transposed to the upper eyelid and fixed to the tarsus by one mattress suture and three interrupted sutures

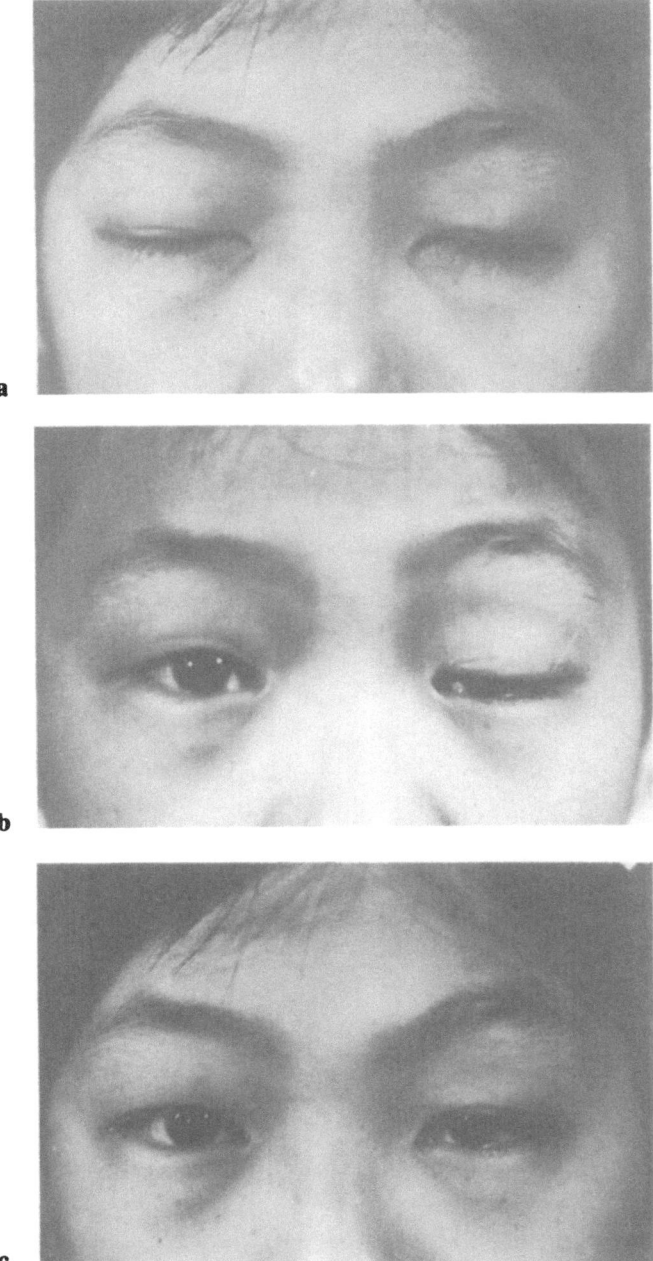

Figure 5.4 **a,** A 13-year-old girl with severe blepharoptosis of the left eyelid. A frontalis suspension operation was performed 6 years before with unsatisfactory postoperative results. **b,** After musculus frontalis rotation flap operation, the girl enjoys cosmetic symmetry of her eyes. **c,** After musculus frontalis rotation flap operation, complete symmetry of the eyes in closed state is obtained.

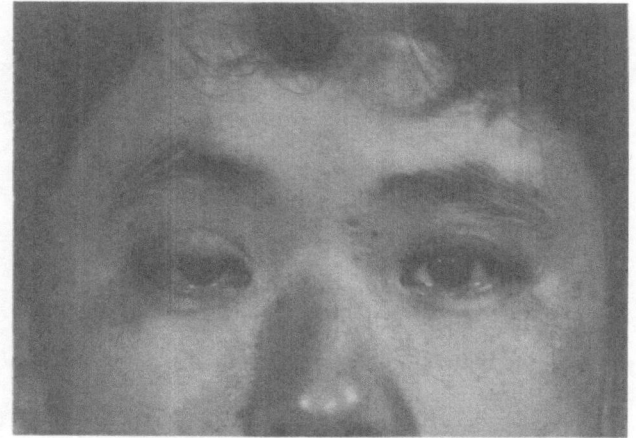

a

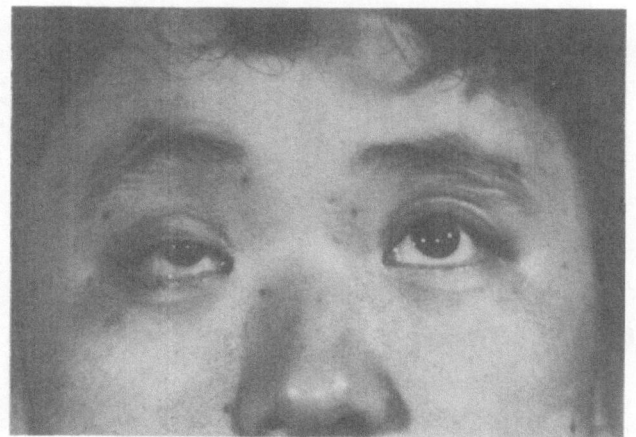

b

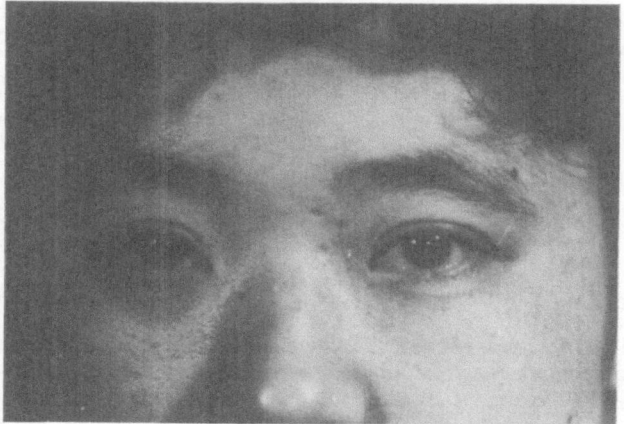

c

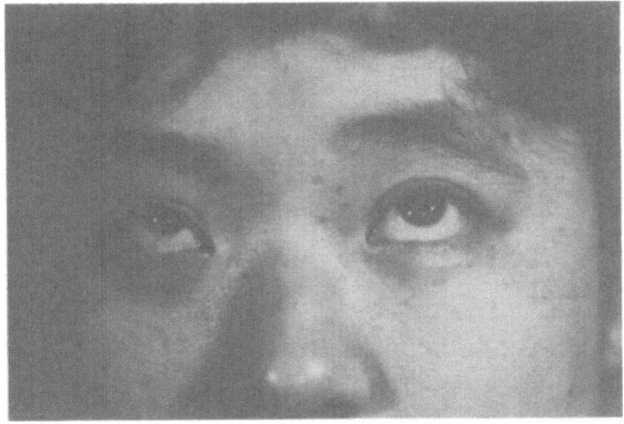

d

Figure 5.5 a, A 24-year-old girl had her congenitally ptosed right eyelid treated by elevator advancement operation 6 years previously with little postoperative improvement. **b,** When she raised her right eyebrow and looked upward, the right eyelid still lagged behind. **c,** Excellent symmetry of eyes after musculus frontalis flap operation. **d,** Good symmetry of eyes when she looks upward

by the rectus superioris. The operative results are often satisfactory in mild cases, less good in severe ones.

The technique of musculus frontalis rotation flap in the treatment of blepharoptosis, first introduced by Professor Song Ru-Yao in the 1960s, merits our attention in that it is suitable not only in mild cases, but in severe ptosis or in cases having unfavorable results from previous plastic surgery.

SURGICAL TECHNIQUES

Technique is as follows.

(1) The upper lid incision is marked out with methylene blue in the position where the suprapalpebral fold should be. The brow incision is marked in a skin crease below the middle third of the eyebrow, lateral to the supraorbital notch (Figure 5.1).

(2) The upper lid incision is made through the skin and musculus orbicularis. The upper margin of the incision is retracted upward. After exposure of the orbital fat, the excess part of which is excised, the musculus levator palpebrae superioris and the tarsus are brought into view. A 2 mm wide strip of the orbicularis muscle is excised from the lower border of the lid incision to facilitate the formation of a double lid.

(3) The forehead skin is pushed upward to shift the brow incision up to the supraorbital ridge. The brow incision is now made and the musculus orbicularis and frontalis incised, care being taken not to injure the

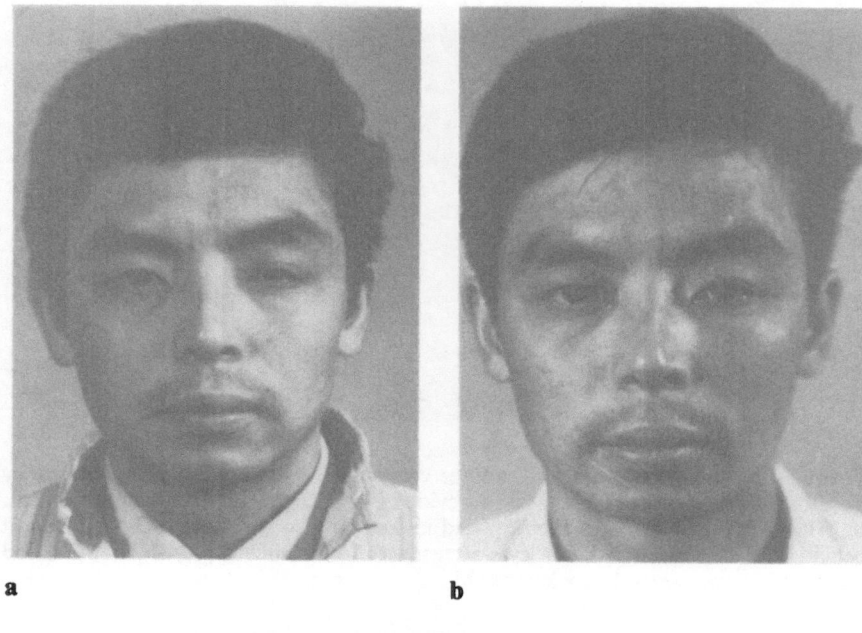

a   b

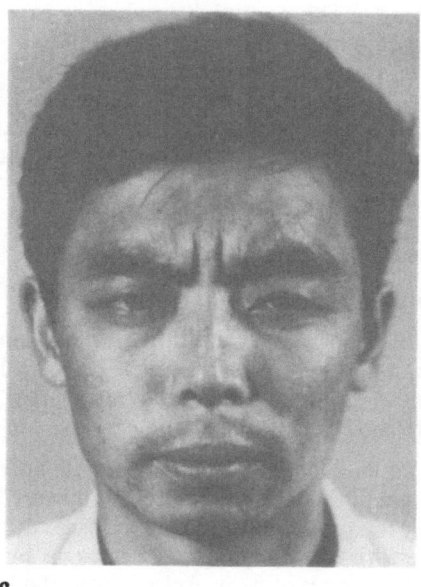

c

Figure 5.6 a, A 27-year-old man had his ptosed left eyelid operated on 20 years previously; asymmetry of eyes is obvious. **b,** Seven months after musculus frontalis rotation flap operation, symmetry of eyes and eyebrow is obtained. **c,** He is able to frown with eyebrow normally

periosteum or damage the supraortical artery and nerve medial to the incision. A thin narrow elevator is introduced into the wound and a 3.5 cm wide strip of musculus frontalis is raised from the periosteum. A pair of small curved scissors is then used to separate the muscle from the overlying skin (Figure 5.2). The freed muscle is transected just lateral to the supra-orbital notch, forming a laterally based musculus frontalis flap.

The musculus frontalis flap is then pulled downward out of the incision and the remaining attachments to the surrounding tissues are freed.

(4) A pair of ophthalmologic scissors is used to prepare a tunnel linking the lid incision and brow incision. The freed musculus frontalis flap is now passed downward through the tunnel and fixed to the tarsus with a mattress suture. The patient is now told to open his eyes and to look straight ahead, and the upper lid will be raised due to contraction of the musculus frontalis. The muscle is then fixed to the tarsus firmly with three sutures placed side by side (Figure 5.3).

(5) From the start of the musculus frontalis dissection, the assistant should constantly apply pressure to control bleeding.

(6) The lid incision is closed using the double lid blepharoplasty technique. After the brow incision is closed, a compression dressing is applied to the forehead and a light dressing to the upper eyelid.

Postoperatively, the patient is told to rest the operated eye until the edema of the eyelid disappears. Sutures are removed on the seventh postoperative day.

RESULTS

Since 1980, we have employed this technique in more than 30 patients. Nearly all these patients have good and lasting cosmetic and functional results (Figures 5.4–5.6).

REFERENCES

1. Fox, S. A. (1980). *Surgery of Ptosis*. (Baltimore: Williams & Wilkins)
2. Berke, R. N. (1962). Types of operation indicated for congenital and acquired ptosis. In Troutman, R. C. *et al.* (eds.) *Plastic and Reconstructive Surgery of the Eye and Adnexa*. (Washington DC: Butterworths)

6 Reconstruction of Facial Elephantiasis: A Case Report

YIN LI-QIAO

Nanjing Medical College Hospital

It is quite common to see a patient with facial erysipelas, whereas it is very rare to see a patient with facial elephantiasis after recurrent erysipelas attacks. In 1964, a case of facial elephantiasis was admitted to our hospital and treated surgically. The patient has been followed up for 17 years, and found to be in very satisfactory condition.

CASE REPORT

On February 12 1964, a 51-year-old man was admitted with the chief complaint of swelling and coarseness of the face, particularly in the bilateral preauricular region, for 21 years.

Twenty-one years before admission, he had suddenly experienced chills, high fever and pain all over the body. There was redness, swelling and tenderness of the facial skin in the bilateral preauricular regions. The submaxillary lymph glands were affected and became swollen and very tender. Having bedrested and had penicillin injections for some 10 days the patient recovered gradually from all symptoms. These symptoms recurred whenever he was subjected to cold and fatigue. The face began swelling gradually with a heavy feeling and itching in spite of a variety of treatments.

Local condition

Symmetrically rough swelling, 10×7 cm in size, was found in the preauricular region of both sides of the face. The swellings were felt distending with moderate hardness and slight tenderness on pressure but with no fluctuation. The skin surface was considerably keratinized. The earlobes were markedly pulled downward and widened, owing to the weight and swelling of the masses. Submaxillary lymph nodes were enlarged and palpable with moderate hardness and slight tenderness (Figure 6.1a).

Nothing abnormal was found regarding the parotid glands by sialography.

Treatment

On February 18 1964, under general anesthesia, the patient was operated on with partial excision of the affected skin, subcutaneous tissue and deep fascia on both sides of the face. The wound was closed by direct sutures. Subcutaneous drainage was employed. The postoperative course was uneventful.

Pathologic report

Hyperkeratosis of the epidermis, keratotic plug of the hair follicles, and moderate sebaceous hyperplasia were observed. The deep layer of the dermis and subcutaneous tissue showed massive fibrosis and collagenation. Discrete chronic inflammatory cell infiltration was seen with focal massive accumulation of eosinophil leukocytes and tissue necrosis.

Pathologic diagnosis

The diagnosis was facial elephantiasis.

DISCUSSION

Pathogenesis of the facial elephantiasis

The facial erysipelas caused by streptococcal infection in the dermal lymph network is the cause of the facial elephantiasis. Persistent or recurrent lymphedema leads to invasion into the intercellular spaces by fibroblasts followed by overgrowth of connective tissue associated with thickening of the lymphatic capillaries. The adipose tissue may gradually be replaced by the fibrous tissue to an extent that the initial pitting edema may eventually become brownish, associated with thickened nonhair-bearing keratotic skin. Repeated attacks of lymphangitis cause progression of the disease into a vicious circle – chronic lymphangitis may follow after repeated acute attacks if it is not adequately treated, and this in turn causes further blockage of the lymphatic drainage.

Method of treatment and its theoretical basis

Based on experience in the treatment of elephantiasis of the lower extremities, excisional operation of the affected skin, subcutaneous tissues and deep fascia was adopted to treat the facial elephantiasis. A good cosmetic result has been obtained in this case.

After a 17-year follow-up, it is interesting to note that no recurrence of erysipelas occurred after operation. The external appearance of the patient's face is normal. The follow-up result seems very satisfactory (Figure 6.1b).

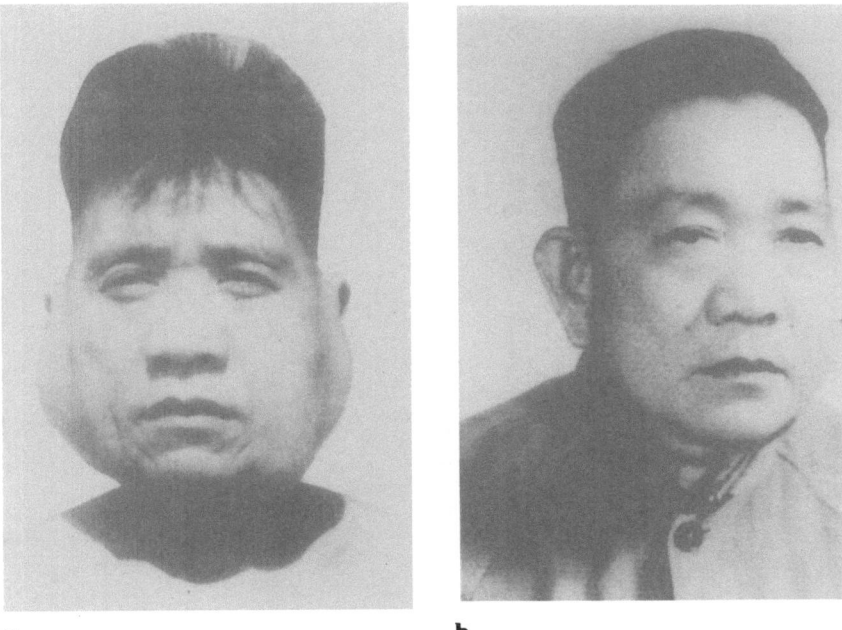

a   b

Figure 6.1 **a,** Preoperative view of the patient with bilateral swelling of the face due to elephantiasis. **b,** View of the patient taken 21 years after operation

REFERENCES

1. Chang Ti-sheng (1979). *Plastic and Reconstructive Surgery*. (Shanghai: Shanghai Scientific and Technologic Publishing Co.)
2. Converse, J. M. (1964). *Reconstructive Plastic Surgery*. (Philadelphia: Saunders)

7 Single Stage Total Ear Reconstruction Without Making Use of the Auricular Skin

SUN YI-LU, LI GUAN-YU and LIN ZEN-LU

Department of Plastic Surgery, Zhongshan Hospital, Shanghai First Medical College

Since the early description of auricular reconstruction by Tagliacozi (1957), Dieffenbach (1845), Szymanovski (1870) and others, Gillies (1920) introduced a technique of embedding a framework of autogenous cartilage under the mastoid skin followed by raising it up to the lateral side of the head, the secondary skin defect being covered by a cervical pedicle flap. A split thickness skin flap was used for this purpose by Pierce (1930). The procedure is reserved for congenital microtia.

In order to prevent local edema and fibrosis secondary to lymphaticovenous stasis which may jeopardize the final result, Fukuda[1] and Ohomori[2] proposed raising the cartilaginous framework from the side of the head in two stages. The operation is usually done in three or four stages, with a 3-month time lapse between the stages.

The reconstruction of the helix by means of a vascular superficial temporal fascial tube should be credited to Dufourmentel[3] and Cosman[4]. Avelar[5] was able to rebuild a congenital microtia in one stage by sandwiching a cartilaginous framework between the posteriorly located fascial flap and the anteriorly placed auricular skin flap.

For the acquired auricular loss, the surgical principle of the reconstruction is similar to that stated by Converse[6], the only difference being the auricular skin replaced by scar tissue which makes the reconstruction more difficult.

The single stage total ear reconstruction without making use of the auricular skin was devised by us and the preliminary clinical application is encouraging.

SURGICAL ANATOMY

The superficial temporal artery, terminal branch of the external carotid artery, bifurcates into the frontal and parietal branches 5 cm superior to the zygomatic arch. A temporoauricular nerve and one or two satellite veins run alongside with the artery to form a neurovascular bundle which gives off a dense plexus of minute perforating vessels between the deep fascia muscularis temporalis and the superficial temporal fascia.

The fascia muscularis temporalis is thin and strong; it covers the whole temporal bone and adheres to the temporal muscle. Undermining of it is easy to carry out, as the perforating vessels are scanty (Figure 7.1).

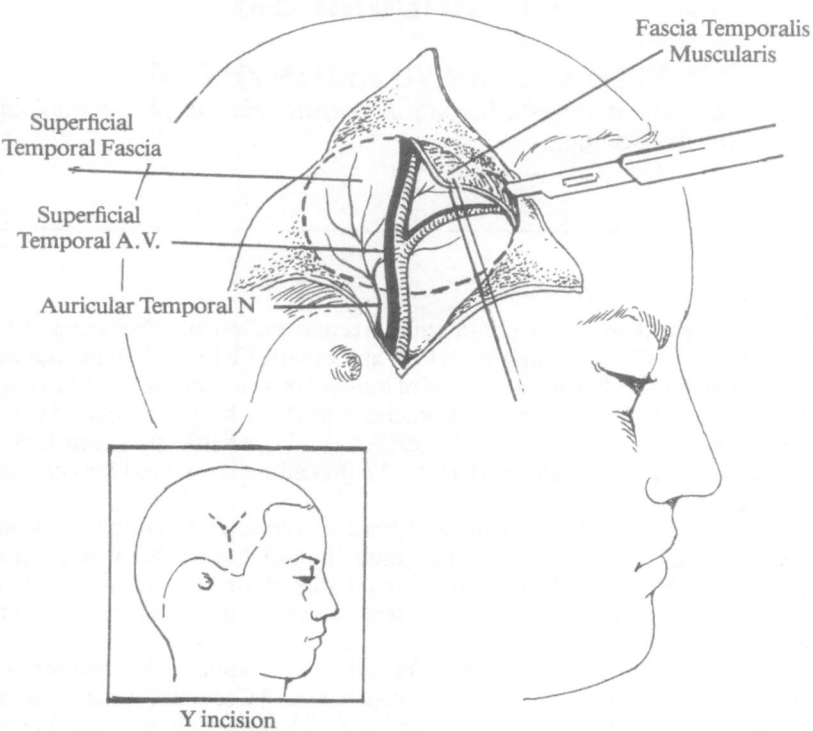

Figure 7.1 Superficial temporal fascia, fascia temporalis muscle and their neurovascular bundle

SURGICAL TECHNIQUE

A contour pattern is made in conformity with the opposite normal auricle as model.

Under local or intravenous anesthesia, a Y skin incision above the zygomatic arch, inside the hairline, along the superficial temporal vessels and their branches is made to expose the superficial fascia.

A one fifth enlargement of the contour pattern is marked with methylene blue on the superficial temporal fascia which is incised in conjunction with the fascia muscularis temporalis to form a composite vascular flap.

An outline of the cartilaginous pattern is laid out on the exposed sixth, seventh and eighth costal cartilages on the contralateral side. These cartilages are removed. The helix should be 5 mm wide and 2 mm thick and the antihelix 8 mm wide and 3 mm thick. The antitragus is carved out.

The layers of fascia are undermined posterosuperiorly at the periphery for 1 cm to include the insertion of the helical cartilage. Mattress stitches are used to fix the inner border to form a depression; the outer edges are then resutured together. Posteroinferiorly a tunnel is made between the two fascial layers of the constructed auricle. Into this tunnel, the antihelical cartilage including the inferior crus is placed obliquely toward the anterosuperior border. By the use of nylon sutures, it is fixed to the helical cartilage remnant. The superior crus of the antihelix is sutured to an appropriate site. The fascia along the border of the cartilage is fixed with mattress stitches (Figure 7.2).

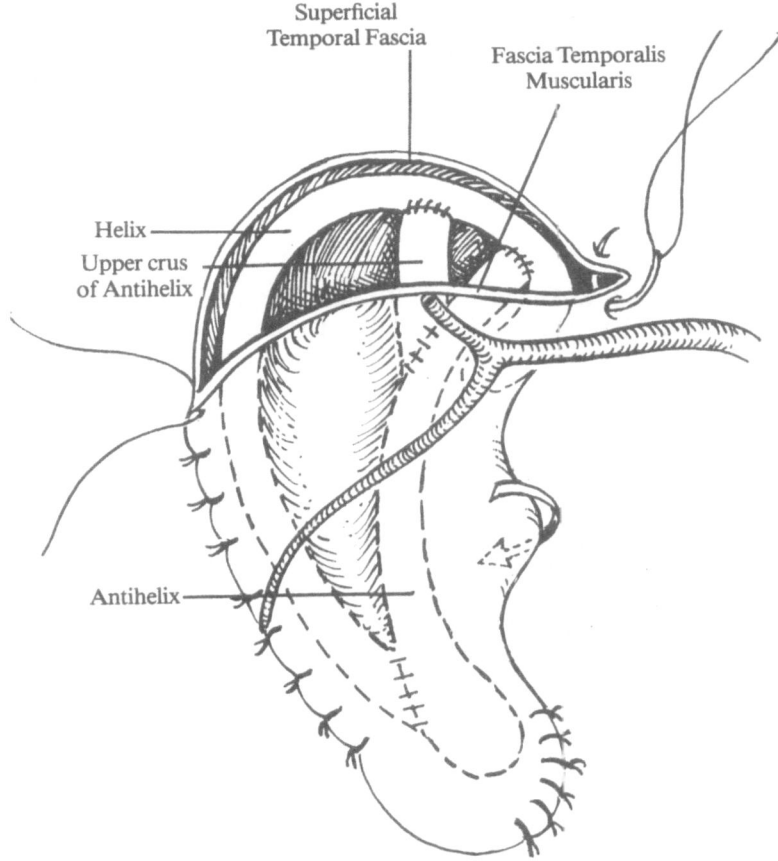

Figure 7.2 The composite island flap with cartilaginous framework

Next, the inner margin of the reconstructed auricle is tailored to conform with the size and contour of the defect and sutured in place. The cartilaginous frame work may be sutured to the remnant cartilage for fixation. Finally, a full thickness skin graft is put to the cartilaginous border with mattress stitches.

In the case of congenital microtia, the auricular lobule is rotated into its proper position and the conchal cavity and tragus must be reconstructed. A vertical incision is made over the remnant ear and an oblique incision made over the lobule to form three flaps. This makes the rotation of the lobule into its normal position easier. At the same time, a tunnel is made in the lobule for insertion of the antihelical tail. The cartilaginous remnant and soft tissues between the mastoid and mandible are excised through an incision in the superior aspect to the periosteum. If the parotid gland is voluminous, its superior portion may be excised to form a broad and deep conchal fossa. The tragus is formed by inserting a small piece of cartilage into the folded pre-auricular skin and maintained in place with stitches. The remaining defect in the conchal fossa is covered with a full thickness skin graft. The cranioauricular angle is restored by a three-point fixation maneuver: the tail of the antihelix is inserted into the lobule, the superior portion of the helix fixed to the periosteum of the temporal bone and the inner margin of the fascial flap sutured to the pre-mastoid periosteum. The more dorsally the latter is fixed, the greater the angle will be.

CASE REPORTS

Case 1

A 20-year-old male was admitted on February 2 1981 for congenital absence of the right ear. The right auricle was absent except for an embedded under-developed irregular cartilaginous appendage with a small lobule. Total ear reconstruction was performed on February 13 1981 by the technique described (Figure 7.3).

Case 2

A 41-year-old male had lost the upper portion of his left ear after a burn injury a year previously. He was admitted on February 2 1981. Under intravenous anesthesia, a fan shaped vascular pedicled fascia temporalis superficialis and fascia muscularis temporalis composite flap was prepared and transferred to the defect. A piece of allogenous cartilage was inserted between the undermined periphery of the composite flap to form the helix. The ends of this cartilage were then fixed to the corresponding ends of the remnant helix by 5/0 nylon stitches. A full thickness skin graft was applied to the raw surface of this composite flap.

Case 3

A 25-year-old male was admitted on January 6 1981 for loss of the right helix and the upper portion of the left ear after burns 2 years previously. Other

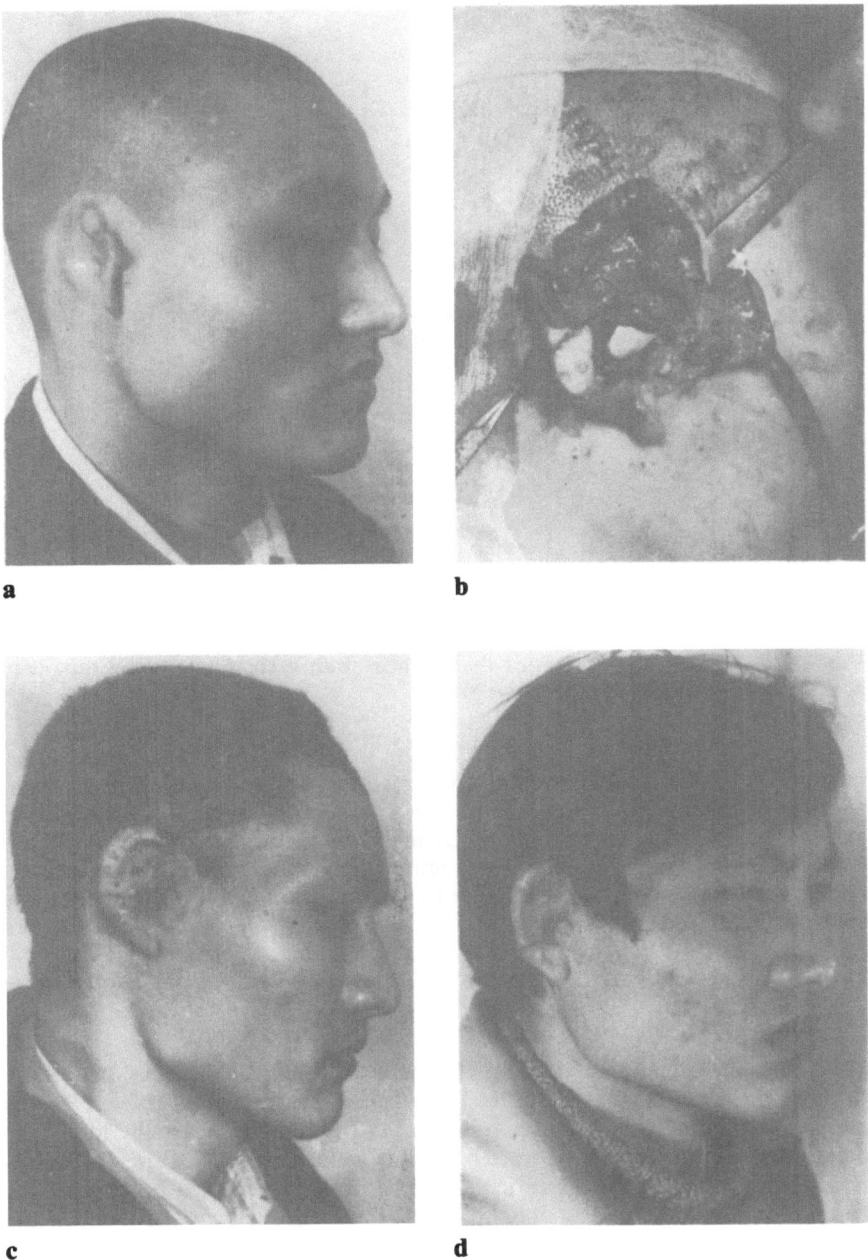

Figure 7.3 Case 1. Total ear reconstruction with composite island flap and rib cartilage. **a,** Before operation. **b,** During operation. **c,** After operation. **d,** Ten months after operation

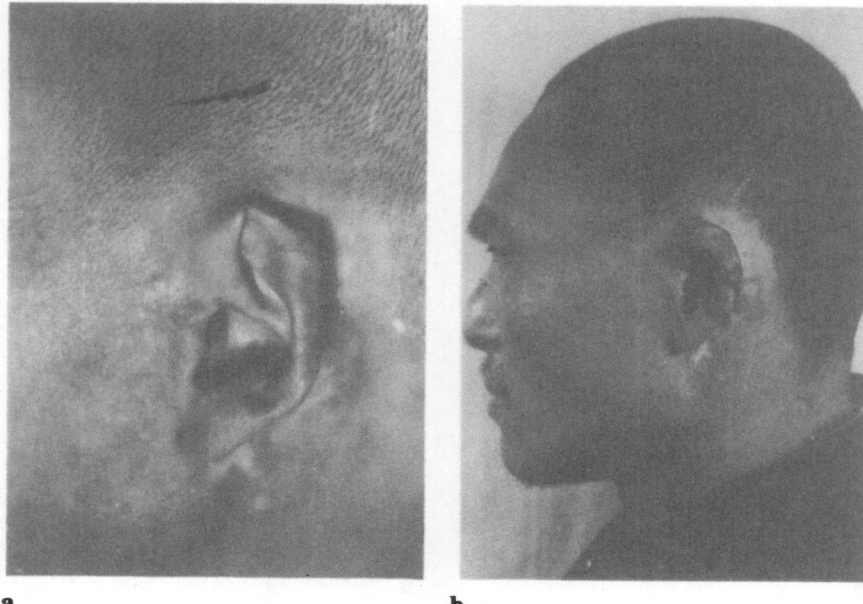

a   b

Figure 7.4 Case 3. Restoration of the left helix with a composite island tube flap. **a,** Preoperative view. **b,** Postoperative view

wounds on the head and extremities were treated primarily with skin grafts in another hospital at the time of the burn accident. Under local infiltration anesthesia, the left ear was repaired by the same method as in Case 2 (Figure 7.4). Two months later, the right ear (Figure 7.5) was repaired by transplanting a composite tissue tube; the raw surface of this tube flap was covered with a free split skin graft.

DISCUSSION

Total auricular reconstruction has been the most unsatisfactory procedure through the years in plastic surgery[1-10]. In case of congenital absence of the auricle, the skin in this region is normal, but the hairline is usually low. This makes restoration difficult because of lack of skin. One stage auricular reconstruction by means of local auricular skin remains a problem because of the compromised blood and lymphatic circulation, especially when the conchal cavity is restored at the same time.

This chapter describes the ear reconstruction with a vascular pedicled composite tissue flap using the superficial temporal fascia and fascia muscularis temporalis. Into it a cartilage is inserted for total auricular reconstruction in one stage. This reconstruction includes formation of the conchal cavity. The

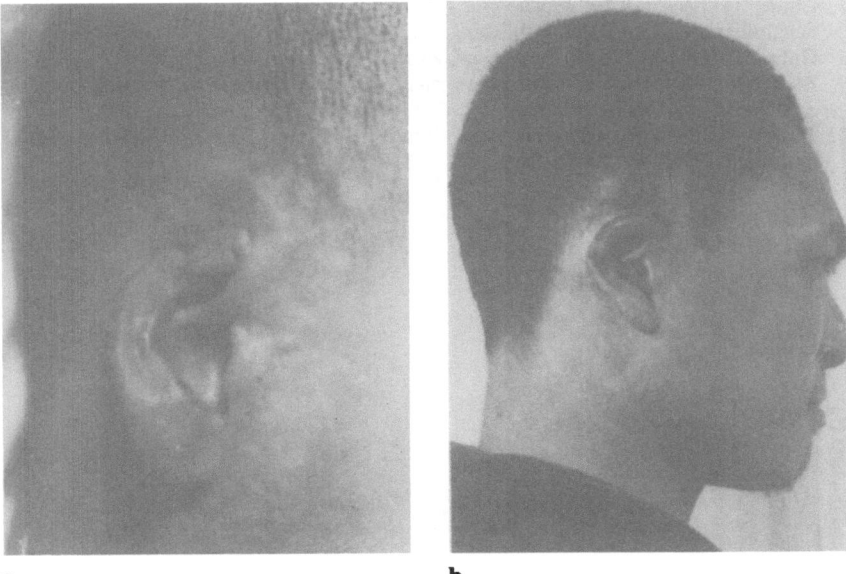

a   b

Figure 7.5 Case 3. Restoration of upper portion of the right ear. **a,** Preoperative view. **b,** Postoperative view.

advantages of this technique are: tissue thinness, rich blood supply, easy molding, sufficient tissue, restoration unlimited by size, no significant edema or contraction of the skin graft, well hidden incision above the hairline and no secondary defect of the donor area. Because the temporoauricular nerve is included in this tissue flap, adequate protective sensation is also restored. This technique is suitable for reconstruction of all forms of total or partial auricular loss, both congenital microtia and acquired ear defects.

REFERENCES

1. Fukuda, O. (1974). The microtic ear: Survey of 180 cases in 10 years. *Plast. Reconstr. Surg.,* **53,** 458
2. Ohomori, S. *et al.* (1974). Follow up study on reconstruction of microtia with a silicone framework. *Plast. Reconstr. Surg.,* **53,** 555
3. Dufourmentel, C. (1958). La greffe libre tubulée: Nouvel artifice pour la réflexion de l'hélix au cours de la reconstruction du pavillon de l'oreille. *Ann. Chir. Plast.,* **3,** 311
4. Cosman, B. *et al.* (1966). The compound tube pedicle in ear, helix reconstruction. *Plast. Reconstr. Surg.,* **37,** 517
5. Avelar, J. M. (1977). Reconstrucão total da pavilhão auricula num único tempo cirúrgico. *Rev. Bras. Cir.,* **67,** 139
6. Converse, J. M. (1977). *Reconstructive Plastic Surgery.* 2nd Edn., Vol. 3, p. 1671. (Philadelphia: Saunders)

7. Chang Ti-sheng (1979). *Plastic and Reconstructive Surgery*. (Shanghai: Shanghai Scientific and Technologic Publishing Co.)
8. Gillies, H. (1920). *Plastic Surgery of the Face*. (London: Stoughton)
9. Brent, B. (1974). Ear reconstruction with an expansile framework of autogenous rib cartilage. *Plast. Reconstr. Surg.*, **53**, 619
10. Tanzer, R. C. (1971). Total reconstruction of the auricle. The evolution of a plan of treatment. *Plast. Reconstr. Surg.*, **47**, 523

8 The Use of Long and Thin Skin Tube to Repair Auricular Defect after Burn – A Report of 42 cases

NIU XING-TAO, KONG FAN-HU, ZHU HONG-YIN and HUI BO-SHENG
Department of Plastic Surgery, The Third Teaching Hospital, Beijing Medical College

In facial burns both ears are often injured simultaneously. However, the concha of the auricle is often preserved, which facilitates the repair of the ear. Adhesion to the mastoid region is commonly seen and should be released by surgical intervention and skin grafting.

The use of long and thin skin tube for reconstruction of the burnt ear is advantageous in restoring the shape of the auricle, and protecting residual or implanted cartilage. This kind of operation was started rather early in our department, first being reported by Kong[1] in 1966. In the present chapter we have summarized 42 such cases operated on within the period March 1963–July 1979. Several points of clinical importance will be discussed.

CLINICAL DATA

The 42 patients were all male, with a total of 58 ears repaired with long and thin skin tubes. In the 28 ears, auto-rib cartilage grafts were transplanted beforehand in the usual way because of the large size of the defect. In one case, silicone implant was used.

Donor sites of skin tube

Donor sites were:

(1) *supraclavicular region*: 23 tubes (39.7%) (Figure 8.1)

(2) *neck region overlying the sternocleidomastoid muscle*: seven tubes (12.1%) (Figure 8.2)

(3) *neck–chest across clavicle*: two tubes (3.4%) (Figure 8.3)

(4) *upper arm*: 25 tubes (43.1%) (Figure 8.3)

(5) *flexor surface of forearm*: one tube (1.7%)

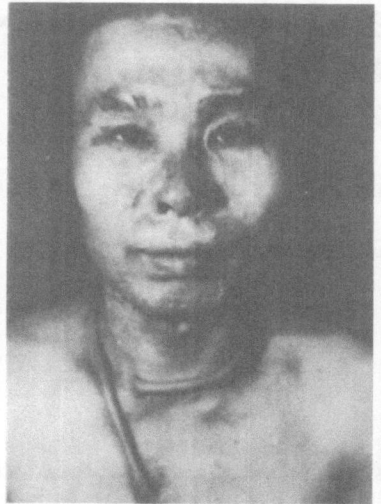 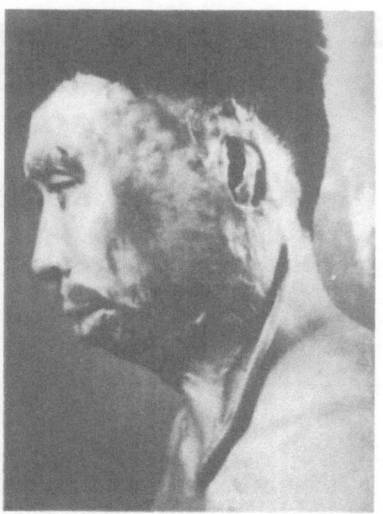

Figure 8.1 Supraclavicular skin tube at the left side of neck. Neck-chest skin tube at right side of neck

Figure 8.2 Sternocleidomastoid muscle skin tube

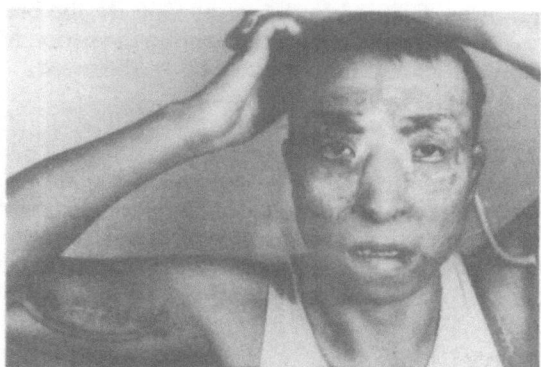

Figure 8.3 Upper arm skin tube

Size of skin tube

Sizes were:

(1) length: 11 cm, the shortest (one tube); 18 cm, the longest (two tubes); average 14.37 cm

(2) width: 1.7 cm, the narrowest (one tube); 2.7 cm, the widest (one tube); average 2.2 cm

(3) length of the 'bridge': 2.5 cm, the shortest; 6 cm, the longest; average 4.1 cm

Complications

Complications during the stage of tube formation were:

(1) central necrosis: one tube (1.7%)

(2) blister formation in the central part: two tubes (3.4%)

Time of 'bridge' severance

Time of 'bridge' severance after tube formation and accompanying complications was as follows. The shortest was 15 days and the longest 217 days, with central necrosis in one case and central blister formation in another after severance of the 'bridge' (1.7% respectively).

Time of tube transfer

The time interval between the 'bridge' severance and the first transfer ranged from 22 to 515 days. The time interval from the first to the second (or the final) transfer ranged from 19 days (the shortest); to 120 days (the longest). However, 13 tubes were lengthened from 2 to 5 cm before transfer.

Eventual results of operation

In this group of 42 cases with 58 ears, one tube was lost owing to central necrosis during its formation. In another case a partial necrosis at the middle part of the tube occurred following separation of the 'bridge'; however, the operation was eventually successful by use of some additional measures. Thus 57 ears were repaired with satisfactory results (Figures 8.4, 8.5).

DISCUSSION

Donor site

The anterior neck and upper arm are the donor areas of choice for tube formation. In this group, 32 tubes were formed at the neck and 25 at the upper arm. The skin of the above sites is loose and thin, with less subcutaneous fat and good texture. So it is easier to form a thin tube, and the donor area can be closed without difficulty. The neck tube is nearer to the ear, so it makes direct transfer easier. The transfer of an upper arm tube necessitates uncomfortable postural immobilization (Figure 8.3). Therefore, we use it only when the skin of the neck has been damaged. The neck tube can be designed at three sites on the neck. One

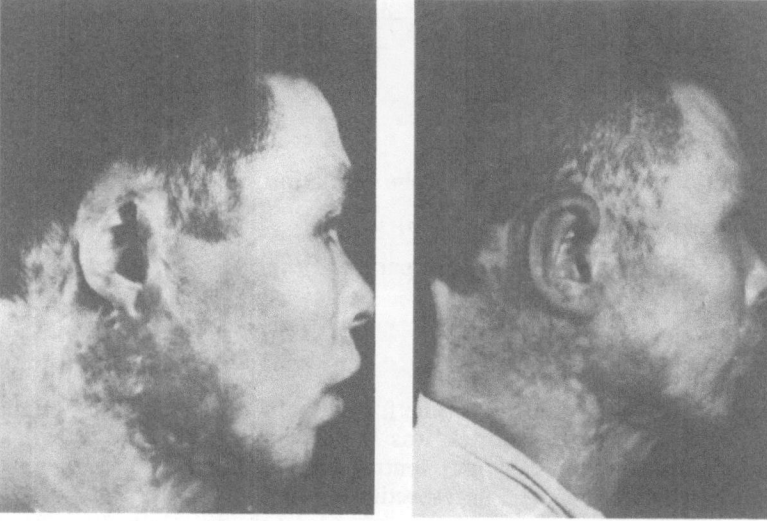

Figure 8.4   **a,** Preoperative view   **b,** Postoperative view

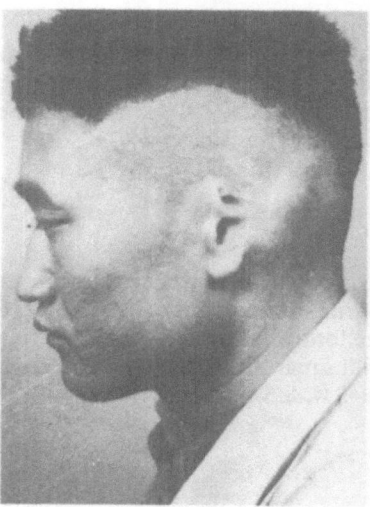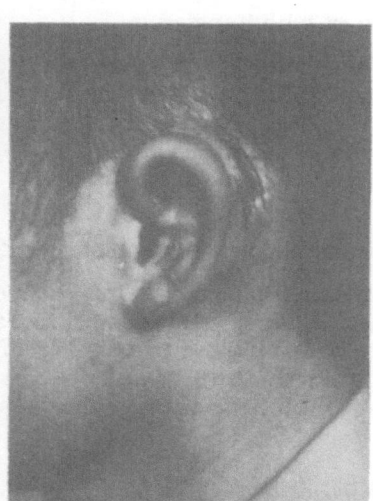

Figure 8.5   **a,** Preoperative view   **b,** Postoperative view

is along the sternocleidomastoid muscle extending from the postauricular region down to the front of the neck. The skin tube at this site is close to the ear. It not only makes direct transfer possible but also provides a longer contact surface between the tube and the damaged ear, the latter being a favorable condition for operation. The shortcoming is that secondary scar on the exposed donor site brings about an untoward cosmetic problem. The second site is the supra-clavicular region. This site is easily concealed by clothing but the skin tube formed at this site is rather far from the ear. As a rule, direct transfer is required. The third site occupies the lower neck and upper chest. It was used only when the above two donor areas were unfavorable, particularly in cases where both ears needed repair.

Size of skin tube

We use long and thin skin tube chiefly for the reconstruction of the helix. Generally, a width of 2–2.2 cm of the tube is required. Skin with superficial scar can also be used, but the width should be increased. For repairing the whole helix, the tube should not be shorter than 14 cm, and for partial repair it should not be shorter than 12 cm, otherwise more stages of transfer are needed.

Length of tube 'bridge' and time of severance

As the ratio of length to width in this kind of skin tube is greater than that normally used (3:1), the 'bridge' left in the middle of the tube is mandatory. In forming a tube 14 cm in length and 2.2 cm in width, we usually leave a 'bridge' of skin on one side, 4–4.5 cm in width. As to the time of its severance, the shortest time in our group was 15 days. We think that an interval of 2–3 weeks is required for a safe transfer, provided no complications such as hematoma or blister formation are present in the tube.

Time of tube transfer

The shortest time for the first transfer was 22 days after division of the 'bridge'. Of course, it is better and safer to wait till 3 weeks and more have elapsed. One week prior to tube transfer, the distal end of the tube is routinely constricted with a rubber band for 5–10 min training, practised twice daily. If there are no un-toward changes in the tube color, the constriction time can be prolonged gradually until a limit of 30 min is reached, because by then the tube can be transferred safely. In this group the shortest time interval between the first and the second (or the final) tube transfer was 19 days. The time interval depends on three factors, i.e. the length of skin tube, the extent of contact surface between the skin tube and the site of its insertion, and lastly the presence or absence of complications following the first transfer. The longest time interval in this group was 515 days. Delay was usually due to intervention of other operations, or the patient being discharged from hospital pending the next operation.

Complications

Necrosis of central portion of skin tube following tube formation

This complication occurred in a patient whose neck skin was not healthy enough to be used as a donor site because of the presence of burn scars. In another case, a skin tube was constructed on the upper arm, 15 cm long and 2.2 cm wide, and the width of the 'bridge' was 3 cm. A part of the subcutaneous fat was removed during operation. Postoperatively, continuous blood oozing occurred at the suture line, resulting in necrosis of the central part of the tube. We attributed the necrosis to inadequate hemostasis during operation, and postoperative formation of hematoma jeopardized blood circulation of the tube.

Necrosis following severance of 'bridge'

A skin tube 16 cm long and 2 cm wide was constructed at the region overlying the sternocleidomastoid muscle, with two 'bridges' left on either side, the width being 4 cm each. The 'bridges' were severed simultaneously on the 36th post-operative day. Cyanosis appeared at the central portion of the tube about 2 cm in length on the following day. Blister and edema followed, resulting in necrosis on the fifth day. The necrotic part was excised and the rest of the tube was inserted to the adjacent normal area. Later, the tube was lengthened and successfully used. This case illustrates the improper design of bridges.

Blister formation

Two skin tubes, one on either side of the neck, were formed. The tube on the left side was 17 cm long and 2 cm wide with a 4 cm 'bridge', while that on the right side was 14 cm long and 2 cm wide with a 3 cm 'bridge'. The donor skin had scars from burns. Blisters developed in both tubes at the central portion after operation. But they disappeared spontaneously on the sixth postoperative day. Blisters reappeared at the central portion of the tube after severance of the 'bridge'. Again they disappeared spontaneously, on the ninth day. This suggests that blood supply of the superficially burnt and scarred skin is poorer than that of the normal skin, so it should be used with great caution.

However, the above complications in our opinion could be avoided by proper design and careful manipulation of the tube during operation.

REFERENCE

1. Kong Fan-ku *et al.* (1966). Experiences in the plastic repair of the burned ear. *Chinese J. Surg.*, **14**, 240

9 One-Stage Total Auricle Reconstruction – A Report of 50 cases

CHEN ZONG-JI and WANG XIAN-LUN

Plastic Surgery Hospital, Chinese Academy of Medical Sciences

Auricles are situated in the middle portions on both sides of the head. Auricle defect causes not only physiological functional disturbances but also mental distress, the latter being much more important than physical trauma. As early as 2500 years ago, in the ancient Indian Veda era, plastic operations for auricle defect had already been described. However, owing to the complexity of the auricle's appearance, total auricle reconstruction was regarded as one of the most difficult operations in plastic surgery and surgeons had to abandon such operations because of their length and multistage technique. More than 20 stages of operation would be needed to achieve a somewhat satisfactory clinical result[1]. Dunton suggested that this kind of multistage technique should be abandoned since it was tedious and time consuming[2]. Therefore, how to achieve a relatively satisfactory result in a shorter course became one of the important problems in plastic surgery.

In 1959, Tanzer reported a six-stage technique of auricle reconstruction, the chief principles of which were demonstrated[3]. Innovations were subsequently introduced, and in 1971 Tanzer further improved it by making it a three to four stage operation[4]. In 1974, we first described a two-stage technique, i.e., a subcutaneous cartilage graft was implanted first and then a new auricle formed by raising the cartilage containing skin flap and completed by free skin graft to cover the donor area behind the auricle and in the mastoid region. However, because of the postoperative fascia contraction, the new auricle tended to change its shape, with an unstable result.

Based on the anatomic characteristics of vessel distribution in the auricular region and the principle of subcutaneous pedicle skin graft, we then planned a skin flap in the auricular region with an anterior pedicle, the chief blood supply being from the posterior perforating branch of the posterior auricular artery. In addition, a piece of subcutaneous tissue flap from the head skin, distal to the pedicle skin flap, with intact subcutaneous vascular net, was carried with it to cover the autogenous cartilage frame. Thus, a new one-stage total auricle reconstruction technique was first completed by the authors and has been used in the Hospital for Plastic Surgery, Beijing, since 1980 in 50 cases with excellent results.

OPERATIVE TECHNIQUE

Modeling

Two pieces of transparent film (Figure 9.1a) were used in modeling, piece A being modeled in the shape and size of the auricle of the healthy side. The modeling was accomplished by reversing the modeled film (piece A) in an opposite direction (face downward) and placing it in an adequate site on the diseased side. The contour of the new auricle would be drawn before operation according to the modeled film (piece A) and the site of the concha cavity designed. The new auricle would be formed according to the modeled film (piece A). Piece B was used to model the helix, counterhelix and fossa triangularis, and was made 2 mm smaller than piece A to be used in the modeling of the cartilage frame during operation.

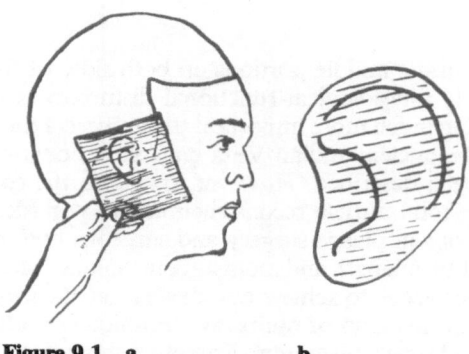

Figure 9.1   a   b

Anesthesia

Local anesthesia is used for adults and general anesthesia for children or the nervous.

Operative steps

Operative steps were as follows.

(1)   Treatment of congenital remnant auricle. The earlobe of the remnant was incised and transplanted caudally to the new position where the earlobe of the new auricle was to be situated by Z-plasty. The rest of the remnant (including shrunken, overlapping cartilage and useless skin) was excised, except the part required for the reconstruction of the tragus. The preauricular incision was closed with sutures or with moderate thick skin graft after wound-deepening to form the external ear orifice.

(2)   An incision was planned parallel to and 2–2.5 cm posterior to the contour line of the auricle as the limit of the skin flap, of sufficient size to enclose the

whole cartilage frame. The hair-bearing portion included in the skin flap should be excised by thick split-thickness skin excision technique and a thin layer of cutis preserved together with the subcuticular vascular net; then, the skin was incised along the planned incision deep to the aponeurotic fascia and a 'skin–subcutaneous tissue flap' containing also a subcutaneous layer of the hair-bearing portion, together with the skin in the contiguous posterior mastoid region, was raised. The aponeurotic or temporal fascia was not included and the skin in the region of the supposed concha cavity not raised, to avoid injuring the posterior auricular artery.

(3) Excision of rib cartilage was performed simultaneously by another team of operators and the auricle cartilage frame made by modeling film piece B to form the helix, counterhelix, fossa helicis and fossa triangularis. The soft tissue in the supposed concha cavity region was then excised. A thin piece of rib cartilage was implanted in the upper margin of the helix to make it more prominent. A piece of arcuate rib cartilage was implanted behind the counterhelix to form the posterior conchal wall, the latter being high enough to form an anterior sloping angle of 30–45 ° when the frame lay flat on a table (varying according to the degree of angle between the auricle and the lateral side of the head on the healthy side). The whole auricle cartilage frame was fixed firmly with steel thread (Figure 9.2).

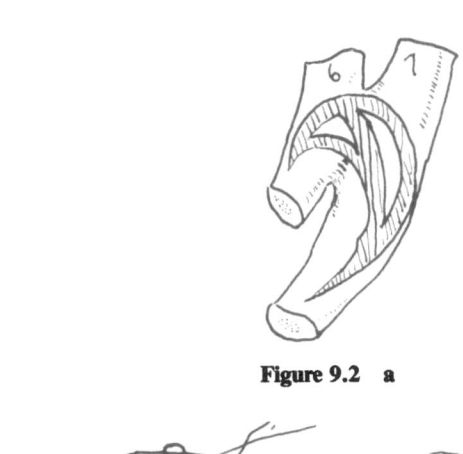

Figure 9.2 a

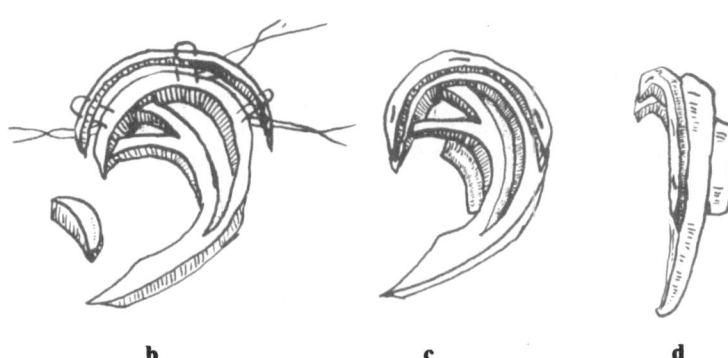

b   c   d

(4)   The auricle cartilage frame was placed beneath the 'skin–subcutaneous flap' in an adequate position according to the plan and the base of the posterior conchal wall was fixed with sutures to the periosteum of the lateral wall of the skull. The limbs of the helix were inserted anterosuperiorly into the subcutaneous layer.

(5)   Wrapping of the auricle cartilage frame with the 'skin-subcutaneous flap'. In order to make the auricle cartilage more prominent, the fixing sutures between the flap and cartilage were placed in the region of the fossae helicis and triangularis. Then the distal end of the 'skin–subcutaneous flap' was brought across the helix to the postauricular region, wrapping round the whole auricle cartilage frame, and sutured to the deep fascia. In the event of the 'skin–subcutaneous flap' not being long enough to wrap around the whole auricle cartilage frame, another flap from the deep fascia, in the mastoid region beneath the cartilage frame, could be raised to cover the exposed cartilage (Figure 9.3).

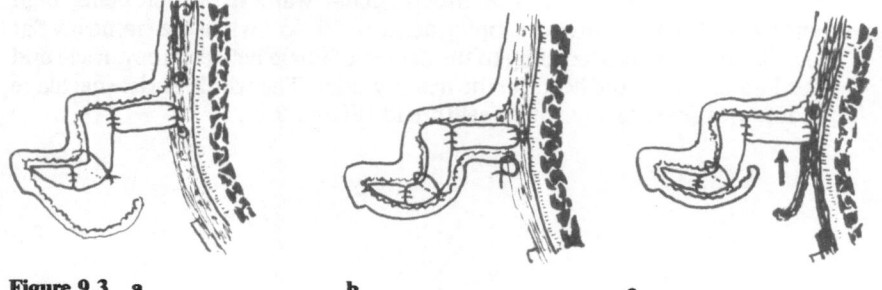

Figure 9.3   a   **b**   **c**

(6)   Free skin graft was used to cover the soft tissue wound of the new auricle without skin in the postauricular or mastoid region. In the event of the remnant ear not being enough to form the tragus, a piece of cartilage implant in the preauricular region might be used instead.

Sutures were removed 2 weeks after operation.

CLINICAL MATERIALS

Since 1980, 50 cases of one-stage total auricle reconstruction have been operated on with this technique – 46 males and four females, patients between the ages of 15 and 40. Causes of auricle defect comprised: congenital microauricle, 43; burn, four; incised wound, one; infection, one; and tumor excision one. Follow-up lasted from 6 to 29 months.

Results

All 50 cases of the reconstructed auricles were alive, with good shape, size and cranioauricular angle, essentially symmetrical with the healthy auricle. The skin

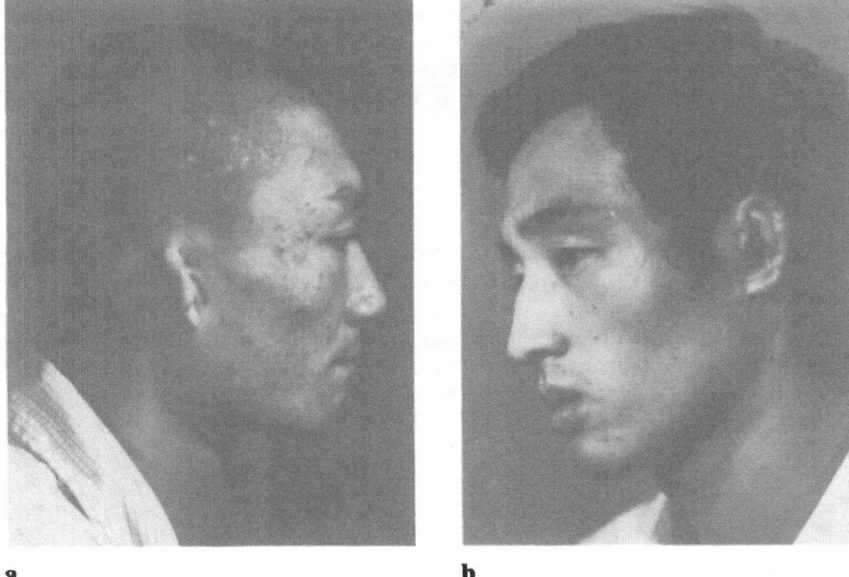

a b

Figure 9.4 Congenital microtia. Case 1. **a,** Preoperative view. **b,** Eleven months after operation

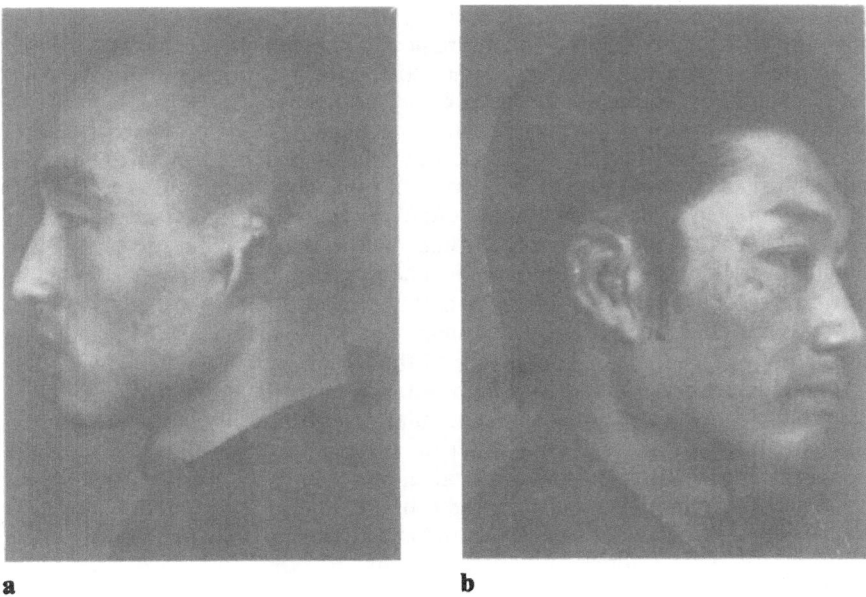

a b

Figure 9.5 Congenital microtia. Case 2. **a,** Preoperative view. **b,** Ten months after operation

color was harmonious, the helix, counterhelix and conchal cavity were well visualized. No dislocation, contraction, transformation of the reconstructed auricle or phenomenon of cartilage absorption was noticed during follow-up observation. The only undesirable result was that the new auricle was somewhat clumsy (Figures 9.4, 9.5).

Complications and their treatment

In nine of the 50 cases, complications were seen. Hematomas under the skin flap occurred in two cases and these were treated with secondary skin graft. Skin perforation due to steel wire occurred in one case and was treated by extraction of steel wire and local plastic management. A small area of exposed cartilage occurred in six patients, four of whom were treated with an islet skin flap containing a branch of the superficial temporal artery or a skin-deep fascia flap, and the others with local skin flap graft. In all the nine cases, the wound healed after secondary treatment.

DISCUSSION

The key to one-stage auricle reconstruction[5-7]

A tissue flap with good blood supply and of good quality, which could be raised in a single step and large enough to wrap around the whole cartilage auricle frame, is essential for one-stage auricle reconstruction. The ideal covering of the cartilage auricle frame would be a skin flap in the postauricular or mastoid region. Unfortunately, the skin in this region is quite limited. Ordinarily, it could be utilized to wrap only the flap anterior surface of the auricle, but it would not be enough to wrap round the deep cavity and protruding structures on the surface of the auricle, especially in patients with a low hair-bearing area. Therefore, there is not enough skin in this region to be used as an ideal covering of the whole auricle. To overcome the difficulty of inadequate skin in this region, the authors adopted a 'skin-subcutaneous flap' raised in this region large enough to wrap any type of auricle cartilage frame, the technique of raising such a flap having been described in detail above. The skin in the mastoid region has the advantages of being harmonious in color, thin and soft in quality, and the different auricle structures are well visualized and give an excellent contour when used for covering the anterior surface of the auricle.

The blood supply of the 'skin-subcutaneous flap' in the mastoid region is chiefly furnished by the posterior auricular artery, and also by the auricular branch of the occipital artery, anterior auricular branch of the superficial temporal artery, anterior tympanic branch of the internal maxillary artery and communicating branches between these branches and the posterior auricular artery, direct anastomosing branches and anastomosing branches between these arteries. All these arteries and their branches together formed a circulatory system. In patients with congenital microauricle, due to atresia of the external ear orifice and auricle defect, some of the above-named deeper anastomotic branches became more superficial and direct. The circulatory system formed by these arteries and their branches provided not only the blood supply of all the different tissue layers, including the skin, subcutaneous layer, periauricular muscles and deep fascia, in a horizontal direction, but also the blood supply in a vertical direction through the vertically communicating branches. Even when the blood supply from the occipital artery is cut off and most of the blood supply from the anterior auricular branches of the superficial temporal artery is obstructed, as often happens during the process of raising the 'skin–subcutaneous flap' and excision of the ear remnant, the bloodstream from the perforating branches of the posterior auricular artery near the posterior auricular muscle would still be sufficient to supply the whole flap through the anastomotic branches. Not one of these 50 cases showed signs of disturbed blood supply of the 'skin–subcutaneous flap'.

The skin in the mastoid region is among the thinnest in the whole body, about 0.79 ± 0.16 mm thick; the subcutaneous layer in this region is also quite thin; the thickness of the 'skin–subcutaneous flap' raised is therefore very thin and almost as thin as the whole-thickness skin at the trunk. In spite of such a thin flap, it still contains abundant subcuticular and subcutaneous vascular nets. Therefore, it is a thin flap with good blood supply and the convex and concave structures of the auricle cartilage frame can be well visualized.

Deep to the subcutaneous layer are situated periauricular muscles and deep fascia, which are continuous upwards with the superficial and deep temporal fasciae backwards with galea aponeurotica; the latter can be raised to wrap the exposed cartilage if necessary and the wound be covered with skin graft afterwards. The temporal fascia can be divided into two layers for reconstructive use so as to lessen its thickness; even then its blood supply will be good. In six of the 50 cases, the deep fascia of the postauricular region was raised as a flap to wrap a portion of the cartilage frame followed by covering the wound surface with skin graft which grew well.

Auricle cartilage frame

In making the auricle cartilage frame, the authors used a piece of arcuate cartilage laid behind the counterhelix as the posterior concha and this technique had the following molding effects in auricle reconstruction: (1) deepening of the concha cavity, (2) formation of a stable cranioauricular angle, (3) stable fixation of the auricle *in situ* and (4) strengthening of stereosensation of the auricle.

The degree of this piece of arcuate cartilage should be made identical with that of the counterhelix and the height identical with that of the normal auricle according to the degree of cranioauricular angle of the healthy side. Ordinarily, the height of this arcuate cartilage is 4–7 mm. The value calculated from the right-angled triangular function might be used for reference (Figure 9.6). The relation of the auricle to the lateral cranial wall in normal subjects is as follows. Should the cranioauricular angle be 30°, then:

ACD would be the line indicating the anterior view of the auricle,
ABF the line of the lateral cranial wall,
CB the line of the posterior conchal wall,

CB $\perp$ AF ($\because$ the angle between the concha and skull $=90°$)
$\angle$ BAC $=30°$ (angle between the auricle and skull),

then, according to geometric analysis, the height of the arcuate cartilage EB would be:

EB $=$ CB $-$ CE
$\because$ CB $=$ sin $30°$ AC $= \frac{1}{2}$ AC ($\because$ sin $30° = \frac{1}{2}$)

AC, the length from the tragus to counterhelix, can be measured on the healthy side; CE, the thickness of the cartilage frame at the site of counterhelix, can also be measured. So, EB can be readily calculated. But during preparation of the posterior concha wall, the height would be:

EB -2 mm (this 2 mm being the thickness of the skin flap enwrapping).

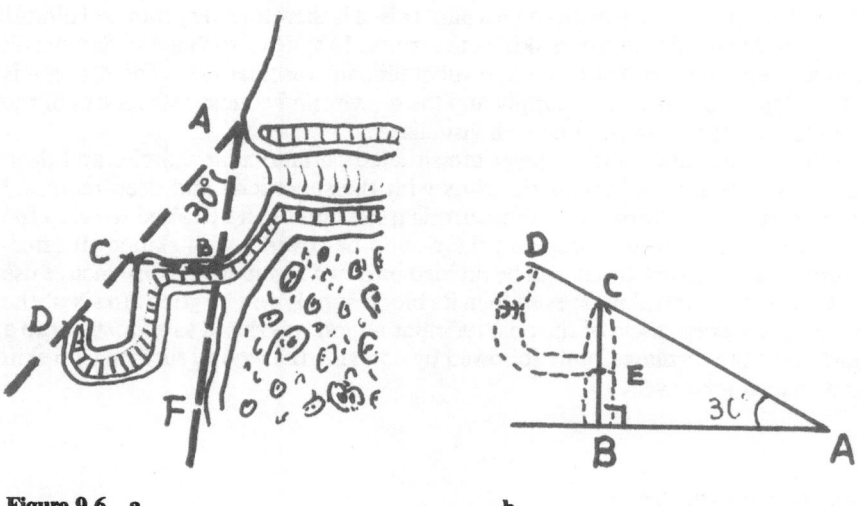

Figure 9.6 a   **b**

Formation of external ear orifice and reconstruction of tragus

In two of the 50 cases, formation of the external ear orifice was performed simultaneously; and in six of them, reconstruction of the tragus with cartilage implant was performed, which made the auricle reconstruction more natural looking. The technique of tragus reconstruction is illustrated in Figures 9.1 and 9.2. In such cases none showed signs of disturbed blood supply of the auricle tissue flap.

REFERENCES

1. Braner, R. O. (1981). Changes in plastic surgery in 36 years. *Plast. Reconstr. Surg.*, **67**, 341
2. Dunton, E. F. *et al.* (1964). A compromise approach to total ear reconstruction. *Plast. Reconstr. Surg.*, **34**, 427

3. Tanzer, R. (1959). Total reconstruction of the external ear. *Plast. Reconstr. Surg.,* **23,** 1

4. Tanzer, R. C. (1971). Total reconstruction of the auricle. *Plast. Reconstr. Surg.,* **47,** 523

5. Arelar, J. M. (1977). Reconstrucão total do pavilhão auricula num único tempo cirúrgico. *Rev. Bras. Cir.,* **67,** 139

6. Arelar, J. M. (1978). Reconstrução total da orelha numa única cirúrgia. *Folha Med.,* **76,** 457

7. Avela, J. M. Microtia – Simplified technique for total reconstruction of the auricle in one stage. *In Proceedings of the VII International Congress of Plastic and Reconstructive Surgery, Rio de Janeiro, Brazil.*

10 Surgical Management of Traumatic Laryngotracheal Stenosis

WANG DA-MEI
The Third Teaching Hospital, Beijing Medical College
YUAN PONG-NIAN, WANG ZHENG-QIANG and WANG WEN-HUI
The First Teaching Hospital, Kunming Medical College

Trauma and infections (tuberculosis, syphilis) are among the commonest causes of cicatricial laryngotracheal stenosis. The patient may breathe freely for a long lapse of time through a relatively narrowed laryngeal or tracheal lumen but may not be able to cope with the difficulties from excessive secretions during the bouts of respiratory infection.

Recent approaches to the problem, especially in the case of severe subglottic stenosis, instead of trying to excise the stenotic portion or to set free the cicatricial adhesions in the laryngotrachea, are aiming at the plastic enlargement of the stricture in order to enhance respiration and phonation.

An autogenous chondromucosal composite flap of the nasal septum or a piece of costal cartilage with intact perichondrium are used by us in the reconstruction of the stenotic laryngotrachea with fairly satisfactory results. Three such cases are reported below.

CASE REPORTS

Case 1

A 37-year-old male worker was admitted in May 1980 with the chief complaints of hoarseness and dyspnea on major exertion for 6 months. The patient had a history of neck stab trauma. Examination revealed a transverse linear scar 12 cm long at the upper border of the thyroid cartilage. Glottic stenosis was confirmed by neck X-ray film, fiberoptic tracheoscopy and direct laryngoscopy. The anterior commissure of the vocal cords was obliterated by a dense membranous scar adhesion, its surface being fairly smooth. The vocal cords had an unclear landmark and motion was limited. The subglottis and trachea were normal. A preoperative diagnosis of traumatic laryngeal web was made. Tracheotomy and laryngotomy were carried out under intravenous administration of γ-OH supplemented by local procaine infiltration anesthesia. An incision was made through the old stab wound scar and the thyroid cartilage was exposed and

65

opened through the midline. The fibrous web was split into two layers along its free margin, and two 60 ° flaps were made as a Z-plasty procedure to repair the vocal cords, enlarge the lumen and cover the raw surface (Figure 10.1). The wound was closed in layers. The postoperative course was uneventful and the tracheotomy tube was removed on the tenth postoperative day. After operation, dyspnea disappeared and phonation improved greatly. Tracheoscopic examination 2 weeks after operation revealed disappearance of the web, and the glottic fissure was nearly normal. This patient was followed 1 year later with a good outcome.

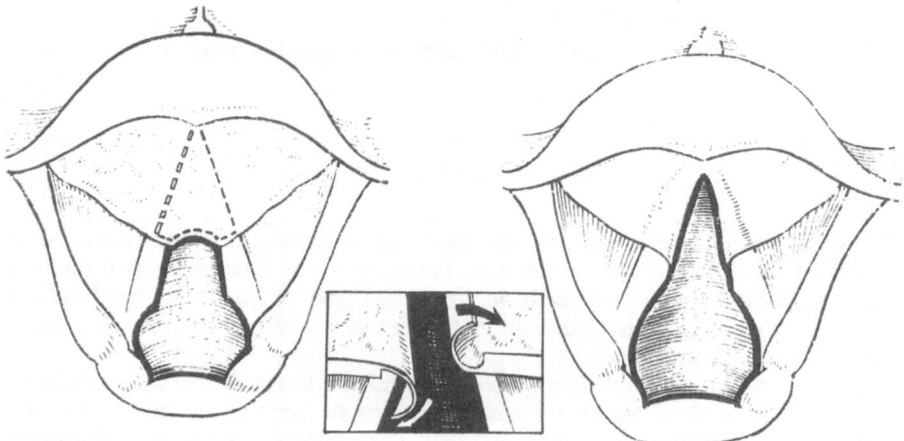

Figure 10.1   Case 1. The fibrous laryngeal web was split at the midline and two flaps were used to reconstruct the vocal cords

Case 2

A 12-year-old boy student was admitted in October 1979 for traumatic tracheal stenosis which originated 8 years before, after a traumatic injury of the neck caused by a cow's horn. Having been fractured and collapsed, the trachea was stenosed in such a way that an urgent tracheotomy was necessary. Repeated dilatations were tried to enlarge the stenosis, but without benefit, and tracheotomy obturation was followed by dyspnea and cyanosis. Fiberoptic tracheoscopy and X-ray film demonstrated a cicatricial ring stenosis of the trachea 4 cm below the glottis, the narrowest luminal diameter being 3–4 mm. Under intravenous γ-OH anesthesia supplemented by local procaine infiltration, plastic enlargement of the tracheal stenosis was done by means of a chondro-mucosal free composite graft of the nasal septum. The cervical trachea was approached through a midline incision with the infrahyoid muscles retracted. The thyroid isthmus was divided. The collapsed second, third and fourth tracheal rings had been replaced by dense fibrous tissues which were excised leaving only a band of tracheal mucosa intact along the posterior tracheal ligament. A $4 \times 4 \, cm^2$ tracheal mucosa defect was estimated, the anterior and lateral tracheal walls being lost. The cut edges of the stenosed trachea were anchored to the sternocleidomastoid muscles to keep them apart.

Under submucous anesthesia of the nasal cavities, the nasal septum was thoroughly exposed via an incision through the right nasal ala. Six millimeters posterior to the columella from the anteroinferior portion of the nasal septum, a curved incision deepened down to the septal cartilage was made. Dissection proceeded into a plane between the septal cartilage and the mucoperichondrium of the opposite nasal cavity in such a way that the mucochondrium of the opposite side should be intact after ablation of the composite flap. The composite chondromucosal flap consisted of a piece of $2 \times 2.5 \, cm^2$ nasal septal cartilage in continuation with a $4 \times 3 \, cm^2$ mucochondrium. Several vertical linear fracture incisions were made on the septal cartilage specimen in order to model a semicircular composite septal graft (Figure 10.2). The incised nasal ala was repaired and the nasal cavities were tamponned with iodoform gauze.

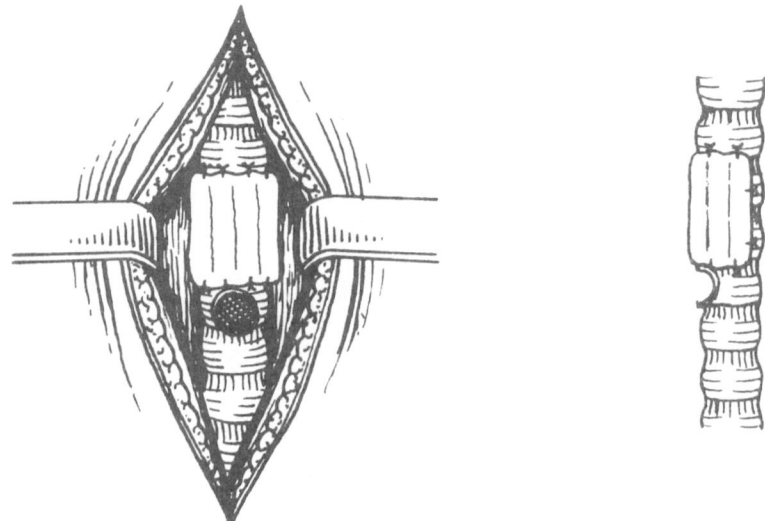

Figure 10.2 Case 2. Contoured nasal septal chondromucosal graft sutured in place of the tracheal wall defect following releasing of the tracheal stenosis

After placing the composite graft in position with its mucoperichondrium facing the tracheal lumen, submucosal No. 1 silk interrupted sutures were used for graft fixation. Care should be taken to avoid exposing the sutures into the tracheal lumen in order to prevent granulation formation within the trachea.

No intratracheal stent was used. A right sternohyoid muscular flap was rotated to cover the graft. The wound was closed in layers with 3/0 interrupted silk sutures. A compressive dressing was applied. Liquid diet was given 48 h postoperatively. Antibiotic therapy was administered for 7 days. The tracheal wound healed without incident.

Twelve days after operation, fiberoptic tracheoscopic examination revealed the composite graft had survived perfectly. There was no evidence of granulation tissues. The diameter of the reconstructed trachea lumen was normal in size. Ablation of the tracheotomy tube was carried out 1 month later and no respiratory distress was observed 40 days after operation. Repeated fiberoptic tracheoscopy and X-ray examination revealed the same features as before (Figure 10.3). The tracheocutaneous fistula 0.6 cm in diameter was repaired under general anesthesia with local hinged and rotation flap. The donor area skin was closed by direct approximation sutures. The patient was discharged 1 week after the fistula repair. Follow-up study 6 months after operation revealed satisfactory result. The patient is free from respiratory distress, even during bouts of respiratory infection.

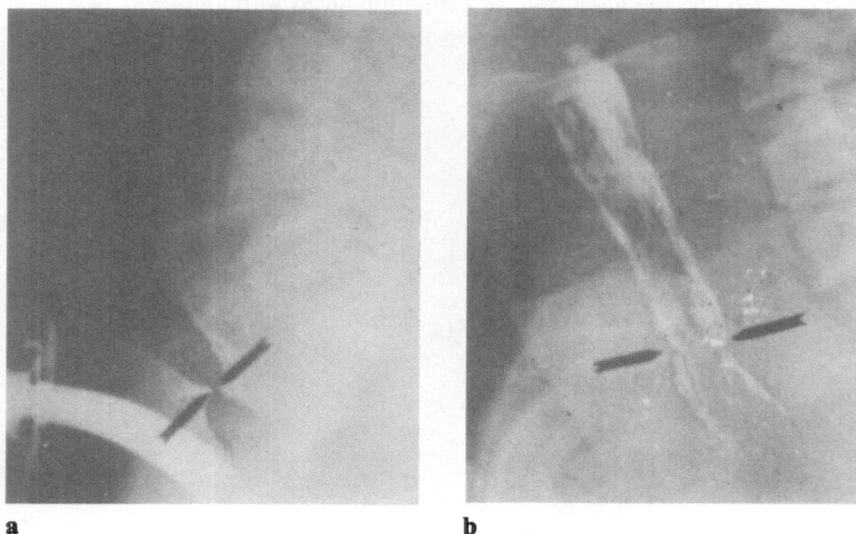

a   b

Figure 10.3 Case 2. **a,** Preoperative X-ray film showing the tracheal narrowing. **b,** Postoperative tomography showing satisfactory correction of the tracheal stenosis

Case 3

A 46-year-old male farmer was hospitalized in February 1981 with the chief complaints of hoarseness for 18 years and shortness of breath for 4 years after a neck blunt trauma. Physical examination revealed inspiratory stridor accompanied by marked retraction of the suprasternal and supraclavicular fossae. Dense fibrotic narrowing below the epiglottis was discovered by laryngoscopy and fiberoptic tracheoscopy. The narrowest part of the trachea was only 3 mm in diameter. Motion of the vocal cords was limited. Cantani and Wassermann tests were negative. Biopsy showed chronic inflammation of the fibrotic tissue. Preparatory tracheotomy was performed under local anesthesia,

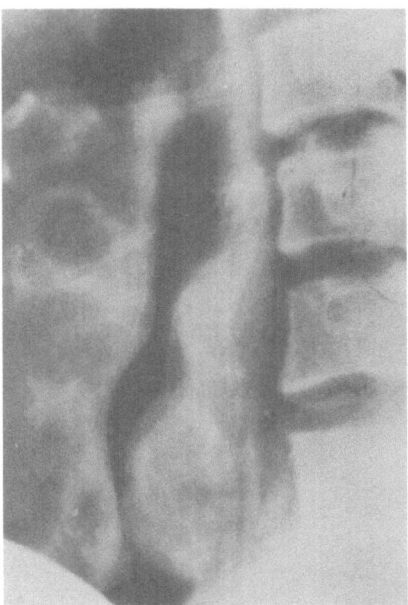

Figure 10.4   Case 3. Preoperative X-ray film showed the presence of subglottic stenosis

the third, fourth and fifth tracheal rings being normal on exploration. X-ray examination of the neck revealed subglottic stenosis (Figure 10.4). A diagnosis of chronic inflammatory subglottic stenosis of the trachea was accordingly made.

Costal cartilage graft with intact perichondrium was used to reconstruct the subglottic tracheal stenosis. Under intravenous anesthesia (2.5% thiopental sodium plus 1% procaine), a vertical neck incision was made to expose the larynx; the thyroid and cricoid cartilage which were markedly thickened and partly calcified were vertically split in the midline. The lumen of the stenotic trachea was in the form of an anteroposterior oval slit which extended from the level of the vocal cords to the first tracheal ring. The stenotic cartilages were longitudinally opened and the cut edges were anchored with No. 1 silk sutures to the sternocleidomastoid muscles to keep them apart (Figure 10.5a). The right eighth costal cartilage was used and a piece of cartilage 5 cm with perichondrium intact was excised. Several linear fracture incisions were made on it in order to shape a semicircular graft which was inserted to the defect in such a way that the broader part of the costal cartilage was interposed between the cut edges of the thyroid and cricoid cartilages, with the perichondrial lining facing the endotracheal lumen (Figure 10.5b). The graft was fixed in position with No. 1 interrupted silk sutures subperichondrially. No stent was used. The wound was closed in layers leaving a rubber tissue drain in place. Compressive dressing was used and meticulous tracheostomy nursing care was carried out.

The postoperative course was uneventful and the rubber tissue drain was

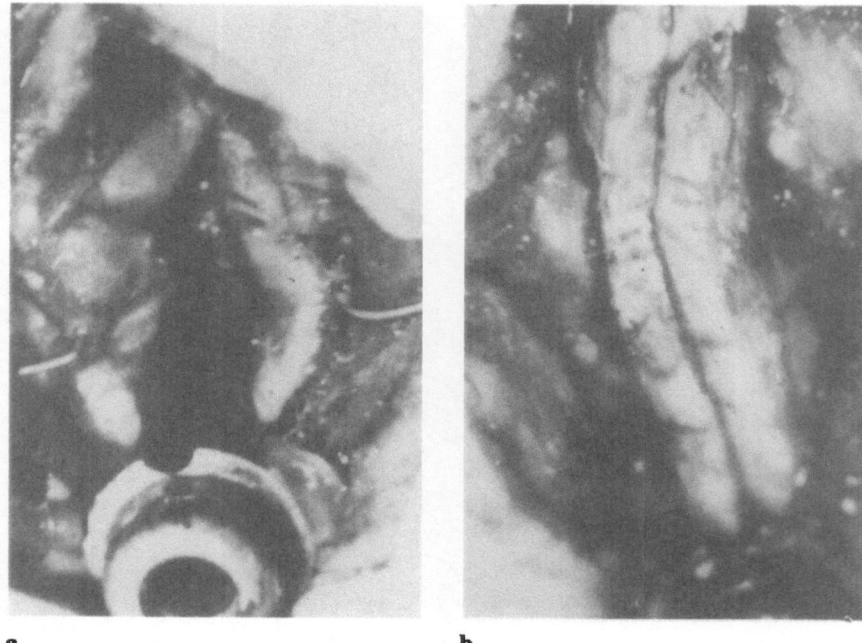

a   b

Figure 10.5 Case 3. **a,** The stenotic cartilages were longitudinally opened and the cut edges were sutured to the sternocleidomastoid muscles to keep them apart. **b,** A piece of costal cartilage with perichondrium intact on one side was inserted into the defect and sutured in position. The perichondrium faces the tracheal lumen

removed 34 hours after operation. Twenty-nine days after operation, fiberoptic laryngoscopic examination demonstrated that the graft was almost completely lined with respiratory epithelium except a grain sized raw surface, no granulation tissue being present. The laryngeal airway was markedly enlarged. The tracheostomy tube was removed without incident and the opening closed without delay. The phonation was much improved. Signs of respiratory distress had disappeared. Repeated laryngoscopic examination 40 days after operation disclosed a complete epithelial lining of the graft. X-ray film examination, 3 months later, showed a subglottic space within normal limits (Figure 10.6).

DISCUSSION

Careful radiologic and endoscopic evaluation is essential for the proper management of laryngotracheal stenosis. In web-like stenosis, even if the stenotic lumen is very much reduced, it can be corrected by judicious dilatations; often only one dilatation will be necessary. The longer the stenotic involvement of the trachea, the more difficult the treatment. Adequate airway and good

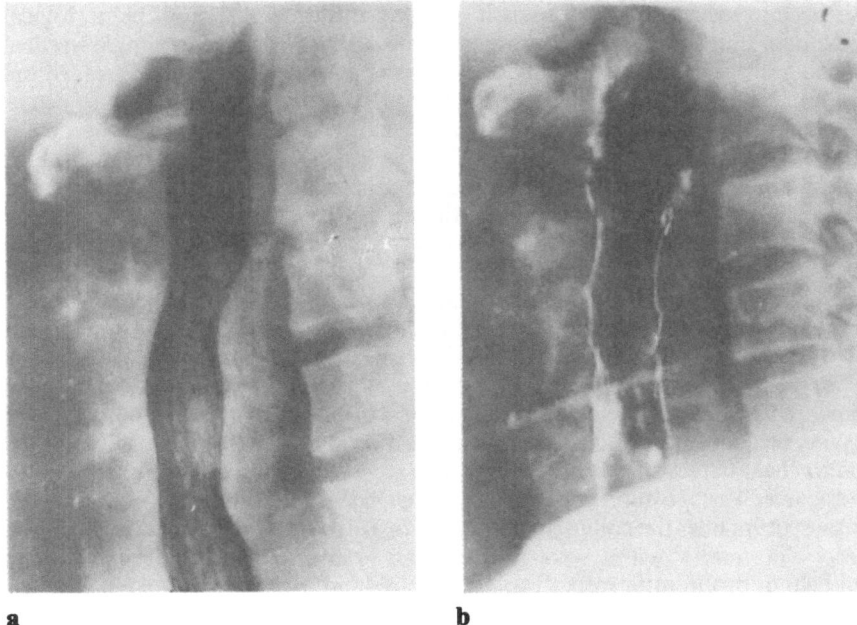

a   b

Figure 10.6   Case 3. **a,** Postoperative X-ray film illustrates adequate correction of the stenosis. **b,** Good result is confirmed on tomography

phonation are the criteria of therapeutic success; the normal growth of the larynx should not be impeded in infant cases.

When subglottic stenosis has not responded to dilatations, an open procedure in an attempt to correct the obstruction is justified.

For supraglottic stenosis, resection of the stenotic part followed by direct suture is recommended. Thin and soft membranous subglottic stenosis can be cured by section of the membrane by use of the fiberoptic laryngoscope followed by repeated dilatations.

In Case 1, the laryngeal web was too firm and thick to respond to the above treatment. Web excision followed by skin grafting necessitates a triangular stent for a long duration. Furthermore, the result is by no means certain. Splitting of the web in two mucosal flaps to reconstruct two vocal cords is a simple and efficacious technique we used in this case, the raw surface being not persisted, and a stent not being used. The postoperative adhesion is reduced to a minimum.

For more extensive subglottic stenosis, surgical resection and end-to-end anastomosis have been advocated. The resection is obligatorily limited and excessive tension to the anastomosis favors subsequent scarring and cartilage resorption with high risk of consequent stenosis. Among other techniques are stenting, steroid injections, auricular composite graft, and costal cartilage combined with buccal mucosal graft.

Plastic reconstruction for such subglottic stenosis should be a logical technique and is now the method of choice. It consists of a simple vertical opening of the stenotic segment and a piece of autogenous cartilage graft (nasal septal cartilage composite graft, thyroid or rib cartilage graft) is used to repair the defect and establish a free airway. Neither stent nor steroid therapy is necessary.

Implantation of an autogenous nasal septal cartilage graft to a defect created on the trachea, cricoid or thyroid cartilages of experimental dogs was done by Fuross and Toohill[1] as early as 1971. The graft was fixed in place by submucosal sutures. Extubation was done immediately after operation. Repeated post-operative laryngoscopic examination and biopsy histologic study revealed that the technique is valuable in the reconstruction of the airway. Clinical application of this technique in the reconstruction of severe laryngotracheal stenosis was reported in 13 cases[1-5]. In Case 2, two cut edges of the stenotic trachea were anchored to the sternocleidomastoid muscles to hold them open, and a nasal septal cartilage composite flap modeled in a semicircular form fit quite well to the tracheal defect with excellent postoperative result. Care should be taken to preserve at least a 6 mm wide septal cartilage in the anteroinferior portion of the nasal septum near the columellar region in order to prevent postoperative saddle nose. The nasal cavities were packed with iodoform gauze. The respiratory epithelium proliferates rather rapidly, about 1 mm per day. In the ten cases of eyelid reconstruction by means of nasal septal graft, no saddle nose deformity was observed.

Cotton (1978)[7] used the autogenous costal cartilage for certain children with severe anterior subglottic stenosis. Fearon and Cotton[6,7], on the basis of experimental data on growing monkeys, indicated that extensive operative procedures in the growing larynx did not interfere with growth potential. It was only necessary to make an incision through the cricoid cartilage to release the stenosis and interpose a graft without removing the scar tissue and without internal resurfacing or stenting to achieve an adequate cricoid lumen. They used autogenous thyroid cartilage for two patients with good results. The logical use of thyroid cartilage as a grafting material is suitable for reconstructing a medium sized cricoid stricture defect. In patients who have little or no identifiable cartilage remaining anteriorly or in whom the stenosis is long, the costal cartilage graft procedure is the method of choice.

When the stenosis is very extensive and is beyond the scope of the operations described above, Fearon and Cotton used a variation of Rethi or Grahne techniques. This consists of a median section of the thyroid and cricoid cartilages as well as the upper tracheal rings. The cicatricial tissue is resected and is followed by a median section of the posterior cricoid lamina down to the esophageal musculature. When necessary, the interarytenoid muscles are divided; an Aboulker type of prosthesis extending from the vocal cords to the level of the tracheotomy is placed in the lumen of the larynx and the trachea beyond the tracheotomy opening. The prosthesis is retained by wiring the tracheotomy tube through a properly placed fenestra in the prosthesis. The prosthesis is maintained in position for 5 months. Our Case 3 belonged to this type. We used the Fearon–Cotton procedure and obtained a satisfactory result.

The definite advantages of autogenous nasal septal and costal cartilage grafts are: (1) the procedure of wedging a graft into a defect is simple to manipulate, neither stent nor steroid therapy are necessary; (2) extensive dissection or section of supportive tissues are avoided; (3) recurrent or superior laryngeal nerve injuries are prevented; (4) good match is achieved between the graft and the laryngotrachea; (5) no functional or esthetic problems arise in the donor site; (6) intratracheal granulation formation is prevented by submucosal sutures.

SUMMARY

Three cases of traumatic cicatricial subglottic tracheal stenosis are presented. Local mucosal flaps, autogenous nasal septal composite graft with intact mucosa and free costal cartilage with perichondrium attached on one side are used in the reconstruction of the stenotic laryngotrachea. A good airway and improved phonation are achieved.

REFERENCES

1. Fuross, J. A. and Toohill, R. J. (1973). Composite nasal septal autograft of the trachea. *Ann. Otol. Rhinol. Laryngol.*, **82**, 2831
2. Toohill, R. J. *et al.* (1976). Repair of laryngeal stenosis with nasal septal grafts. *Ann. Otol. Rhinol. Laryngol.*, **85**, 600
3. Wilflingseder, P. von (1971). Tracheal stenosis reconstruction by means of a nasal-septum graft. In *Fifth International Congress of Plastic and Reconstructive Surgery*, pp. 1219–22. (London: Butterworths)
4. Wilflingseder, P. von (1972). Rekonstruktion der trachea durch ein segment-transplantät vom nasenseptum. *Sonderdruck Wien. Klin. Wochenschr.*, **84**, 226
5. Fearon, B. and Cotton, R. (1974). Surgical correction of subglottic stenosis of larynx in infants and children. *Ann. Otol. Rhinol. Laryngol.*, **83**, 428
6. Fearon, B. *et al.* (1978). Subglottic stenosis of the larynx in the infant and child. Method of management. *Ann. Otol. Rhinol. Laryngol.*, **87**, 645
7. Cotton, R. (1978). Management of subglottic stenosis in infancy and childhood. Review of consecutive series of cases managed by surgical reconstruction. *Ann. Otol. Rhinol. Laryngol.*, **87**, 648

11 Second Toe to Thumb Reconstruction – Long Term Observation on a Child

GAO JING-HANG, XU ZHEN-KUEN and ZHENG HUA-XIANG

Department of Surgery, Zunyi Medical College

The second toe to thumb reconstruction is a classic method for adult patients[1-5]. Here we report a child having had his thumb reconstructed with his own second toe. A 4-year follow-up study revealed satisfactory esthetic and functional results.

CASE REPORT

An 8-year-old boy was admitted in September 1978 for electric burn sequelae in his left hand. Examination revealed complete thumb loss with cicatricial contracture of the index and middle fingers (Figure 11.1). Under endotracheal anesthesia, the second toe to thumb reconstruction was carried out by two surgical teams.

Donor site

After the first digital web skin incision and division of the first plantar artery, the extensor hallucis brevis muscle was divided at the level of the metatarso-phalangeal (MTP) joint. The medial skin flap was dissected from deep fascia to the extensor hallucis longus muscle. The dissection proceeded proximally along the ligated plantar artery to expose the first metatarsal dorsal artery. The first dorsal interosseous muscle and lumbrical muscle were divided.

After the second web skin incision and division of the third plantar artery, the second interosseous muscle was divided and the second metatarsal bone was exposed and divided with a wire saw.

The incisions of the first and second webs were extended to the sole and the deep and superficial flexor tendons of the second digit along with the common plantar neurovascular bundle were exposed. After division of the tendons, the second toe was turned dorsally and the deep branch of the dorsalis pedis artery was exposed. The deep branch along with the arteria tarsea lateralis and arteriae

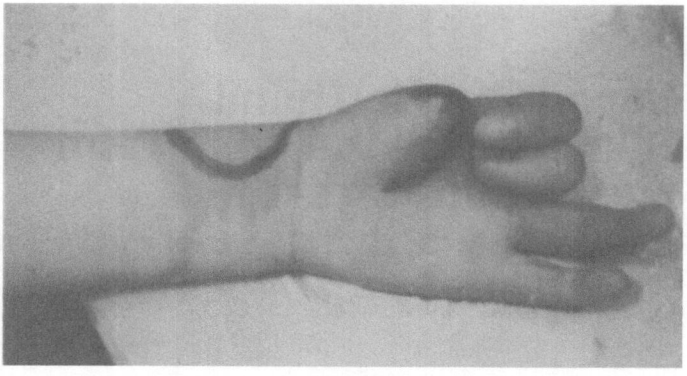

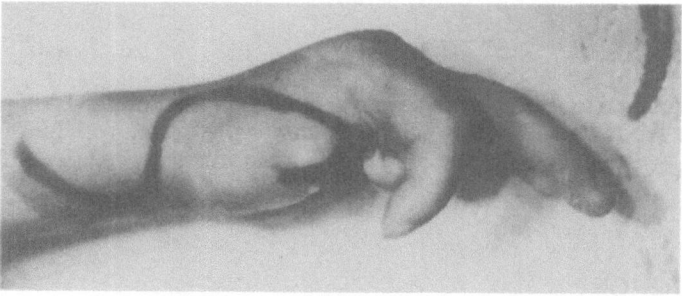

Figure 11.1   Loss of left thumb, and flexion deformity of index and middle fingers due to scar contraction

tarseae mediales were divided and tied and the bulk of extensor hallucis brevis divided. Now only the dorsalis pedis artery with its satellite vein remained attached to the transplant.

Recipient site

After scar excision on the thumb stump, the extensor pollicis longus and brevis, adductor pollicis and the sensory nerve of the thumb were exposed. The thenar muscles, superficial flexor muscle of the index and the proper nerve of the thumb were identified in the volar aspect of the hand. The cephalic vein and radial artery were exposed and ready for anastomosis.

Toe to thumb transplantation

The stumps of the second metatarsal and the first metacarpal were fashioned into an L shape and fixed by circular steel wire. The circulation of the transplant was reestablished by anastomosing the ankle vein (1.5 mm) to the cephalic vein

(1.3 mm) and the dorsalis pedis artery (1.2 mm) to the radial artery (1 mm). The transplant was reinnervated by suturing the superficial peroneal nerve and common plantaris nerve to the dorsal sensory nerve and the proper nerve of the thumb. The first dorsal interosseous and lumbrical, the extensor digitalis longus and the flexor profundus of the transplant were sutured respectively to the thenar muscles, extensor pollicis longus and flexor superficialis of the index.

The postoperative course was complicated by a subcutaneous hematoma which was evacuated without incident. Callus formation was found 5 weeks after operation. Nearly normal range of motion of the reconstructed thumb was obtained (Figure 11.2). The epiphyseal development and bone growth of the transplant were normal 4 years after operation (Figure 11.3).

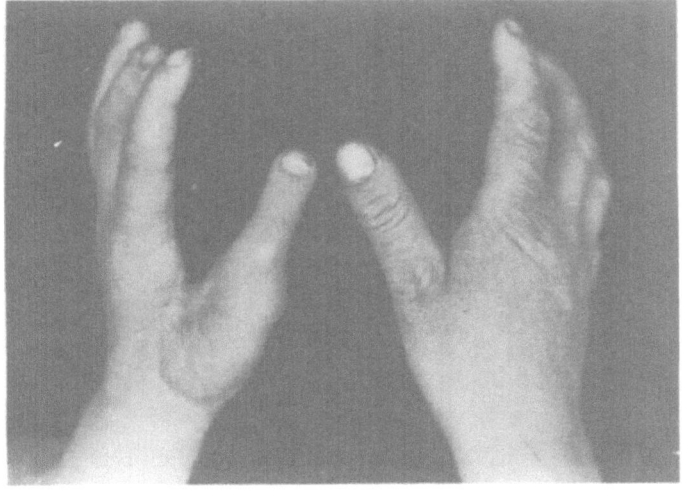

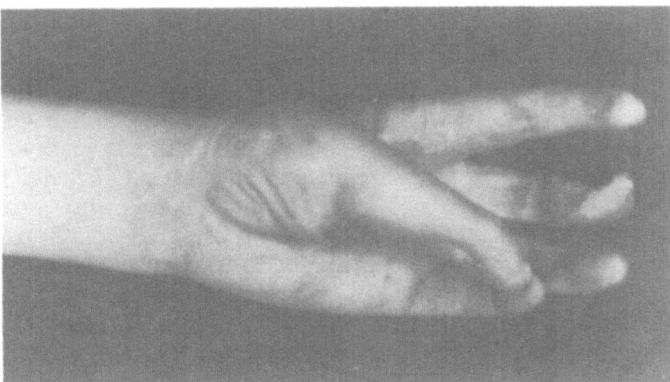

Figure 11.2 Function of the new thumb nearly normal and its configuration satisfactory. The new thumb was slightly longer than the right thumb

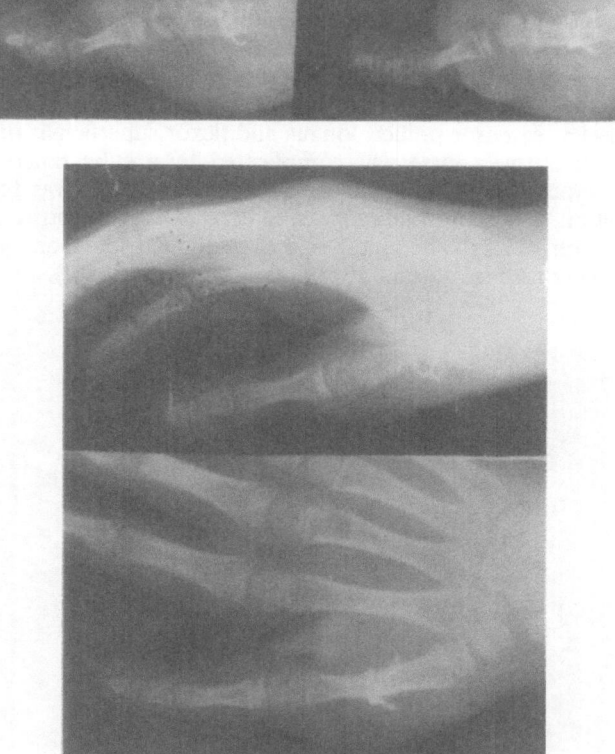

Figure 11.3 Epiphysis enlargement and normal growth of the bone graft were revealed in the roentgenograms

DISCUSSION

Growth of the transplant in childhood

In the toe to thumb transplantation, the MTP joint and its epiphysis should be included in the transplant to assure its normal growth (O'Brien[3]). In this case report with normal growth of the transplant, the following measures were carried out to protect the integrity of the epiphysis: (1) the middle section of the second metatarsal leaving the epiphysis intact; (2) circular steel wire fixation of the L-shaped bone stumps instead of using Kirschner wire, which may damage the epiphysis.

Integrity of the pedis dorsalis vascular bundle

This is the key to success of transplantation. To have an intact dorsalis pedis vascular bundle for anastomosis purposes, the dorsalis pedis flap and the second toe dissection should proceed alternately. The plantar dissection should be carried out first and the plantar neurovascular bundle is easy to approach; after section of the second metatarsal bone, the deep branch of the dorsalis pedis artery is easy to expose and tie; this makes the dissection of the dorsalis pedis vascular bundle much easier.

Strict postoperative surveillance

Strict postoperative surveillance should be undertaken within the immediate 24 postoperative hours. Any signs of disturbance in transplant circulation should be detected and treated in time. In this case, the evacuation of a subcutaneous hematoma was all that was necessary to overcome the circulation disturbance of the transplant.

REFERENCES

1. Yang, T. Y. (1977). Second toe to thumb reconstruction – a report of 40 cases. *Chinese J. Surg.*, **15**, 13.
2. Chang, T. S. (1979). In *Symposium of Microsurgery*, p. 66. (Shanghai)
3. O'Brien, B. McC. (1977). *Microvascular Reconstructive Surgery*. p. 182. (Edinburgh: Livingstone)
4. Cobbett, T. R. (1969). Free digital transfer. *J. Bone Jt. Surg.*, **51**, 677
5. Buncke, H. J. (1973). Thumb replacement. Great toe transplantation by microvascular anastomosis. *Br. J. Plast. Surg.*, **26**.

12 The Reverse Island Forearm Flap

WANG WEI and CHANG TI-SHENG

Department of Plastic and Reconstructive Surgery, Shanghai Second Medical College

In the past ten years, as a result of the growth in use of microsurgical techniques in the field of plastic and reconstructive surgery, more and more myocutaneous flaps and island flaps of different designs have emerged. Based on findings in anatomic study, we first designed an island dorsalis pedis flap in a clinical case in 1977, followed in 1980 by an island medial plantar flap (based on the medial plantar artery) and a reverse island forearm flap. These newly designed flaps together with microsurgical techniques have brought in a new era in our department. In this chapter we present our experiences in the use of the reverse island forearm flap, which was first performed on June 7 1980. This reverse island flap may be utilized to cover either the dorsal or the palmar side of hand defects. It can moreover be used for the purpose of reconstructing a lost thumb. Up to December 1982, a total of 18 cases (mostly hand injury) were carried out with 100% success.

ANATOMIC BASIS

The reverse island forearm flap, based on the distal part of the radial artery, receives a retrograde blood flow from the ulnar artery via the deep and superficial palmar arterial arches, and the venous blood returns through the cephalic vein and venae comitantes of the radial artery.

Anatomic features of the forearm arteries

The humeral artery courses down the upper arm to lie beneath the biceps branchial tendon at the cubital fossae of the elbow joint whence it divides into radial and ulnar arteries. These two arteries then run separately down along the radial and ulnar aspects of the forearm and send out the palmar interosseous artery and others. At the wrist region, each of these three arteries gives off tiny branches to communicate with each other, while in the hand, the radial and ulnar arteries meet to form the superficial and deep palmar arches in a closed circuit, with a caliber of about 1 mm. Therefore, the bloodstream can flow in a reverse direction in either of the arteries if it is cut proximally. The radial artery lies more superficially just beneath the skin at the lower third of the forearm where it sends between four and seven subcutaneous branches to supply the forearm skin. At the middle third of the forearm it traverses within the loose connective tissue between the brachioradialis and extensor carpal muscles, giving off two or three branches to nourish the skin. At the upper third, the artery is covered by the belly of the brachioradial muscle, supplying the over-lying skin through one to three tiny myocutanous branches.

Based on these anatomic features, a reverse island forearm flap may therefore be safely designed at the lower half of the forearm, if these subcutaneous branches are well preserved. But when the flap is placed at the upper half of the forearm, the surgeon must keep some of the myocutaneous branches intact. In order to achieve this, it is advisable to include a small belly of brachioradial muscle, about 2–3 cm wide, with the flap. Should need arise, one can also include the forearm lateral cutaneous nerve within the flap. Resection of this nerve usually brings no problems, as it produces only a small area of numbness at the lower half of the forearm.

DESIGN OF THE FLAP

Design principles are as follows.

(1) Draw with ink the course of the cephalic vein on the forearm.

(2) Define the course of the radial artery. Fix a point at the insertion of the biceps humeral tendon and a second point at the skin crease of the wrist intersected by the radial artery. Connect these two points with a line which represents the course of the radial artery. The size of the flap should be estimated according to individual need, and is outlined on both sides of this line. In order to include the cephalic vein enclosed in the flap, the radial half must be greater than the ulnar half (Figure 12.1)

(3) The length of its vascular pedicle should be well considered according to the requirements of the defect. There should be no overtorsion present when the flap is turned upside down by 180°.

OPERATIVE STEPS

The incision is made along the outline and carried down to the plane just superficial to the forearm fascia. Dissection of the flap begins from the two lateral margins and then carefully proceeds towards its center. When dissection approaches near the sulcus between the brachioradial muscle and radial extensor carpal muscle, it is deepened to include the forearm deep fascia and then carried on along this plane underneath the radial artery. At this stage, care should be taken to keep the artery and its branches as closely attached to the flap as possible. If the flap is placed at the upper half of the forearm, a thin belly of brachioradial muscle must be included within the flap. The proximal segment of the artery is then divided underneath the brachioradial muscle and the dissection is completed.

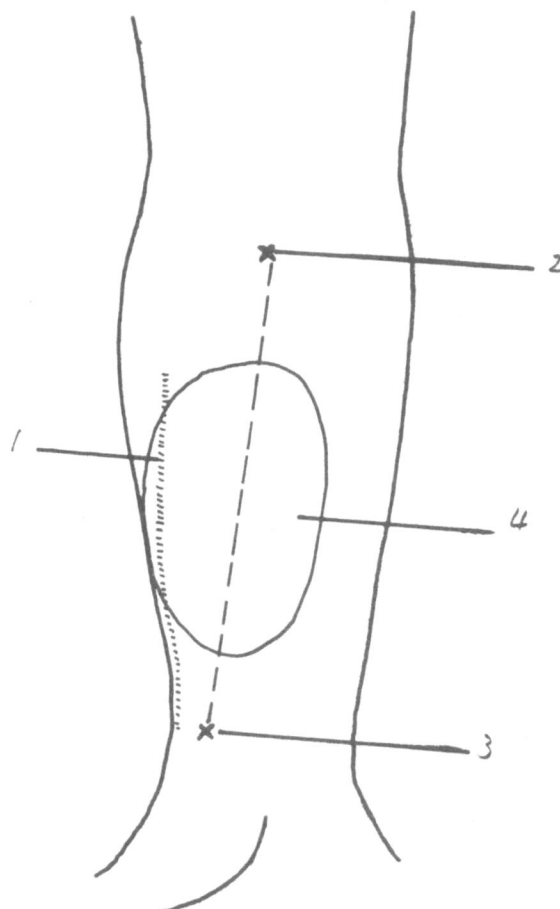

Figure 12.1 Plan of forearm island flap. The skin incision and the vessels outline. 1, Cephalic vein; 2, a point at the insertion of the bicep humeral tendon; 3, point where radial artery crosses the skin crease of the wrist; 4, the forearm island flap outline on both sides of the line of radial artery

It is important to keep intact the venae comitantes of the artery as well as the cephalic vein as a whole vascular bundle during dissection, and finally they are divided and ligated at the proximal end of the flap.

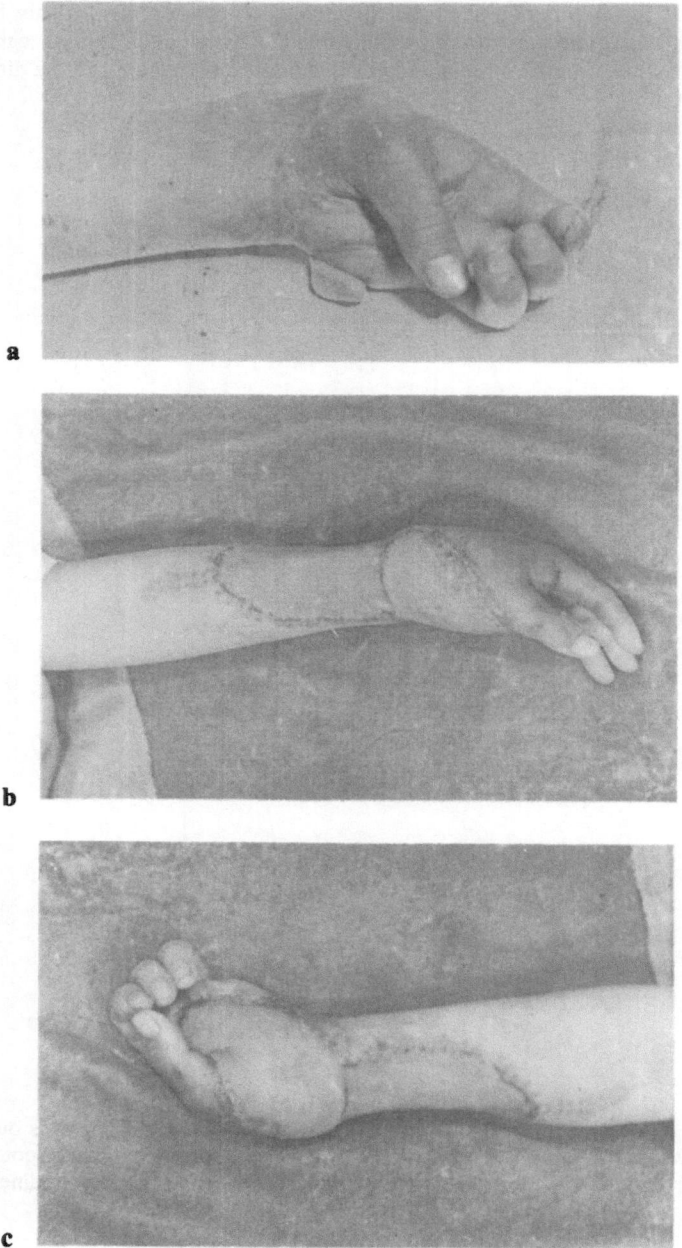

Figure 12.2   Case 1. **a**, Preoperative palmar view. **b**, Postoperative lateral view. **c**, Postoperative palmar view

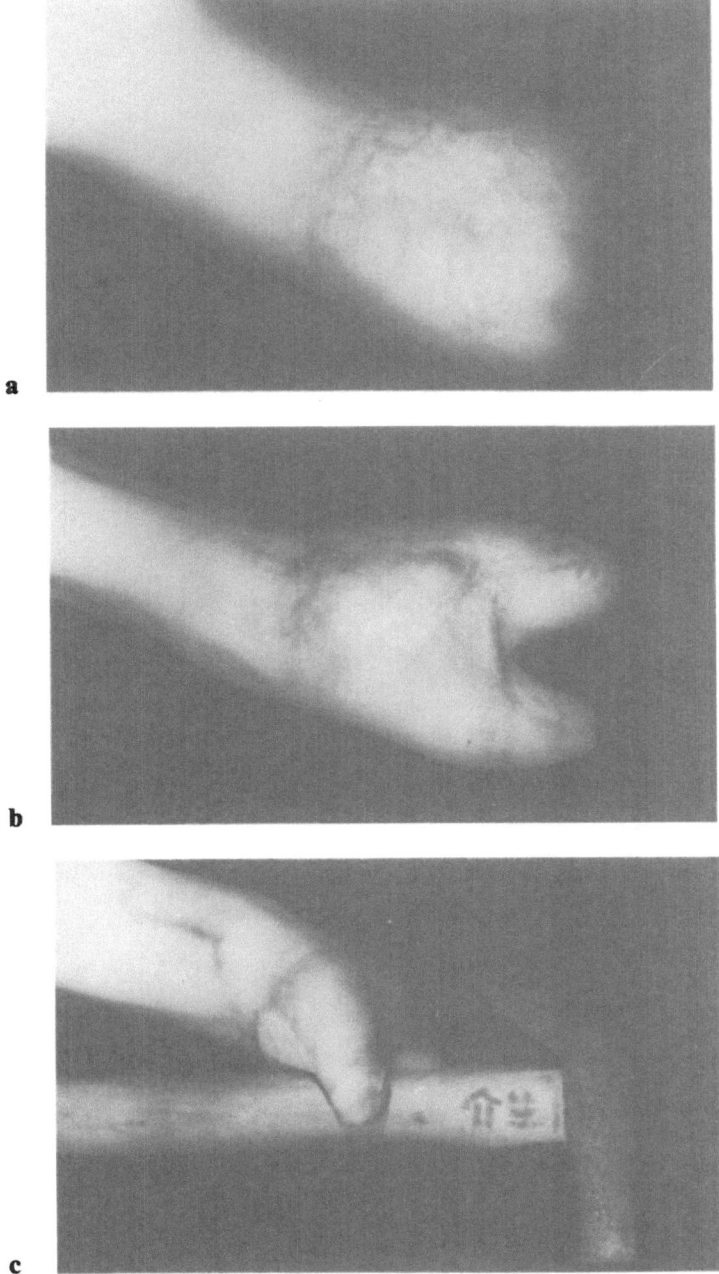

Figure 12.3 Case 2. **a**, Preoperative dorsal view. **b**, Postoperative palmar view. **c**, The patient can use the hammar

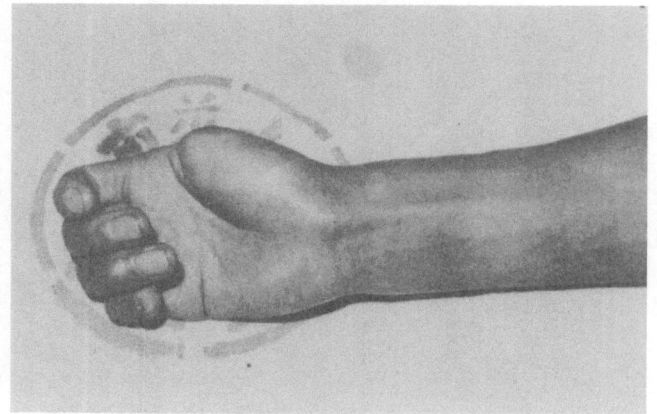

a

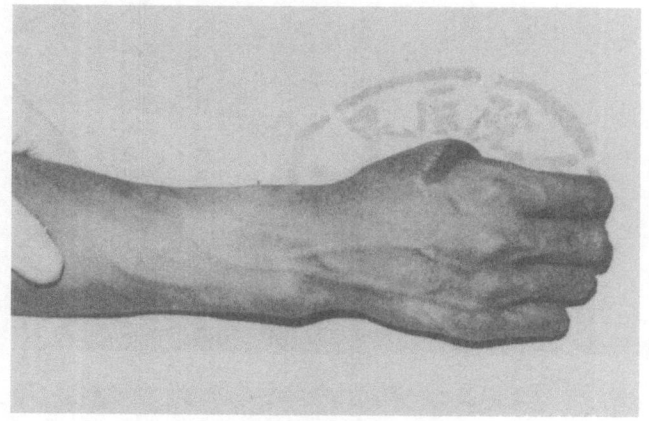

b

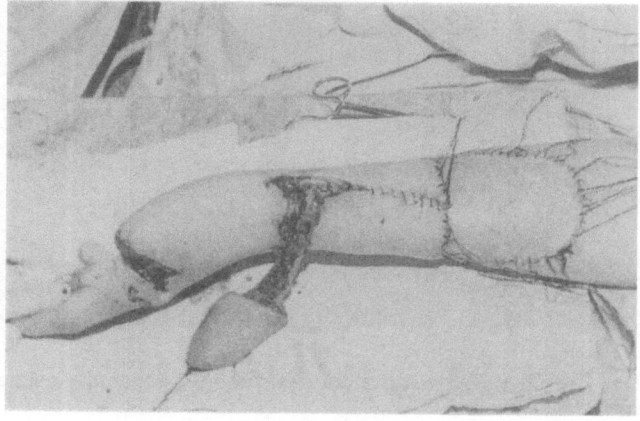

c

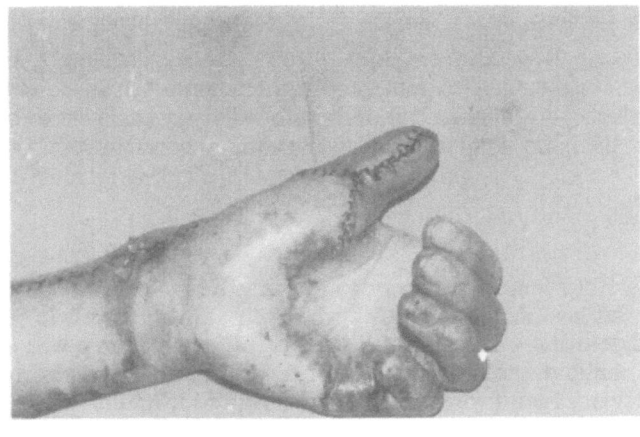

d

e

Figure 12.4 Case 3. **a,** Preoperative dorsal view. **b,** Preoperative palmar view. **c,** A forearm island flap was ready for transfer. **d,** Postoperative palmar view. **e,** Postoperative dorsal view

Management of the nerve

In this reverse flap, the forearm lateral cutaneous nerve may be included so as to make this a sensory flap. Partial recovery of sensation can usually be expected after nerve anastomosis. However, the superficial branch of the radial nerve must be preserved intact on the donor site.

Skin graft

This is usually required for coverage of the donor site.

CLINICAL CASES

In a period of 2½ years from June 7 1980 to December 1982, this flap was performed in 18 cases, ten male and eight female. Of these, ten cases were palmar defects with adducted thumb deformity, six cases were defects of the dorsum of the hand and two cases were thumb reconstruction.

Case 1

This 38-year-old female suffered from a severe scar contraction on her right palm and lost her small finger postburn. The right thumb was in severe adduction flexed deformity. The scar over the patient's right palmar was removed and the adduction and flexed deformities of the right thumb were corrected in one stage. A reverse island forearm flap measuring 13×7.5 cm^2 was designed and turned over to cover the wound on the palmar. The donor site of the forearm was covered with split thickness skin graft (Figure 12.2).

Case 2

A 22-year-old male had all the fingers and thumb of his right hand amputated at MP joint level, after postburn and avulsion injury. The right palmar and dorsal scar contraction are shown here. A surgical procedure was performed including removal of the second and third metacarpals and an island forearm flap measuring 6×8 cm^2. The patient is shown using a hammer after the operation (Figure 12.3).

Case 3

A 28-year-old male suffered from amputation of his right thumb at MP joint level. This patient was referred to us after failure of a toe-to-hand free transplantation. A forearm flap 7×7.5 cm^2 was designed and used to rebuild a thumb with iliac bone graft in one stage (Figure 12.4).

DISCUSSION

Firstly, due to its accessibility, the reverse island forearm flap is easily available for reconstruction of hand deformities, and the procedure is simple and safe. It can be completed in one stage even for quite a large defect. So far no postoperative functional disturbances with the donor site have ever been observed. The flap contains thin subcutaneous tissue overlaid by a rather tough skin, and therefore, when judged from the esthetic viewpoint, it seems to be an ideal flap for most cases of hand injury. It can be used either in acute injury or late cases. It is especially indicated for complicated cases when deep structures are exposed, such as damage to the tendon, bone and joint. It has also been used for the correction of first web contracture and adducted thumb, and also for the reconstruction of a missing thumb, etc.

Secondly, the reverse island forearm flap is nourished by a retrograde blood blow from the ulnar artery and therefore the capability of backblow in these two arteries must be confirmed by the Allen test preoperatively. Of course, this by no means implies that the integrity of veins can be ignored. However, physical examination can verify the status only of the superficial venous system, not the deep system. This problem can only be solved by a presumption – and this does work well in our hands, – ie, a detectable forceful pulsation of the artery in a patient who is not badly injured always speaks of the soundness of the venae comitantes. Moreover, it should be stressed that a normal artery if accompanied by two sound returning venous systems provides a smoother postoperative course for the flap than only one.

Thirdly, the island forearm flap can be safely designed as large as 12×8 cm^2, but when this limit is exceeded there will probably be problems in venous return. The following precautions are taken to alleviate this adverse outcome.

(1) If possible, avoid a flap larger than 12×8 cm^2.

(2) Never strip the nourishing vessels bare, but instead preserve carefully a thin layer of loose tissue around them to facilitate venous return.

(3) When a larger flap is inevitably needed for an extensive defect of the hand, a vein graft between the cephalic vein and that of the hand to enhance venous return may be helpful.

(4) Apply appropriate light pressure dressing postoperatively to overcome excessive edema of the flap.

Fourthly, generally the donor site requires a thick split-thickness skin graft for its coverage. A tieover dressing is applied to ensure a 100% take of the skin graft so that no functional interference with the donor forearm will follow.

REFERENCE

1. Yang Guo-fan et al. (1981). Forearm free skin flap transplantation. Natl. Med. J. China, 61, 139

13 Reconstructive Surgery for Postburn Hand Deformity

GAO XUE-SHU, HE QING-LIAN and ZHANG HUI-LAN

Department of Plastic and Reconstructive Surgery, Second Army Medical College

Superficial burns of the hand leave hardly any deformity after healing, but deep burns, especially those that have not been properly treated or just left to heal without skin grafting, will result in deformities with marked functional disturbances owing to scar contraction. Therefore, proper postburn reconstruction for these deformed hands is urgent and paramount. Since 1955, a total of 416 cases with postburn hand deformity has been admitted into our hospital for reconstruction; 317 patients were male and 99 female; 336 patients were adults and 80 children. Of the total patients, 40% (167 cases) were between 20 and 30 years old. In this chapter, we discuss the principles of treatment and methods adopted in our hospital.

CHARACTERISTICS OF CLAWHAND DEFORMITY

The hand consists of many small joints and tendons and is covered dorsally by a thin sheet of loose skin and subcutaneous tissue. The bony structures are so arranged that they form two important arches, namely the transverse and the longitudinal arches (Figure 13.1a) which are closely related to the hand's delicate functions of pinching, lifting, grasping etc.

Deep burn, especially third degree burn on the dorsum, usually ends up with severe scar contraction with overextended metacorpophalangeal joints and an adducted thumb lying in line with the second metacarpal. The so-called 'clawhand deformity' is thus established. In such a deformity, the hand's two fundamental functions – pinch and grasp – are usually impaired significantly (Figure 13.1b). With passage of time, the functions deteriorate progressively when secondary deformities of the joints (rupture of capsule and dislocation), tendons (adhesion), and muscles (atrophy) set in owing to infection, persistent edema and prolonged immobilization. The most complicated type – the so-called frozen hand – may sometimes result, with complete loss of functions of the hand.

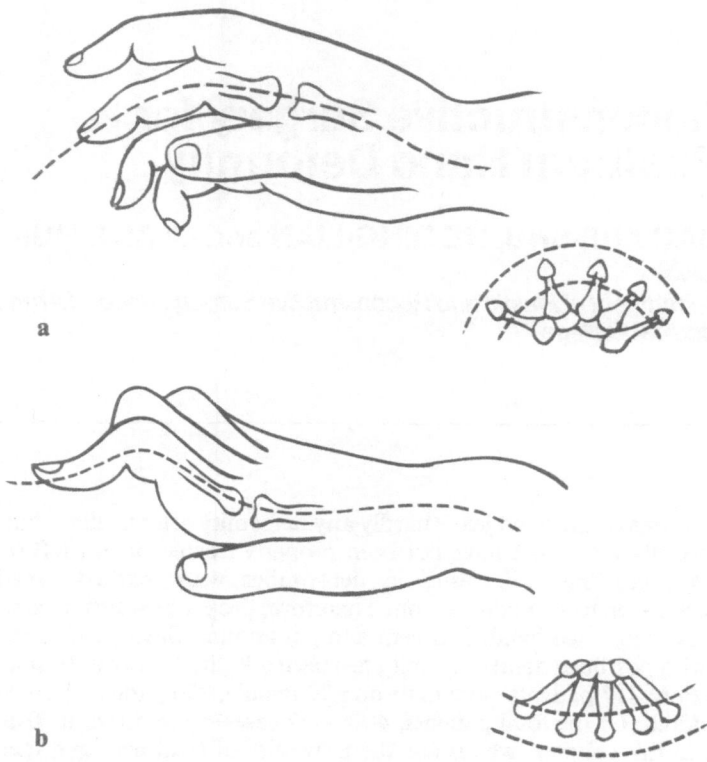

a

b

Figure 13.1 Longitudinal and transverse arches of the hand. **a**, Normal. **b**, Abnormal

PRINCIPLES AND METHODS OF TREATMENT

Complicated and diversified as the deformity may appear, any approach to it should be aimed exclusively at recovery of the two fundamental functions – pinch and grasp. To achieve this end, the first consideration should be given to the restoration of the two arches, the key technical points of which are:

(1) excise the scar and repair the skin defect;
(2) reduce all the joints especially the MP joints – restoration of the longitudinal arch;
(3) release the first web contracture and reposition the thumb in opposition and abduction – restoration of the transverse arch.

Repair of skin defect

A mild deformity with only the skin involved can be satisfactorily treated by excising the scar on the dorsum and covering the raw surface with a medium split

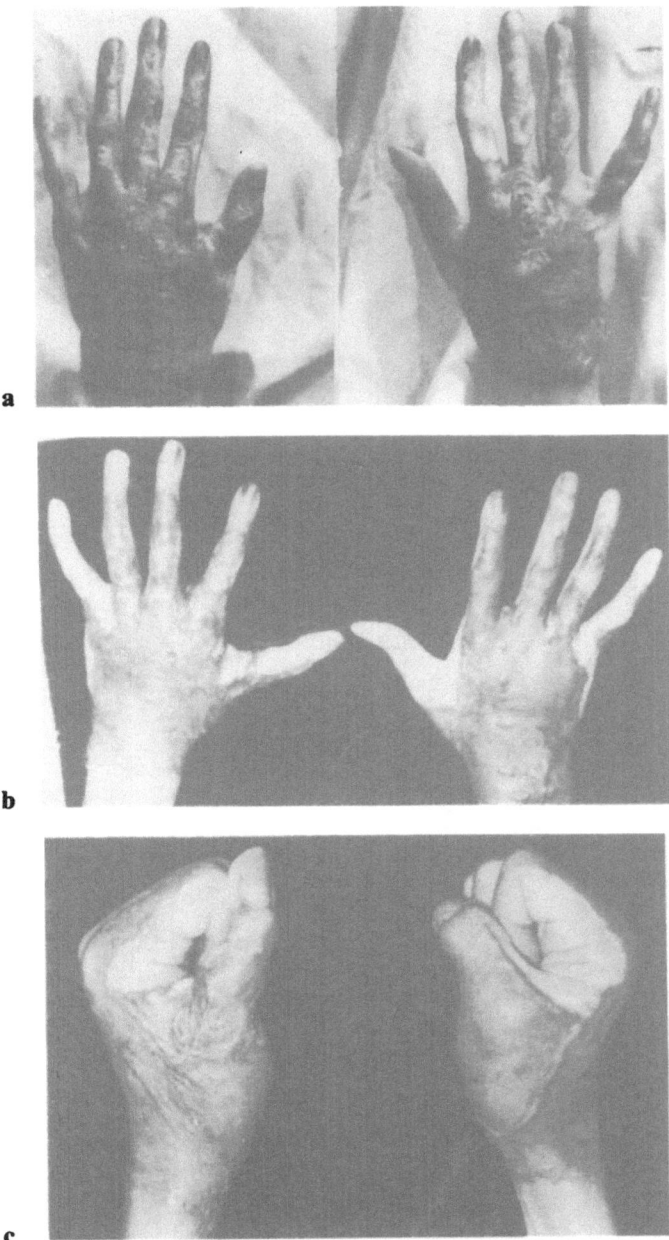

Figure 13.2 Deformity of both hands due to contracture of hypertrophic scar on the dorsum. Repaired with split thickness skin graft. **a**, Preoperative view. **b,c**, Postoperative views

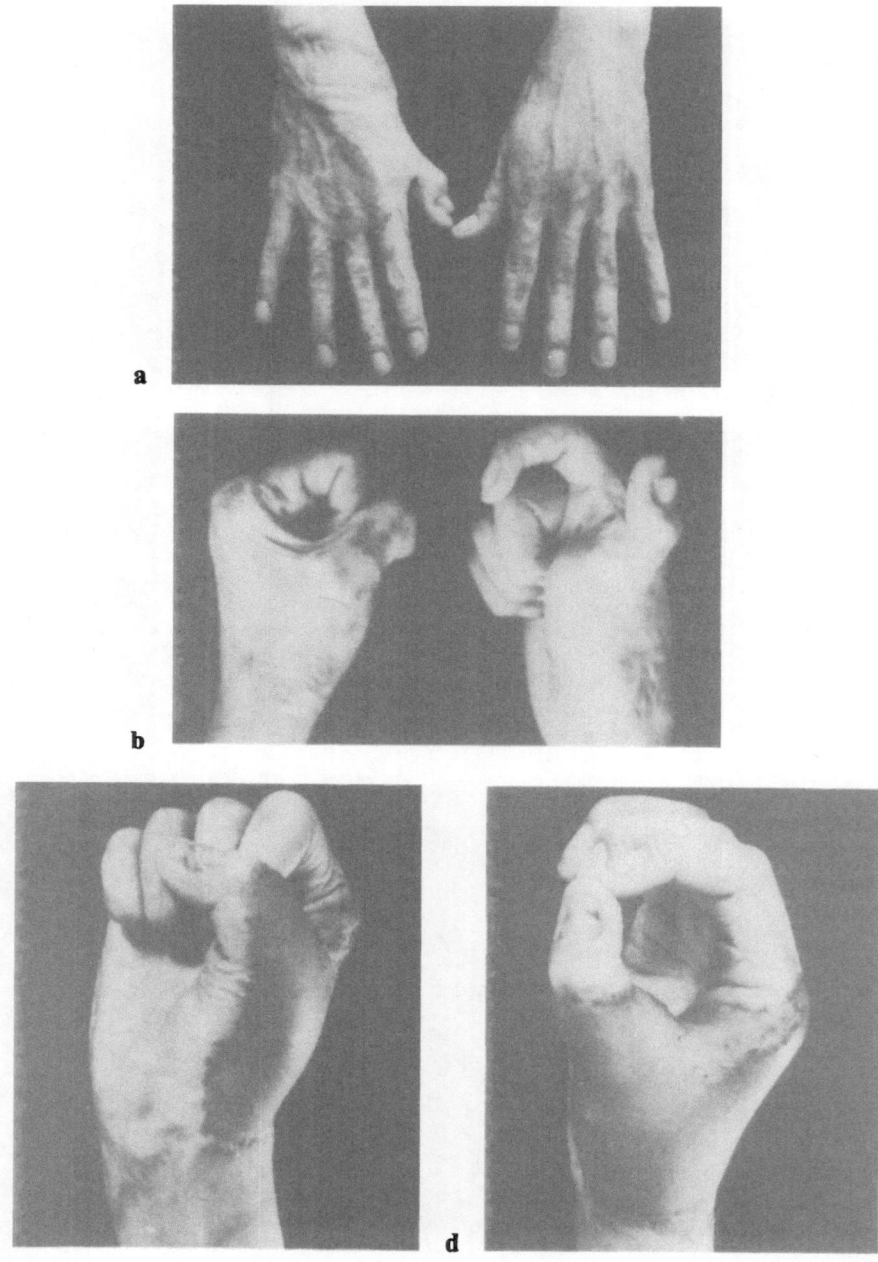

Figure 13.3 Dorsoflexion and adduction deformity of the right thumb MP joint. Reconstructed with skin tube after tackling of deep structures. **a,b,** Preoperative views, **c,d,** Postoperative views

thickness skin graft (Figure 13.2). However, in the later 109 cases of this series, a better result was achieved by utilizing a full thickness graft taken from the abdominal flank, instead of a split thickness graft. Usually a strip of skin, 6–7 cm wide and 20 cm long, was removed from this region and then defatted. Such a piece of skin was large enough for complete covering of the whole wound on the dorsum or the palm, and at the same time its donor site could be closed by direct approximation. The procedure is so simple that a general surgeon may be competent to perform it. This procedure is also effective for a severe type deformity in children or young adults, as their overextended MP joints and adducted thumb could readily be corrected after excision of the contracted scar. A more complicated tube or flap procedure was reserved for those cases requiring synchronous correction of secondary deformities of the bone, joint and tendon in addition to skin covering. Tube or flap procedures are also indicated for a severely adducted thumb with overextended MP joint or a little finger with similar deformity (Figures 13.3, 13.4). Thirty-one cases in this series required a tube or flap reconstruction.

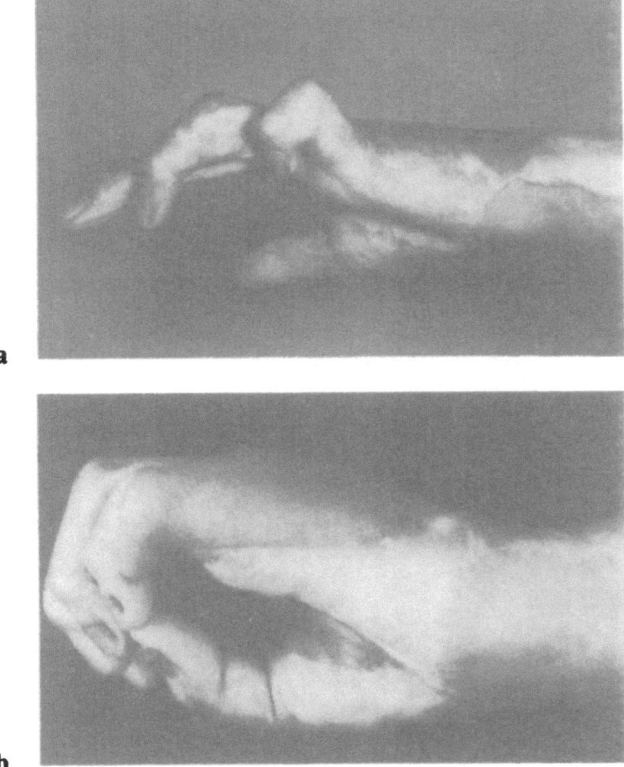

a

b

Figure 13.4   Dorsoflexion deformity of the left little finger. Reconstructed with skin flap after tackling of deep structures. **a**, Preoperative view. **b**, Postoperative view

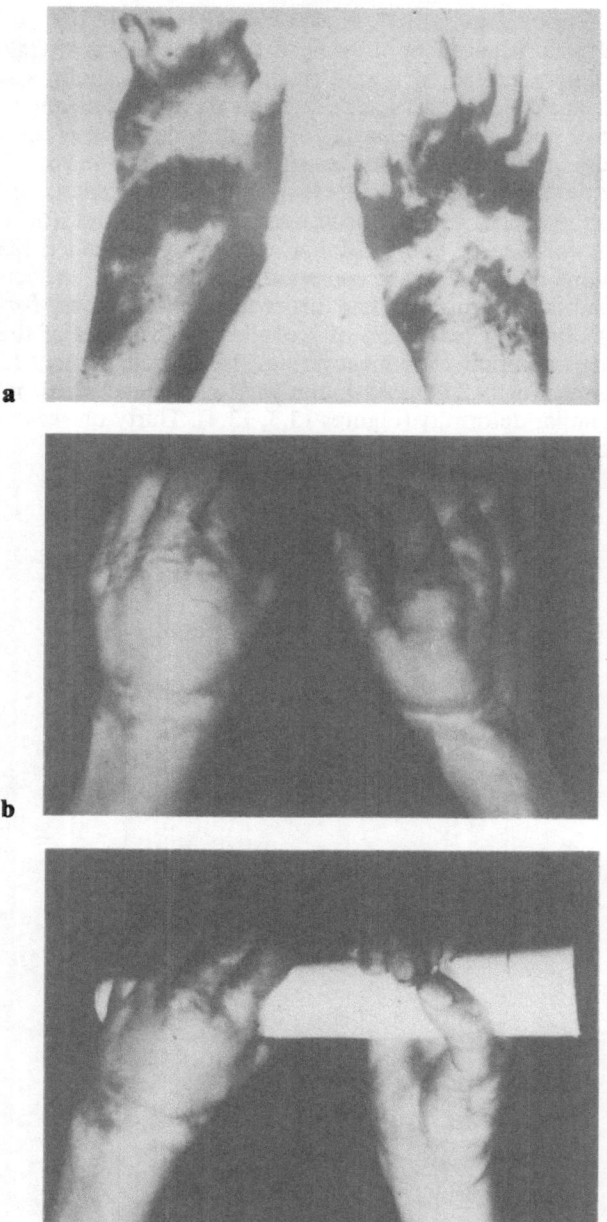

Figure 13.5 Severe clawhand deformity of both hands due to burn on the dorsum. Reconstructed with skin tube after tackling of the joints and tendons. **a,** Preoperative view. **b,c,** Postoperative views

Correction of joint deformity

Reduction of an overextended MP joint is the essential step for restoration of the longitudinal arch of the hand. Severe flexion of the proximal interphalangeal (PIP) joint due to rupture of the extensor hood is corrected by functional joint fusion if there is no chance for the recovery of flexion and extension movements. Choice of treatment for the PIP joint, whether fusion is indicated and how many degrees the flexion should be, depends largely on the status of the MP and PIP joints as well as the position of the thumb. A mild overextended MP joint can be easily reduced by mere excision of contracted scar tissue, but a severe type usually necessitates a combined treatment of the tendon, joint and bone in addition to skin coverage. The whole reconstructive procedure is better carried out in the following order: resect the collateral ligament on both sides except the thumb, divide the adhesion between the tendon and joint capsule, release the dorsal joint capsule and lengthen the tendon if necessary. Should all these efforts fail to reduce the MP joint, then arthroplasty is undertaken. The latter procedure, if supplemented by postoperative elastic splinting, has proved capable of producing an acceptable result of MP joint reduction (Figure 13.5).

Correction of adducted thumb deformity

Z-plasty is indicated for a mild case where there is still sufficient normal skin available in the surrounding region. In a severe case, where contracture of the adductor pollicis has existed and mere division of the transverse head of the latter failed to yield a satisfactory result, the additional detachment of the first dorsal interosseus muscle from its insertion should be attempted. However, in a still more severe case, where there is fibrosis or atrophy of the adductor pollicis

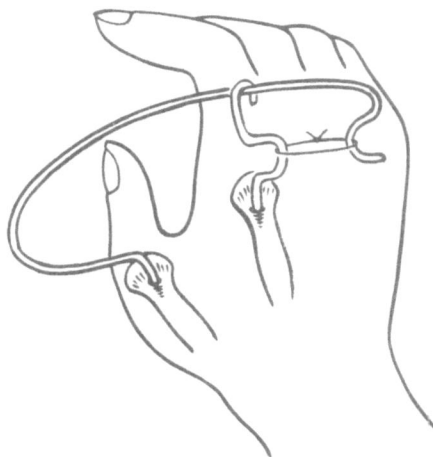

Figure 13.6 Traction splint made of two pieces of Kirschner wire. Rubber band is applied to maintain the width of the first web and oppositional position of the thumb

and the first dorsal interosseus muscle with the thumb assuming a position in line with the other metacarpals, the above procedures are seldom able to maintain the thumb in an opposing and abducting position after operation. This problem could only be solved by application of an elastic splint postoperatively for about 2 weeks. Two types of elastic splint have been used in this series. The first is made of two Kirschner wires inserted separately into the distal part of the first and the second metacarpals, with the wire in the first metacarpal bent at its distal end to make a hook. A rubber band is then placed between the two wires to effect traction (Figure 13.6). The second type is the Anderson appliance (Figure 13.7) often used in maxillofacial patients. Though the former device has a traction effect, it is not as reliable as the latter in terms of immobilization.

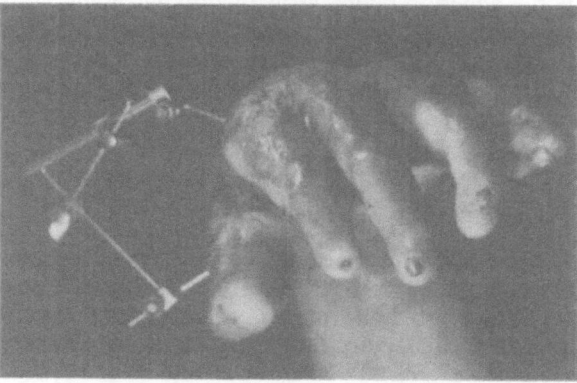

Figure 13.7 Anderson splint to maintain the width of the first web and oppositional position of the thumb

14 An Analysis of Operative Results on Late Deformities of Burnt Hands

YU BAO-LIANG, REN LIN-SEN, HUANG GANG-FU, ZHANG DE-CHAO and ZHOU JI-LIN
Affiliated Hospital of Sichuan Medical College, Sichuan Medical College, Chengdu

Between 1973 and 1981, 289 hands (225 cases) with late burn deformities were operated upon in our clinic. Satisfactory long term results were obtained in 196 hands (153 cases) (Figures 14.1–14.4). For further enhancement of the therapeutic effect, the relationship between the degrees and duration of deformities, ages of patients and survival rate of skin grafts to operative results has been reviewed, and is discussed here.

CLINICAL MATERIALS

There were 102 males and 51 females, aged 2 to 50 years, with 85 hands in 67 children and 111 hands in 86 adults.

Course of hand deformities: 67 hands were seen within 1 year after burns; 63 in 1–2 years; 35 in 2–5 years and 31 in more than 6 years.

Dorsal deformities occurred in 93 hands and volar deformities in 103.

CLASSIFICATION OF HAND DEFORMITIES

Dorsal and volar deformities are recognized anatomically, while mild and severe cases are divided morphologically and functionally (Table 14.1).

Table 14.1 Classification of hand deformities

Degree of deformity	Dorsum of hand		Palm of hand	
	Number	%	*Number*	%
Mild	51	54.8	70	68
Severe	42	45.2	33	32
Total	93	100.0	103	100.0

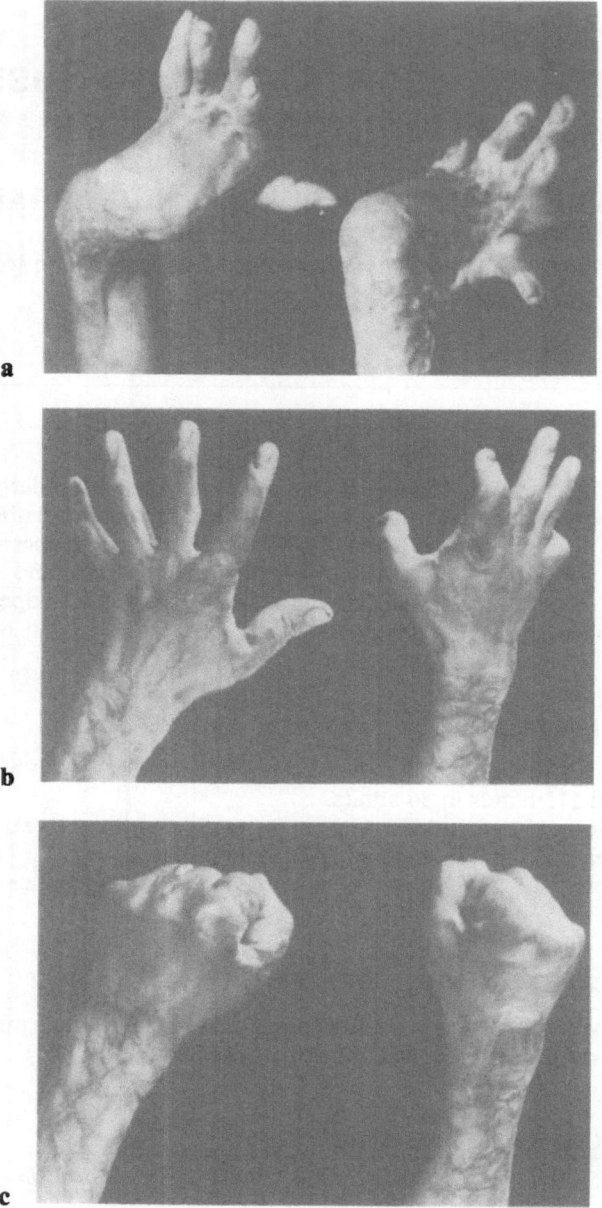

Figure 14.1 Case 1. **a,** Severe dorsal contractures of both hands before operation. **b, c,** Seven years after two reconstructive operations including PIP joint arthrodeses of the thumb, index and little finger in the right hand. Excellent functional recovery of both hands

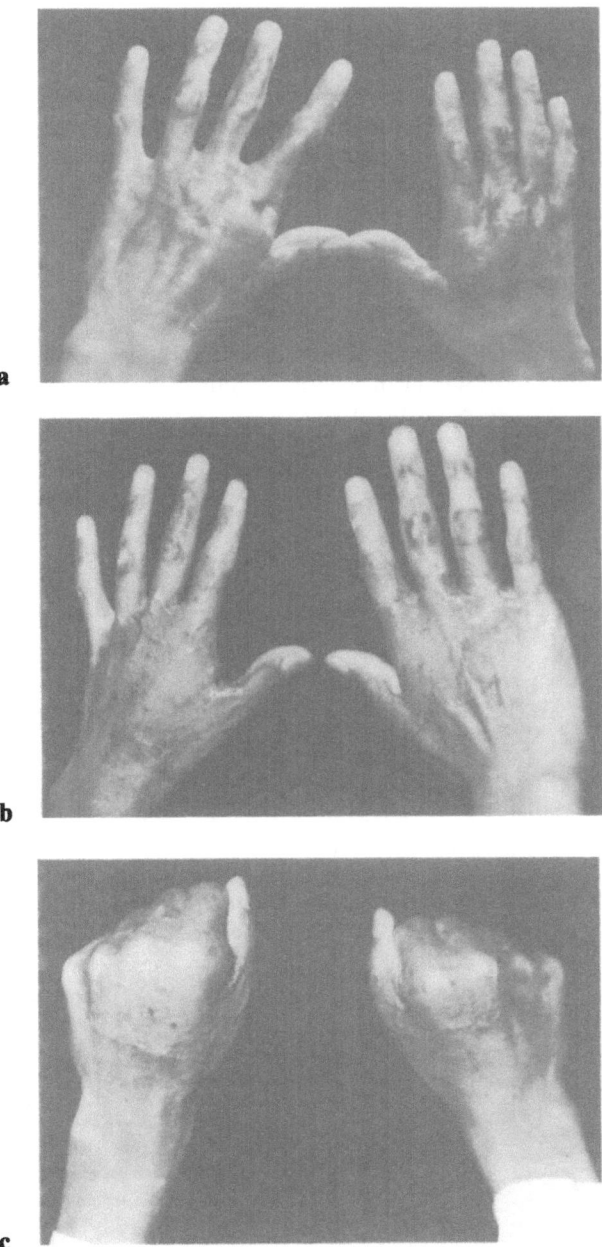

Figure 14.2 Case 2. **a**, Dorsal hypertrophic scars in both hands. **b, c,** Excellent functional recovery 6 months after operation

Dorsal deformities

Mild cases (54.8%)

The superficial tissue layers of the dorsum of the hand are involved, with hypertrophic scarring of the skin and subcutaneous tissues. The cicatricial retraction of the dorsal skin resulted indirectly and functionally in disturbance of deep tissue components, the range of motions of MP and IP joints being limited with the thumb mildly adducted.

Severe cases (45.2%)

Deep structures involved are the joints, ligaments and tendons with resultant secondary joint stiffness and intrinsic muscle contracture of the hand. The burnt 'clawhand' is a typical morbid entity.

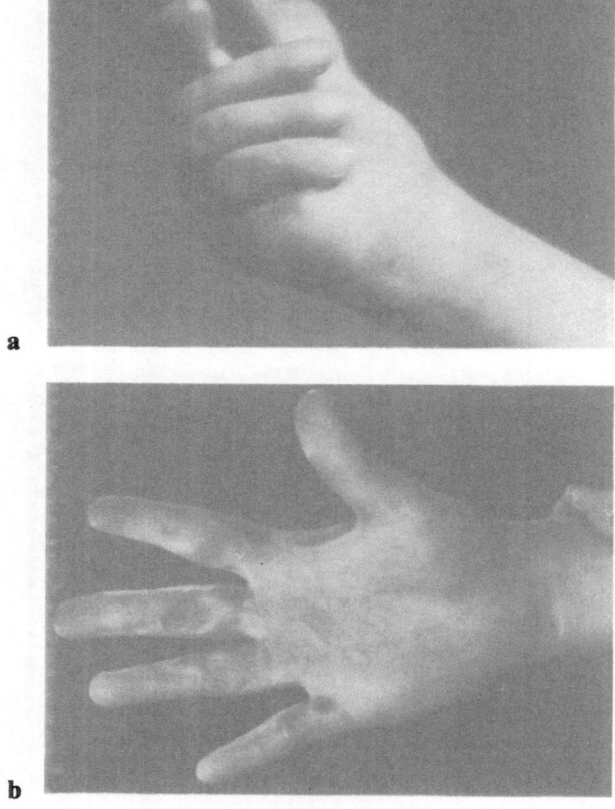

a

b

Figure 14.3 Case 3. **a**, Severe volar contracture of the right hand. **b**, Five years after two successive free skin grafting operations with excellent functional result

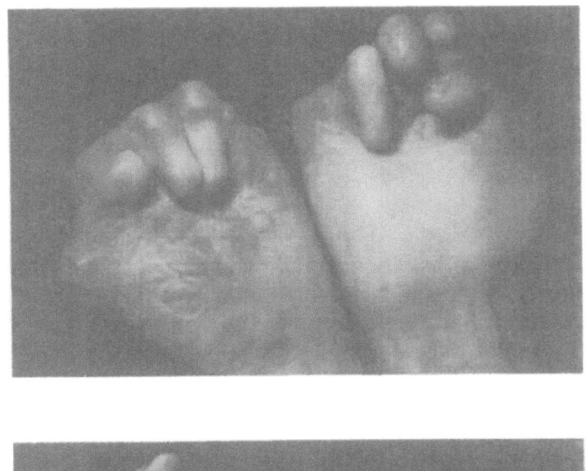

a

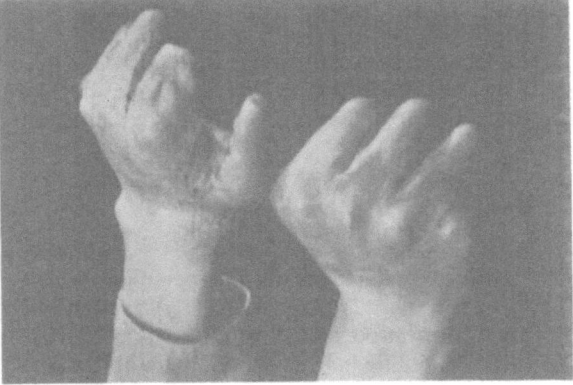

b

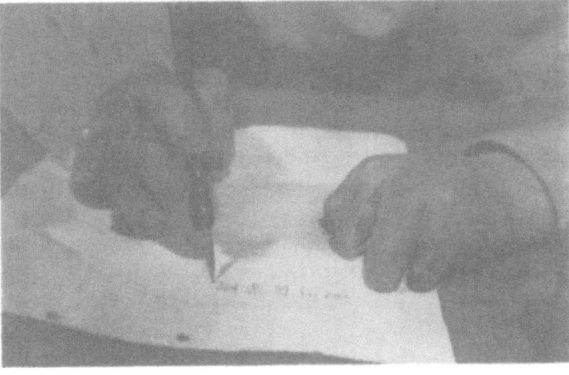

c

Figure 14.4 Case 4. **a,** Severe volar contracture deformities of both hands before reconstructive surgery. **b, c,** Good functional result of both hands 1 year after operation

Volar deformities

Mild cases (68%)

The cicatricial retraction of the palmar skin is responsible for the deformities, the movements of the tendons and joints being hampered, especially finger extension movement.

Severe cases (32%)

Deep involvement of the tendons and joints makes the fingers deformed, the thumb being adducted and web spaces obliterated. In the case of first deformity, functional loss of the hand is complete.

SURGICAL MANAGEMENT

Skin defect coverage

Secondary skin defects after scar excision are covered in the majority of cases by split thickness or full thickness skin grafts (192 hands), skin flaps were used in four hands, and skin flaps plus split grafts in four others.

Web space plasty

A vertical incision on the obliterated web space is commonly used. A split thickness skin graft, shaped into one or two triangular flaps, in the form of a V or W, is inserted to cover the secondary skin defect to widen the web space. Adduction deformity of the thumb is corrected by Z-plasty or triangular skin graft to the secondary skin defect following releasing of the obliterated first web space. In the case of cicatricial retraction of the adductor pollicis muscle, its transverse head near the MP joint has to be sectioned. In some cases, the first dorsal interosseous muscle must be partially cut off as an adjunctive procedure.

MP joint deformities

Manual reduction to flexion in 90° is all that is necessary to correct the mild hyperextension deformity of the MP joint. In severe cases, it is hard to achieve reduction manually, and surgical reduction including partial excision of the collateral ligaments, thorough excision of extracapsular scar tissues and complete lysis of intracapsular adhesion of the MP joint is necessary. Kirschner wire fixation of the reduced MP joint functional or hyperflexed position for 2 weeks is necessary to prevent it from recurrence.

IP joint deformities

Stiff IP joints, resulting from either palmar or volar deformities, are treated by

arthrodesis as a routine procedure, the PIP joint being fixed in flexed 45–60 °
and distal interphalangeal (DIP) in 30 ° for 6 weeks. The angle of the fixed IP
joint is variable in accordance with the hand function as a whole.

Extensor tendon lengthening

In order to maintain the stability of the reduced MP joint, any contracted
extensor tendon should be lengthened or its dorsal aponeurosis sectioned.

FOLLOW-UP STUDY

Follow-up study from 6 months to 8 years was done in 196 hands (153 patients).
   Functionally, operative results are classified into three grades.

(1) *Excellent*. Hand functions including thumb opposition, finger extension
    and fist clench are recovered in great measure. Good fist clench represents
    an excellent result in dorsal deformity and full finger extension signifies the
    best operative result in palmar deformity.

(2) *Good*. There is quasinormal recovery of thumb opposition, finger exten-
    sion and fist clench. In this grade, thumb opposition is recovered in dorsal
    deformity and finger extension recovered to the functional position in
    palmar deformity.

(3) *Poor*. No functional amelioration has been obtained even if there is some
    esthetic improvement. The fingers cannot be flexed to the functional posi-
    tion in dorsal deformity, or extended to the functional position in volar
    deformity.

ANALYSIS OF OPERATIVE RESULTS

Degrees of deformities and operative results

It can be seen, from Table 14.2, that the overall operative results of hand dorsal
deformities are satisfactory (92.5% of the total are excellent–good results, with
96.1% in mild cases and 86.1% in severe cases). However, the excellent rate

Table 14.2   Degrees of dorsal deformities and operative results

Results in grades	Mild cases		Severe cases		Total	
	Hands (n)	%	Hands (n)	%	Hands (n)	%
Excellent	31	60.8	15	35.7	46	49.5
Good	18	35.3	22	52.4	40	43.0
Poor	2	3.9	5	11.9	7	7.5
Total	51	100.0	42	100.0	93	100.0

(35.1%) in severe cases is too low to be satisfactory and further enhancement should be expected. In severe cases, the tendons and joints are often involved in the early stage of deep burns and cicatricial contracture with serious joint deformities in the late stage. The classical surgical treatment, including excision of collateral ligaments, intracapsular and extracapsular lysis of adhesions, did not yield a satisfactory result; IP joint deformities can be satisfactorily corrected by arthrodesis.

The recovery of hand function as a whole is largely determined by the degree of functional recovery of the MP joint. The results are always unrewarding in seriously deformed cases, in which surgical correction would be very difficult if not impossible, kinesitherapy having been useless. Of the seven patients graded as poor operative results, five are cases of serious MP joint deformities, with the hands deformed in a hyperextension position and with MP joint dislocation surgically noncorrectable. The thumb opposition could not be restored even though IP arthrodesis had been performed. The two mild cases consisted of two child patients. The poor postoperative immobilization, and the impracticability of kinesitherapy after successful surgical reduction of MP joint dislocation, are the main factors for postoperative recurrence, and further surgical reduction has to be done.

Table 14.3 Degree of palmar deformities and operative results

Results in grades	Mild cases		Severe cases		Total	
	Hands (n)	%	Hands (n)	%	Hands (n)	%
Excellent	43	61.4	18	54.6	61	59.2
Good	26	37.2	11	33.3	37	35.9
Poor	1	1.4	4	12.1	5	4.9
Total	70	100.0	33	100.0	103	100.0

It can be seen in Table 14.3 that the overall operative results in hand volar deformities were satisfactory (91.5% of the total are excellent–good results, with 98.6% in mild cases and 87.9% in severe cases). The severe volar deformities were the sequelae of deep burns in early childhood. In childhood growth, the burnt scar retraction impeded the normal development of hand joints, resulting in joint deformities which are surgically noncorrectable. Generally speaking, in volar deformities it is the cutaneous contracture with subsequent entrapment of the underlying tendons and neurovascular bundle that is responsible for the functional disturbance of the hand, the MP joints being rarely involved. In some severe cases, two operations at an interval of 6 months to 1 year are necessary to achieve a complete correction. In the five cases graded as poor results, four were of electrical burns with the tendons and joints involved and surgical corrections were difficult. Another poor case was a 5-year-old child whose hand growth was seriously impeded by burn skin contracture; the flexed finger deformities cannot be completely corrected by surgery, and the inefficient postoperative immobilization and impracticability of kinesitherapy make finger extension very limited.

Duration of dorsal hand deformities and postoperative results

It is seen in Table 14.4 that the results of surgical correction of dorsal hand deformities performed within 1 year after burn healing are better than after 1–2 years, the former accounting for 97.7% of the total excellent–good results and the latter 83.9%. The 'excellent' percentage is also higher in the former series. The difference is statistically significant ($p < 0.05$). In regard to the degree of deformities, there is no statistical difference between the two series (Table 14.5). The optimum operative time of less than 1 year after burn healing in our series is quite in accord with Chang's experience[1] that 3–6 months after burn healing is the optimum operative time, when secondary joint deformities are mild and surgical correction is easy, to obtain a fine operative result.

No difference in results can be seen between the degrees and duration of volar hand deformities (Tables 14.6, 14.7). It is worth noting that 15 out of 25 hands with volar deformity duration of more than 6 years (the longest being more than 30 years) had excellent results. Most of the patients have had their hands burnt in early childhood, the scars being softened and joint deformities less serious, favoring surgical correction. As to the optimum operative time, we prefer early operation within 1 year after volar burn healing.

Age of patients and operative results

In dorsal deformities (Table 14.8), the adult group has a higher 'excellent' result rate (60%) than the child group (34.2%), the difference being statistically significant ($p < 0.05$). No difference in degree of deformities is seen in the two age groups (Table 14.9). The possible factor accounting for the better result in the adult group is the postoperative kinesitherapy which is impracticable in children.

In the volar deformities (Table 14.8), the adult group has a 66.6% excellent result as compared with 51.1% in the child group; there is no statistical significance ($p < 0.1$). In addition, there are more severe cases (37.5%) in the adult group than in the child group (25.5%) (Table 14.9); no statistical significance existed. One may deduce that if two 'no significances' can make a significance, that is to say, the operative result in the adult group is better than in the child group, here the kinesitherapy plays an important role.

Note that, in the 93 dorsal hand deformities, split thickness skin grafts are used to cover the secondary skin defect in 89 hands and skin flap in four.

A high skin graft survival rate is a prerequisite for the enhancement of immediate and long term results (Table 14.10). Most of the hand deformities, either dorsal or volar in type, having a skin graft survival rate of over 90%, fall in the excellent–good result grades. In the case of low survival rate, an excellent–good result can be expected should the necrotic skin graft, usually the result of an underlying hematoma, be replaced by another skin graft within 2–3 days after the graft accident. The major joint deformities are the main factors responsible for the poor results in eight hands having a skin graft survival rate of over 95%.

Table 14.4 Duration of dorsal hand deformities and postoperative results

Result in grades	Duration of deformities						
	1 year		1–2 years		3–5 years		6 years	
	Hands (n)	%	Hands (n)	%	Hands (n)	%	Hands (n)	%
Excellent	25	58.1	11	35.5	7	—	3	—
Good	17	39.6	15	48.1	5	—	3	—
Poor	1	2.3	5	16.1	1	—	0	—
Total	43	100.0	31	100.0	13	—	6	—

Table 14.5 Degrees and duration of dorsal hand deformities

Degree of deformity	Duration of deformities						
	1 year		1–2 years		3–5 years		6 years	
	Hands (n)	%	Hands (n)	%	Hands (n)	%	Hands (n)	%
Mild	26	60.5	17	54.8	6	—	2	—
Severe	17	39.5	14	45.2	7	—	4	—
Total	43	100.0	31	100.0	13	—	6	—

Table 14.6 Duration of volar hand deformities and postoperative results

| Results in grades | 1 year | | Duration of deformities | | | | | |
| | | | 1–2 years | | 3–5 years | | 6 years | |
	Hands (n)	%	Hands (n)	%	Hands (n)	%	Hands (n)	%
Excellent	14	58.3	19	59.4	13	59.1	15	60.0
Good	8	33.4	12	37.5	8	36.4	9	36.0
Poor	2	8.3	1	3.1	1	4.5	1	4.0
Total	24	100.0	32	100.0	22	100.0	25	100.0

Table 14.7 Degrees and duration of hand deformities

| Degree of deformity | 1 year | | Duration of deformities | | | | | |
| | | | 1–2 years | | 3–5 years | | 6 years | |
	Hands (n)	%	Hands (n)	%	Hands (n)	%	Hands (n)	%
Mild	17	70.8	22	68.7	15	68.2	16	64.0
Severe	7	29.2	10	31.3	7	31.8	9	36.0
Total	24	100.0	32	100.0	22	100.0	25	100.0

Table 14.8 Age of patients and operative results

Results in grades	Dorsal deformities				Volar deformities			
	Child		Adult		Child		Adult	
	Hands (n)	%	Hands (n)	%	Hands (n)	%	Hands (n)	%
Excellent	13	34.2	33	60.0	24	51.1	37	66.1
Good	21	55.3	19	34.5	21	44.7	16	28.6
Poor	4	10.5	3	5.5	2	4.2	3	5.3
Total	38	100.0	55	100.0	47	100.0	56	100.0

Table 14.9 Age of patients and degrees of deformities

Degree of deformity	Dorsal deformities				Volar deformities			
	Child		Adult		Child		Adult	
	Hands (n)	%	Hands (n)	%	Hands (n)	%	Hands (n)	%
Mild	22	57.9	29	52.7	35	74.5	35	62.5
Severe	16	42.1	26	47.3	12	25.5	21	37.5
Total	38	100.0	55	100.0	47	100.0	56	100.0

Table 14.10 Skin graft survival and operative results

Results in grades	Survival rate of skin grafts											
	Dorsal aspects of hands						Volar aspect of hands					
	95%		90–94%		89%		95%		90–94%		89%	
	Hands (n)	%	Hands (n)	%	Hands (n)	%	Hands (n)	%	Hands (n)	%	Hands (n)	%
Excellent	35	51.5	10	55.6	1	—	47	58.8	12	57.2	2	—
Good	28	41.2	8	44.4	2	—	30	37.4	7	33.3	0	—
Poor	5	7.3	0	0	0	—	3	3.8	2	9.5	0	—
Total	68	100	18	100	3	—	80	100	21	100	2	—

DISCUSSION

Early treatment of hand burns

The degrees of deformities are the determinants of operative results of burn sequelae. In severe cases, only a third of the dorsal and a half of the volar deformities are graded as 'excellent'. To obtain a good hand function, it is essential to protect the hand joints from injury, especially the MP joints which, as emphasized by several authors[2-4], should be immobilized in functional or hyperfunctional positions in the early stage of treatment. In dorsal hand burns, one should immobilize the wrist in mild extension, the MP joint in semiflexion, IP in full extension and the thumb in abduction position; in volar burns, the wrist, MP and IP joints in extension positions. More recently, many have advocated[5-7] early eschar excision or tangential excision by immediate skin graft to prevent joint deformities and enhance operative results. Elastic compressive dressings and kinesitherapy are recommended.

Optimum operative time for hand burn sequelae

It is generally agreed that burnt scar should not be excised before it has become softened and stabilized, which demands an interval of 1-2 years after burn healing. In hand deformities, this time interval is too long for surgical correction without encountering secondary joint deformities. In the present authors' view, the optimum operative time is within 1 year after burn healing for dorsal deformities and 1-2 years for volar deformities.

Replacement of necrotic graft

In low skin graft survival rate, an excellent-good result may be expected should the necrotic graft be excised and replaced by another skin graft within 2-3 days after the failure of the original graft.

Severe first web space adduction deformity

In severe cases of the first web space adduction deformity, split thickness skin graft after space widening often makes the postoperative result esthetically and functionally unacceptable. The adduction deformity of the thumb recurs easily and secondary surgical correction is always necessary. Recently, the free dorsalis pedis skin flap and forearm island flap have been used to cover the secondary skin defect of the first web space after its widening, with encouraging immediate postoperative results. The long term result deserves further observation.

REFERENCES

1. Chang Ti-sheng *et al*. (1982). Experience in the treatment of postburn scar contractures: An analysis of 713 cases. *Chinese J. Surg.*, **20**, 447

2. Corlett, R. J. (1979). The treatment of deep burn of the hand. *Aust. J. Surg.*, **49**, 567
3. Bunke, J. F. *et al.* (1976). Primary surgical management of the deeply burned hand. *J. Trauma*, **16**, 593
4. Huang, T. T. *et al.* (1978). Ten years of experience in managing patients with burn contractures of axilla, elbow, wrist and knee joints. *Plast. Reconstr. Surg.*, **61**, 70
5. Mahler, D. *et al.* (1975). Tangential excision and grafting for burns of the hand. *Br. J. Plast. Surg.*, **28**, 189
6. Shi De *et al.* (1980). Late results of auto-skin-grafting in treatment of deep burns of hand. *Chinese J. Surg.*, **18**, 139
7. Sun Yong-hua *et al.* (1980). Analysis of 156 cases of deep burns of the hand treated by tangential excision of eschar. *Chinese Med. J.*, **60**, 358

15 The Forearm Radial Arterial Turnover Flap and its Clinical Application

LU KAI-HUA, ZHONG DE-CAI, CHEN BI and LUO JIN-HUI

Department of Plastic Surgery and Burns, The First Affiliated Hospital, The Fourth Military Medical College, Xi'an

The free forearm flap technique with its anatomic basis and clinical applications was reported by Yang Guo-fan *et al.*[1]. Drawing inspiration from this type of free flap, we developed a forearm radial arterial turnover flap to repair acute hand injuries and late deformities (including burn deformities) in 1980. The shape and size of the flap are designed according to the defect of the wound. The flap is reversibly placed on the radial side of the midpart of the forearm with a narrow skin pedicle on the distal end which is along and including the course of the radial artery. The blood supply of the flap is from the ulnar artery through the palmal arch reversibly. The venous return is by way of three channels: (1) the accompanying radial vein and its collaterals, (2) the small venule in the skin pedicle and (3) one or two veins of the flap anastomosed to the recipient site. The width of the pedicle is about 1.5 cm. It does not matter what the length is, and it would not do any harm to the flap if its size extended even to the length of half of the upper forearm.

OPERATIVE TECHNIQUE

Design the flap reversibly on the radial side of the forearm with the pedicle on the distal part, the shape and size of the wound being measured and marked with methylene blue. The incision is made along the blue line. The dissection is carried out along the plane under the deep fascia. The radial artery and its accompanying veins of the proximal ends are ligated and divided separately. The flap may be larger beyond the point of ligation. The whole flap is elevated, with the narrow strip of skin pedicle and the underlying blood vessels connected distally to the wrist region (Figure 15.1). Turn the flap 180° reversibly to the wound for the coverage or reconstruction of the degloved or severed thumb. The flap is sutured in position. The wound is dressed with fluffed gauze and splinted in the functional position. The hand is put in an elevated position with two pillows.

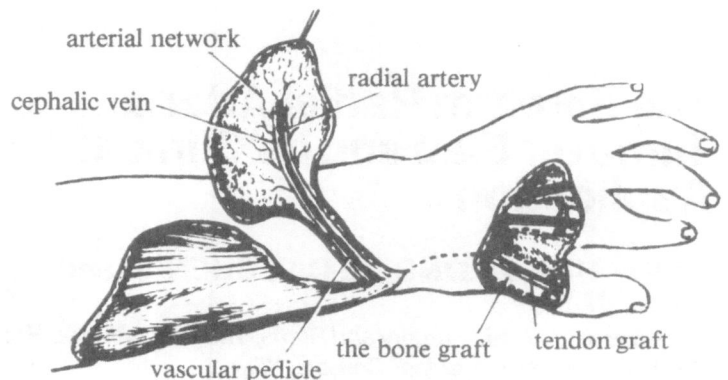

Figure 15.1   Schematic drawing of the forearm radial anterior turnover flap

CLINICAL APPLICATIONS

We have applied this kind of flap in 12 cases of severely injured hands. There have been six cases of finger reconstruction (including five thumb–hand) and two cases of the wrist region. In nine of the 12 cases, deep structure repair has been made, such as bone grafts, tendon transplantation and anastomosis of the nerves. Good results were achieved in all 12 cases.

REPORTS

Case 1

This female, 21, had a history of severe injury of the left hand, leaving a scar contracture of the dorsum of the hand and first web space, defect of the first and second metacarpals and extensor digitorum tendons for 4 months (Figure 15.2a,b). Under brachial block anesthesia, the scar of the hand was excised and the contractures were completely released. The exploration showed that there were defects of the extensor tendons by 6 cm of each thumb, the second and third fingers, and defects of the first and second metacarpals by 2 cm and 3 cm respectively (Figure 15.2c). A bone block of $5.2 \times 1.5 \times 1.5$ cm was taken from the left iliac crest. Then the bone block was divided transversely into two pieces, which were put into the two defects separately and fixed with Kirschner wires (Figure 15.2d). Tendons of the palmar longus and flexor carpi radialis were taken for the repair of the defect of extensor of the thumb and the other two fingers. After all these repairs were completed, a forearm turnover flap 12×7.5 cm in size was designed with a pedicle of 1.5×6 cm, which was attached to the wrist region. The incision was made along the designed line. The flap is elevated by careful dissection just about the myolemma or just under the deep fascia. The radial artery and its branches were preserved and kept attached with the flap by careful dissection under direct vision. The proximal part of the radial

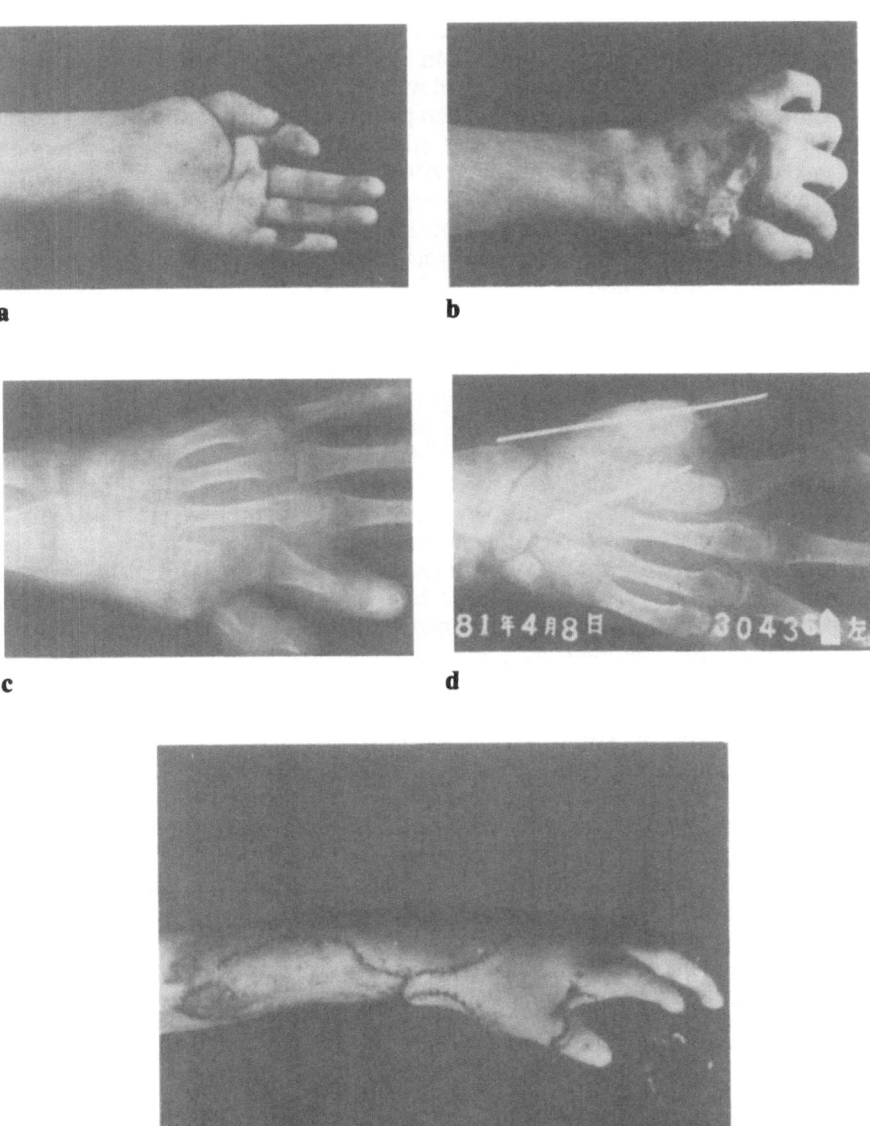

Figure 15.2 Patient Xue, male, 21, was admitted for scar of 40-day duration over dorsum of left hand, resulting in contracture of first web space. There were also defects in first and second metacarpals and extensors. **a,b,** Preoperative condition. **c,** Preoperative X-ray film demonstrates defects in the first and second metacarpals. **d,** Postoperative X-ray film demonstrates bone grafts stabilized with Kirschner wires. **e,** Postoperative view, the forearm radial arterial turnover flap and the skin graft on the donor site survived well

artery and its accompanying veins were ligated and divided under the flap. The flap was then turned over to the dorsum of the hand and sutured into position. A vein of the flap end was anastomosed with the neighboring vein of the dorsum of the hand. The skin flap was sutured in place and a rubber drain was put under the flap. The donor site was covered with free whole thickness of skin with preserved subdermal vascular plexus. All the wounds were dressed with fluffed gauze with some pressure. Both the flap and donor site healed per primam (Figure 15.2e). After 1 year follow-up, the texture of the flap was fine and the sensations of tactility and pain were restored; however, the web space was not wide enough. An addition revision was done to widen the web space by a rotation skin flap. The function of the left hand was then almost fully restored.

Case 2

This male, 21, had severe injury to the left hand resulting in severed thumb and skin avulsion. He was admitted as an emergency case 6 hours after the accident. Examination showed the thumb was badly crushed and severed, with only a narrow strip of skin attached to the index finger. The skin of the dorsum of the hand and web space was avulsed with extraction of tendons and digital nerves, leaving an irregular 9×7 cm wound. The muscle of the thenar eminence was exposed. The wounds were badly stained with coal dust and smeared with dirt (Figure 15.3a,b). The hand was thoroughly cleaned with saline and peroxide solution. Emergency operation was done under brachial block anesthesia. The severed thumb was skinned, leaving the digital nerves and tendons intact. It was fixed to the remaining stump with Kirschner wire (Figure 15.3c). The extensor tendon was sutured and the nerves were anastomosed with 9/0 nylon suture. Then a turnover flap was designed and elevated for reconstruction of the thumb (Figure 15.3d). In this case, the pedicle of 2×5 cm carried a flap of 9×7.5 cm without vein anastomosis. The skin flap survived well (Figure 3e,f). Six months follow-up showed some restoration of sensation of the flap, except the tip of the thumb. The first web was somewhat narrower. A further operation was performed. A neurovascular island flap was transferred from the ring finger to the tip of the thumb. At the same time, the first web was widened by full thickness graft. The function of the left hand improved (Figure 15.3g,h).

Case 3

A 22-year-old female was admitted with stump deformity of loss of all digits of the right hand after a severe burn. All the metacarpals were encased by scar tissue (Figure 15.4a,b). By careful examination, the tiny remnants of proximal phalanx were found, with some motion. During operation an incision was made on the first web space and the metacarpal of the thumb was released. A piece of bone was taken from the left iliac region and transferred to the stump of the proximal phalanx of the thumb. It was transfixed by two Kirschner wires. Then the flap was transferred, enclosing the bone graft and web space for reconstruction of the thumb. The wounds on the palm and donor site were covered with

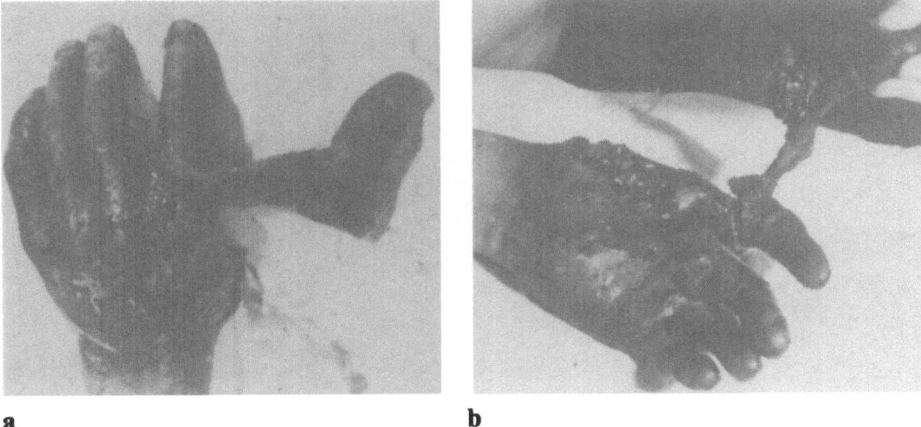

a   b

Figure 15.3 Patient Fan, male, 24, sustained skin avulsion injury to the left hand resulting in amputation of thumb. **a,b,** Views immediately after injury, taken before cleansing of wound

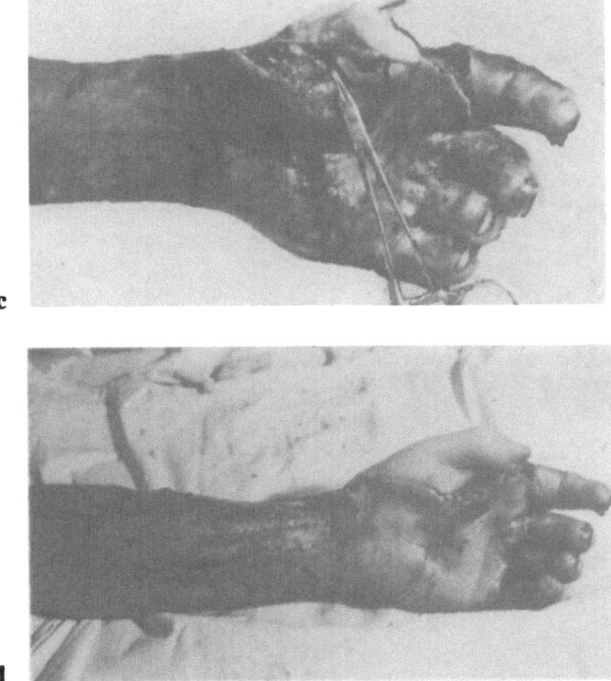

c

d

Figure 15.3c, d During operation. The two phalanges of the thumb, after peeling off of the soft tissue, were held in place with Kirschner wire. After repair of the nerve and tendon, the thumb was reconstructed with a forearm radial arterial turnover flap

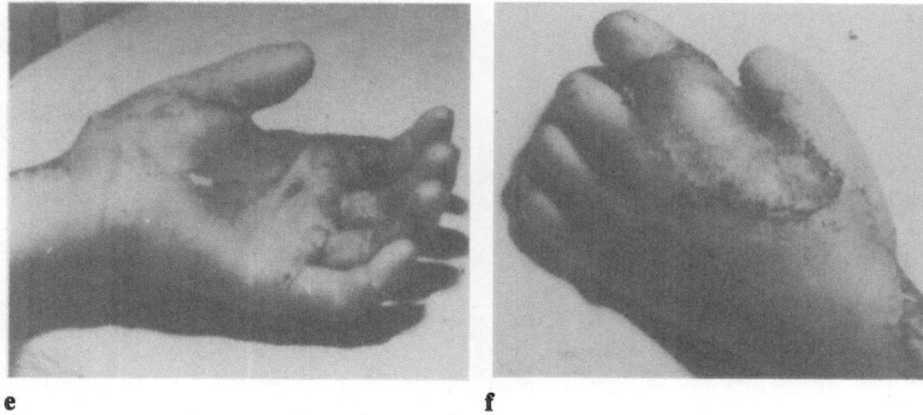

e   f

Figure 15.3   **e,f** Twelve days after operation, the flap and the skin graft on donor site survived well

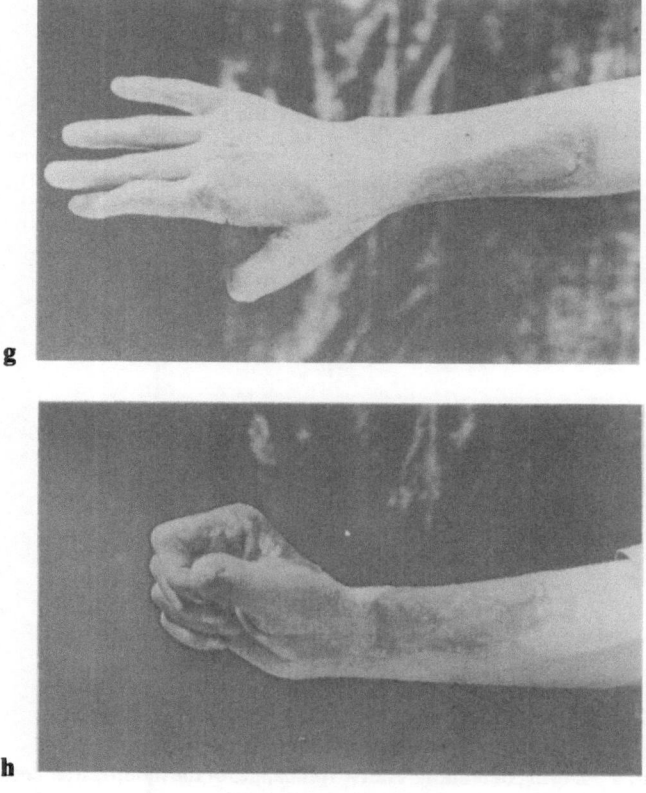

g

h

Figure 15.3g, h   Good functional recovery 2 years after operation

full thickness skin grafts (Figure 15.4c,d). On the 12th postoperative day, the skin flap and free skin graft showed complete survival. After six months follow-up, some function of the hand had been restored (Figure 15.4e,f) and a lot of daily housework could be done, such as washing and cooking, as well as buttoning up clothes and even riding her bike. However, sensation has not been completely regained in the thumb, especially the distal end.

DISCUSSION

Forearm radial arterial turnover flap: indications and advantages

This skin flap with fine texture, feasible thickness and an abundant blood supply is a very suitable skin coverage for deep tissue repair in one stage. It is technically safer and simpler, as the microsurgery of vascular anastomosis is no longer required.

Indications

Indications are

(1)   immediate reconstruction of acute hand injuries such as crushing, avulsion or severance of thumb;

(2)   repair of late cases of traumatic or burn deformities with deep tissue loss in the hand and wrist region;

(3)   the flap may be used to repair deformity of the face, trunk and lower limbs without any delay as an ordinary random flap.

With this type of flap we have satisfactorily repaired a case of deep burn of the mandibular region with exposed mandible.

A new method for thumb reconstruction

There are many methods for thumb reconstruction[2] such as pollicization of the first metacarpus, pollicization by the adjacent finger, free transposition of the second toe, the local flap, or tubed flap bone graft. However, the forearm turn-over flap was viable for most cases of thumb reconstruction, and has not hither-to appeared in the literature. In this article we have reported five cases of thumb reconstruction with good results. Sensation and motion could be restored in the thumb if the nerves and tendons were left in the severed digit. The method of skinning the severed thumb leaving the nerve and tendon in place to reconstruct the thumb by skin tube has appeared in the literature[3]. In our case we did the same, as described in Case 2, except that the coverage was a forearm turnover flap, not a skin tube. An additional advantage is that the limb does not need to be fixed to other parts of the body as the tubed flap does.

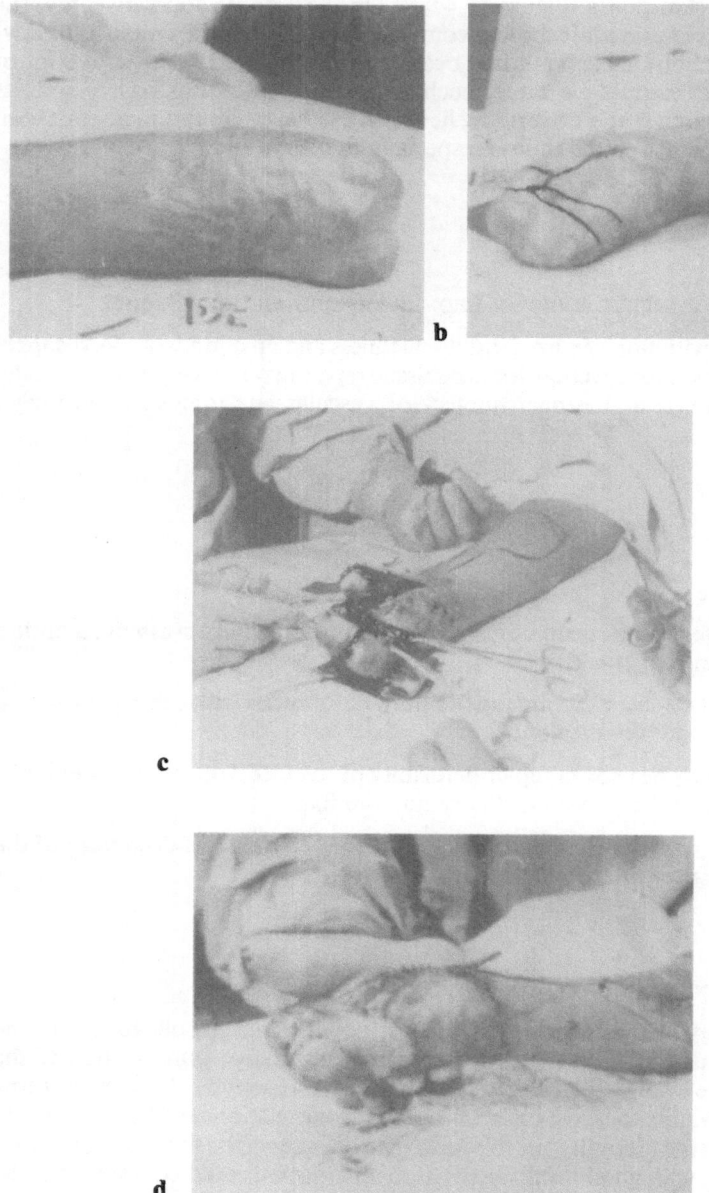

Figure 15.4   A 22-year-old female was admitted with stump deformity of the right hand.
a,b, Preoperative views, design of incision. **c,d,** Views during operation, the first web and
palm had been opened up. A piece of iliac bone graft was inserted into the stump of
proximal phalange of the thumb and covered with a forearm radial arterial turnover flap.
The donor wound was skin grafted

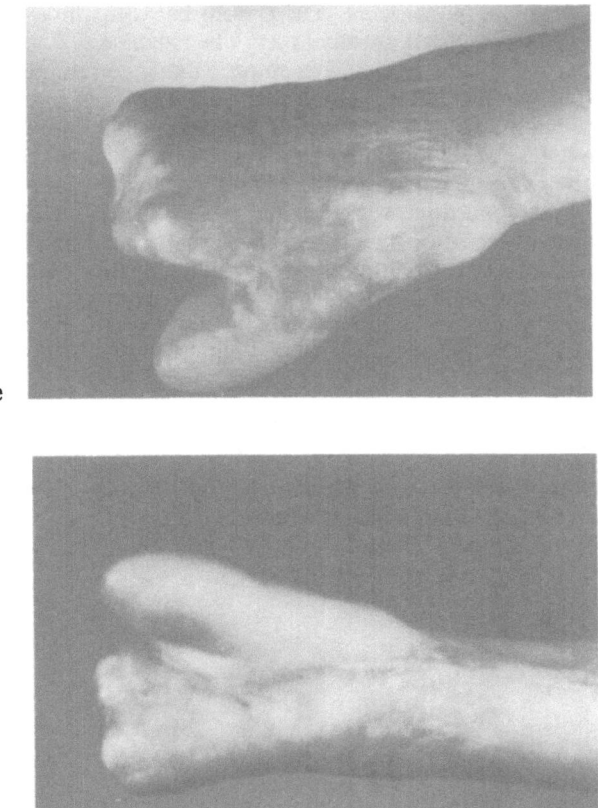

Figure 15.4e, f   Postoperative view, appearance and function were improved

The crux of operative success

There are many factors affecting operative success. From the technical point of view, during the operative procedure, the key point is that the level of dissection of the flap should be carried out in between the deep fascia and myolemma. The flap and the radial artery with its accompanying veins and their branches should be protected carefully, and one should see that they are always kept in contact with the flap. The blood supply of the flap and fingers should, of course, be watched and tested before the severance of the artery at the proximal end, if the patient has a history of injury of the ulnar side of the hand or forearm. In that situation, the radial artery should be clamped at the site of severance for a few minutes and the color of the digits and the flap watched. The operation should not be continued unless the blood supply of the flap is sure to be in good condition. As regards the venous return, we had studied ten radial veins under the operating microscope in cadavers. There were between three and six venous valvulae in a 15–20 cm length of radial vein. The valvulae of two accompanying veins were not on the same level and there were many communicating branches in between. The perfusion tests show that a solution could pass through easily against the direction. This shows the blood could return reversibly through the collateral branches of the accompanying veins in spite of the presence of valvulae. This has also been confirmed by the clinical cases where the flap remained in good condition even without anastomosis of veins (six cases). In brief, the clinical observation over one or more years showed that the short term result was satisfactory, without any complication. Further observations of this technique are of course indispensable.

REFERENCES

1. Yang Guo-fan *et al*. (1981). Forearm free skin flap transplantation. *Natl. Med. J. China*, **61**, 139
2. Chang Ti-sheng. (1979). *Plastic and Reconstructive Surgery*. 1st Edn., pp. 437–50. (Shanghai: Scientific and Technologic Publishing Co.)
3. Gillies, H. and Millard, D. R. (1957). *The Principles and Art of Plastic Surgery*. Vol. II, p. 492 (London: Butterworths)

16 Reconstruction of Metacarpophalangeal Joint by Free Vascularized Autogenous Metatarsophalangeal Joint Transplant

GUO EN-TAN, JI ZHENG-LUN, ZHANG MING-LI and ZHAO YUE-ZHEN

Department of Plastic Surgery, Changhai Hospital, The Second Military Medical College, Shanghai

The metacarpophalangeal (MP) joint is essential to hand function, which will suffer severe deterioration in the event of traumatic or arthritic stiffening. Early this century, a stiffened MP joint was replaced by autograft of a small joint which was subjected to degenerative changes within 1–2 years. Since Buncke's[1] second to third MP joint transplantation on an intact vascular pedicle was proved to be successful without any late degenerative changes in long term observation in 1967, experimental small joint transplantation was undertaken independently by Buncke[1] and Hurwitz[2], with the same conclusion: long term survival of the vascular graft without any degeneration and severe degenerative alteration in nonvascular transplant.

At the beginning of 1980, on the basis of a detailed study on the blood supply and innervation of the metatarsophalangeal (MTP) joint, free transplantation of revascularized MTP joint in two cases was successfully carried out in our clinic[3]. Since then, four more cases (five joints) have been treated by this method, with three transplants reinnervated. Satisfactory postoperative results were obtained in all cases during a follow-up study of 6–30 months.

SURGICAL ANATOMY OF THE SECOND MTP JOINT

The MTP joint, with the largest range of motion, has a solid capsule, a thick and tough ligament on the sole side and two strong collateral ligaments on both sides. The anatomically matched structure of MTP to MP is characteristic with the exception of its dominant dorsal extension which is opposite to the dominant palmar flexion of the MP.

According to our autopsy study, the blood supply of the second MTP is based mainly upon the articular branch of the first dorsal metatarsal artery (FDMA) with its two accompanying veins for venous drainage (Figure 16.1).

123

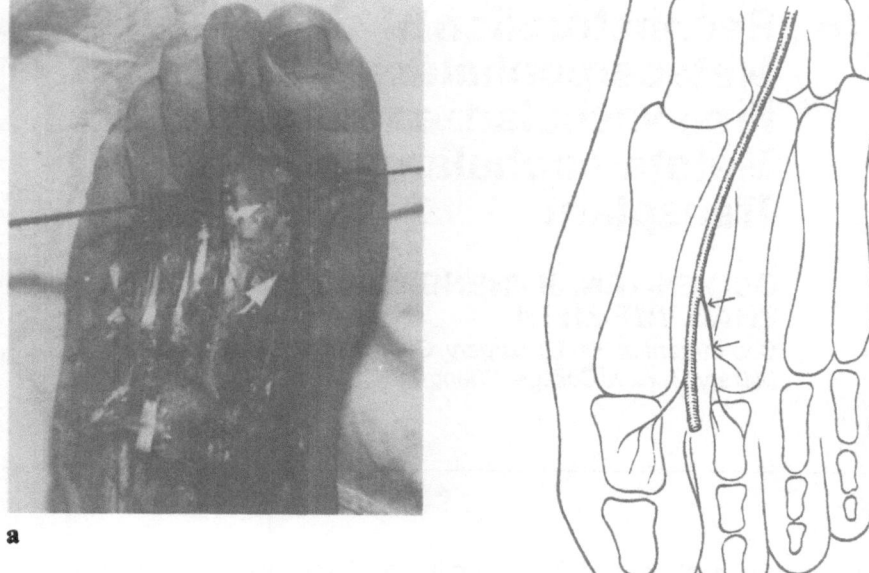

Figure 16.1 a, The first metatarsal artery originates from the second metatarsophal-angeal articular branch (arrow). **b,** In diagrammatic form

The articular branch of the FDMA may be classified into three types in regard to its origin and course.

In *Type I* (80%) the articular branch originates from the interosseous portion of the FDMA at the junction of the distal and middle thirds of the metatarsus bone, 1.5 cm proximal to the MTP in adults (Figure 16.2).

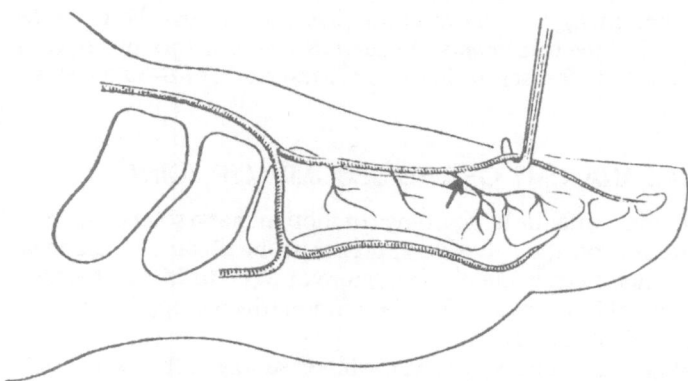

Figure 16.2 The first type of articular branch

In *Type II* (18%) it detaches from the origin of the FDMA and then penetrates the deep fibers of the interosseous muscle to supply the joint (Figure 16.3). Some small branches are given out on its way to supply the interosseous muscle. The FDMA, having crossed the interosseous muscle, proceeds along the fibular side of the first metatarsus bone.

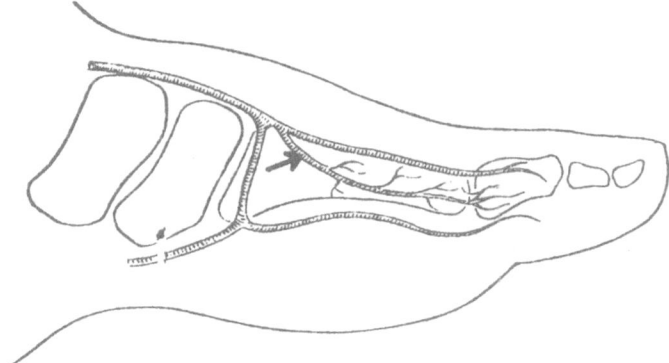

Figure 16.3   The second type of articular branch

In *Type III* (22%) the FDMA passes underneath the first dorsal interosseous muscle giving out the articular branch in immediate contact with the joint (Figure 16.4).

Besides this constant articular branch, a supplementary MTP joint branch is present in 78% of cases and communicates with the main dorsal articular branch via collateral anastomosis. The origins of the supplementary articular branch are the first plantar metatarsal artery and the deep plantar branch of the dorsalis pedis artery (DPA).

The second MTP joint is innervated by the terminal branch of the peroneus

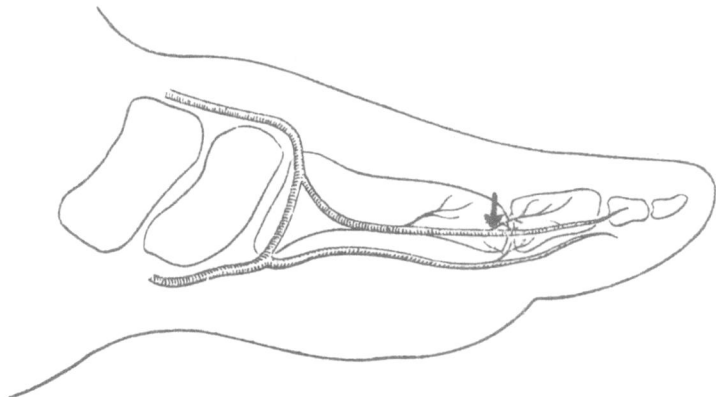

Figure 16.4   The third type of articular branch

profundus nerve which proceeds between the DPA and the cutaneous dorsal medial nerve of the peroneus superficialis nerve.

SURGICAL TECHNIQUE

There are four surgical steps.

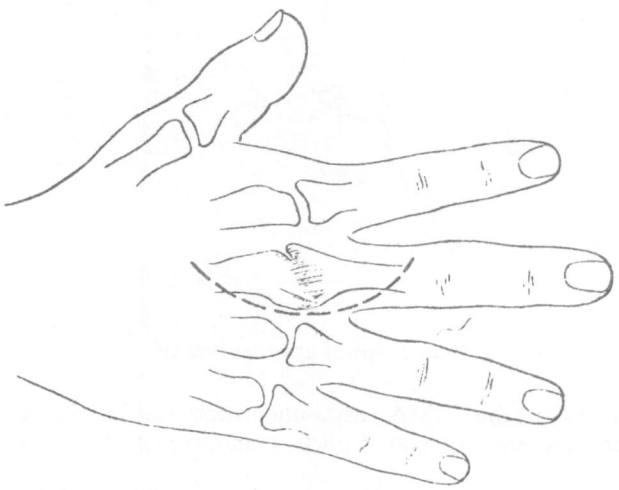

Figure 16.5   Incision for excision of damaged joint

1.   Resection of the diseased joint

A curved or 'S' incision (Figure 16.5) is made on the dorsal aspect of the finger crossing either side of the MP joint. The incision is deepened through the subcutaneous layer to the deep fascia which is incised and carefully dissected from the underlying tissues, and the lesions of the MP joint are explored. The ulnar side of the hood of the digital extensor is opened and the tendon is retracted to the radial side. The diseased joints including the head of the meta-carpus and the base of the proximal phalanx are resected. The radial artery lying in the floor of the Snuffbox and the commencement of the cephalic vein are dissected for anastomosis purposes with the donor vessels. The small branch of the superficial radial nerve located at the dorsal side of the wrist is also dissected out for the innervation of the transplant.

2.   Dissection of the graft

The long saphenous vein and the DPA along with its FDMA are exposed. During the dissection of the FDMA in the interosseous portion, care should be taken to protect the articular branch from any injury. The terminal branch of the peroneus profundus nerve concomitant with the DPA must also be preserved with caution. A skin island overlying the joint is preserved as a marker to determine the viability of the transplant. After dividing the extensor and flexor tendons, the MTP including its capsule and ligaments are isolated from the surrounding tissues. The metatarsal and phalanx are then osteotomized. The

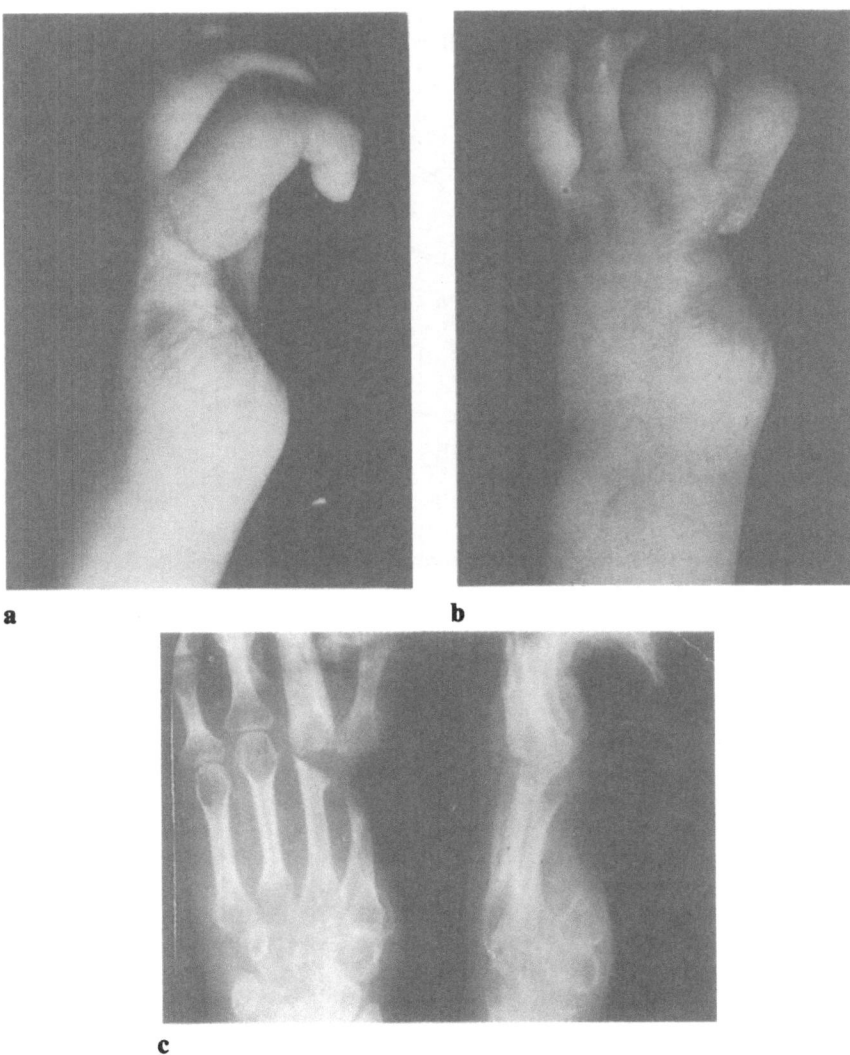

a   b

c

Figure 16.6   Case 3, 22, female, sustained crush injury to her left hand, resulting in total loss of left thumb and most of the first metacarpus, and also damage to the index and middle finger MP joints. **a**, Preoperative radial view. **b**, Postoperative posterior view. **c**, Preoperative X-ray film

whole joint is then detached from its neurovascular bundle when the recipient area is ready for transplantation.

In the reconstruction of two continuous MP joints as a one-stage operation (Figures 16.6–16.8), the second and third MTP joints are prepared as a single composite transplant unit. In such a case, the arcuate artery (Figure 16.1), and the main branch of the PDA supplying the third MTP joint should be included in the vascular bundle to ensure the blood supply of both the third and second MTP joints, and the combined vascularized joints as a single unit can be used for the reconstruction of the second and third or third and fourth MP joint defects.

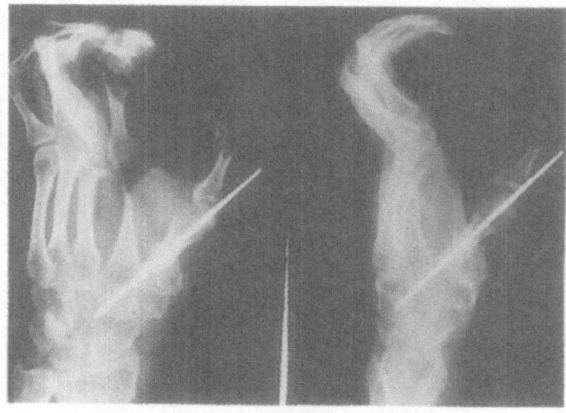

Figure 16.7 Case 3. Revascularized second toe to repair the missing left thumb

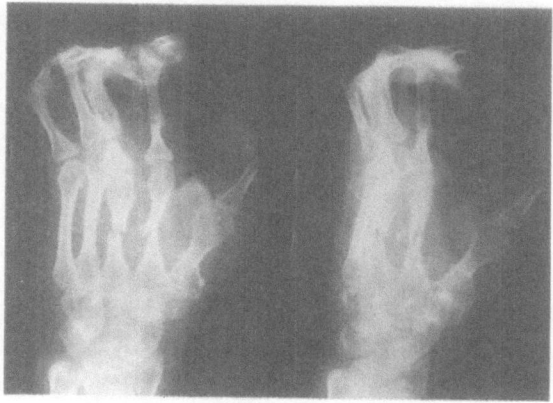

Figure 16.8 Case 3. The destroyed MP joints of index and middle fingers were replaced by the left second and third metatarsophalangeal joints with tendons and a piece of skin attached, one-stage procedure (dorsal artery as the common pedicle).

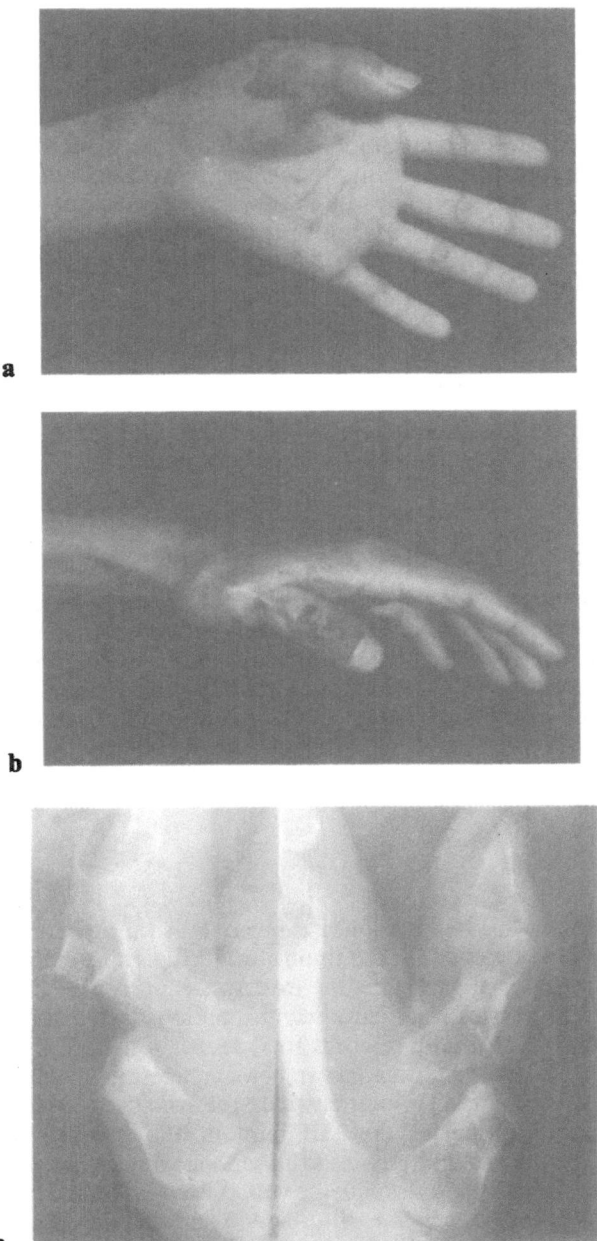

Figure 16.9 Case 1. Crush injury to left hand, resulting in loss of thumb MP joint together with soft tissue around base of the first metacarpus. **a,** Preoperative palmar view. **b,** Preoperative radial view. **c,** Preoperative X-ray.

3. Transplantation of the joint

The transplant is turned 180° around its longitudinal axis. Then the solar aspect of the MTP joint is turned to the dorsal side of the hand. The head of the metatarsal is connected with the shaft of the metacarpal bone, and the base of the proximal phalangeal bone of the toe with the shaft of the phalangeal bone of the hand. After fixation with Kirschner wires, anastomosis of the DPA to the radial artery, the long saphenous vein to the cephalic vein, and the nerve of the transplant to the superficial branch of the radial nerve at the dorsal side of the wrist is accomplished by microsurgical technique. After repair of the tendons, the skin incision is closed.

4. Treatment of the donor site

The defect created by the dissection of the MTP joint can be replaced by the resected MP joint or by a piece of spongy bone tissue.

Postoperative management

This includes elevation of the hand which has been operated on, prophylactic use of antibiotics and daily infusion of low molecular weight dextran for several days. The Kirschner wire is removed 4 weeks after operation and functional exercises are encouraged. After immobilization of the donor site in a cast for 4 weeks, walking is permitted. No apparent disorders of the donor foot have been noted.

CASE REPORTS

Case 1

A 24-year-old peasant had sustained a severe crush injury to his left hand 6 months prior to admission. The left thumb lost its function because the MP joint with the adjacent bone as well as the extensor tendons were destroyed in the initial injury. There was also dense scar formation on the radial, dorsal and palmar aspects of the thumb (Figures 16.9, 16.10). On January 9 1980, under epidural and brachial plexus nerve block anesthesia, the autogenous vascularized left second MTP joint based on the articular branch of the FDMA was transplanted to replace the MP joint of the thumb. The DPA was anastomosed to the radial artery and the saphenous vein anastomosed to the cephalic vein. The anastomosis of all the vessels was performed under the operative microscope. The transplant carried tendon and skin flap to repair the defect of the recipient site.

Six months postoperatively the function of the thumb was restored (Figure 16.10d). During the follow-up of $2\frac{1}{2}$ years, the transplanted joint was stable with an active range of motion (ROM) of 0°/50° and passive ROM of 0°/60°, and no obvious degenerative changes were observed on radiography (Figure 16.10c).

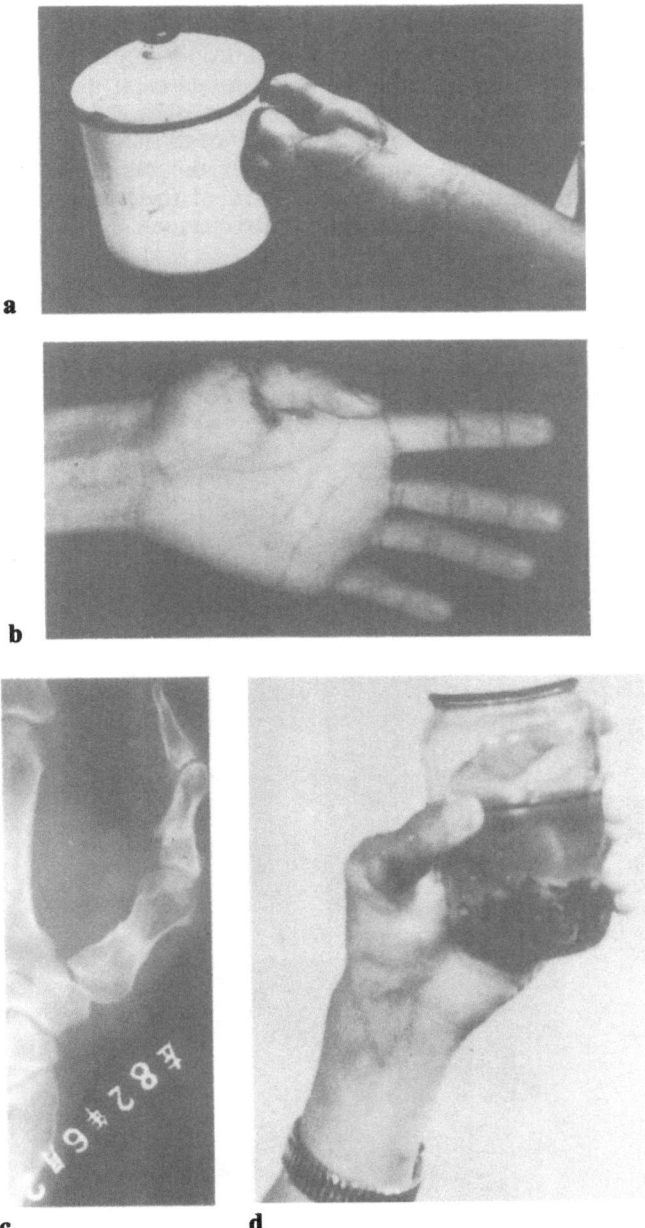

a

b

c   d

Figure 16.10 Case 1. **a,** Postoperative palmar view. **b,** Postoperative posterior view. **c,** Two and a half years after operation. Good union of bone. Articular surface and interarticular space are normal. **d,** Six months after operation, the function of left thumb nearly normal

Case 2

A 38-year-old worker had sustained a crush injury to his left hand 6 months prior to admission. The index finger was amputated at its base in the initial injury. The MP joint of the long finger was damaged, resulting in bony ankylosis. The vascularized second MTP joint of the left foot was transplanted to repair the MP joint of the long finger. During the follow-up of 2 years, active ROM of 0°/30° and passive ROM 0°/45° of the transplanted joint were found. Radiography showed no degenerative changes.

Case 3

A 22-year-old female had suffered severe crush injury to her left hand 1½ years prior to admission. The initial injury consisted of traumatic amputation of the

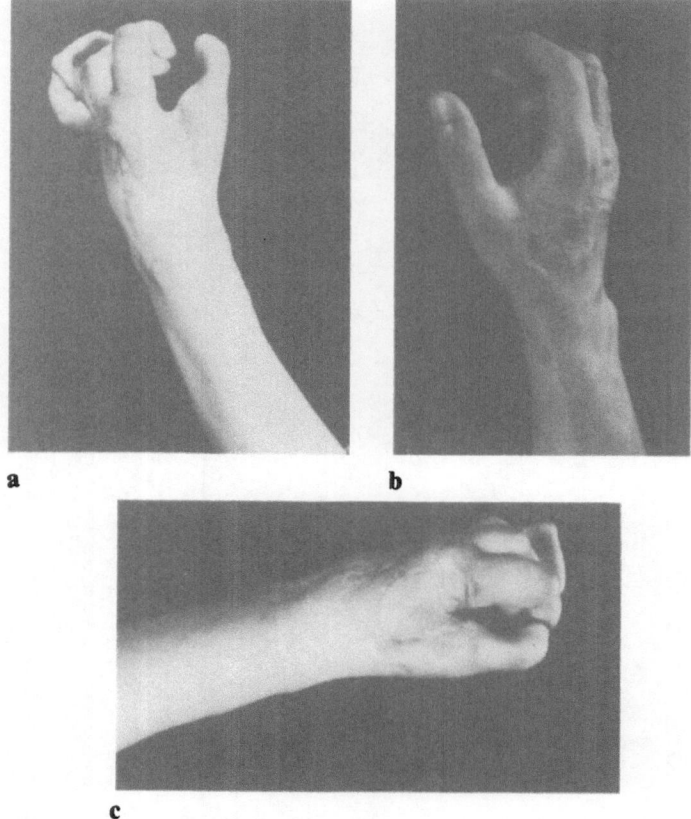

a

b

c

Figure 16.11 Case 3. **a**, Postoperative view. Good oppositional function. **b**, Postoperative view. Abduction of the new thumb. **c**, One year after operation, showing partial recovery of function

thumb and the main part of the first metacarpus, and damage to the MP joints of the index and long finger (Figure 16.6). Reconstruction of the thumb was carried out by transplantation of a vascularized right second toe, and the transplantation of combined left second and third MTP joints, with the tendons and skin island overlying the joints still attached, to repair the MP joints and soft tissue defect of the index and middle fingers. The latter procedure was carried out in the second operation. Follow-up study of 1 year revealed an active ROM of 0 °/50 °, passive 0 °/20 ° of the index and active 0 °/5 °, passive 0 °/10 ° of the middle finger (Figure 16.11).

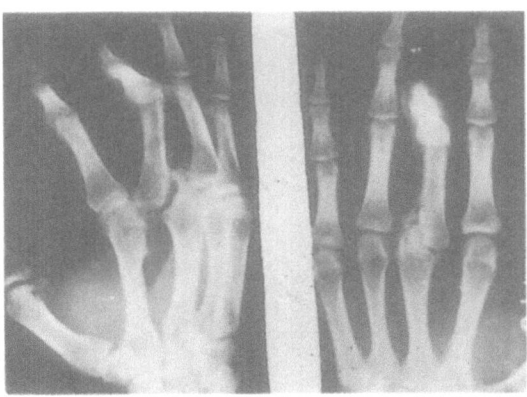

Figure 16.12   Case 4. Preoperative X-ray shows defect of the middle finger MP joint.

Case 4

A 23-year-old worker had sustained comminuted fracture of the third metacarpus due to crush injury to his right hand resulting in bony ankylosis and deformity of the third MP joint (Figure 16.12) 1 year prior to admission. The transplantation of the second left MTP joint with nerve, which anastomosed to the superficial branch of the radial nerve in the snuffbox area, was carried out to repair the damaged MP joint of the middle finger in April 1981.

During the follow-up of 1½ years, active ROM 2 °/90 ° and passive 2 °/90 ° of the transplanted joint was observed (Figure 16.13). Radiography showed no degenerative changes (Figure 16.14)

Case 5

A 51-year-old worker had sustained a severe injury to his left hand 1 year prior to admission. The injury consisted of compound comminuted fracture of the thumb and index finger, traumatic amputation of the middle finger, and fracture of the proximal phalanx of the fourth and fifth fingers. There were also ankylosis and deformity of the thumb MP joint and dysfunction of the left hand. The transplantation of the free vascularized second left MTP joint with

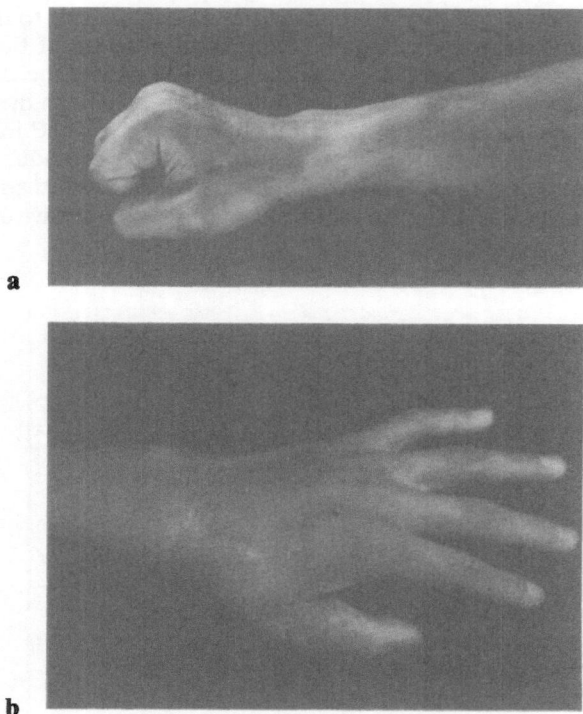

Figure 16.13 Case 4. Follow-up 1½ years after operation. **a,** Flexion of fingers. **b,** Extension of fingers

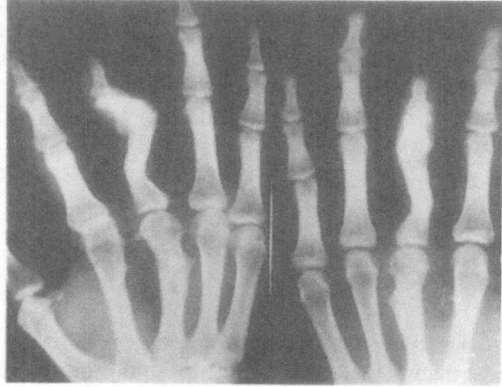

Figure 16.14 Case 4. One and a half years after operation. X-ray reveals no degenerative changes in transplanted joint. (Malunion of the proximal phalanx corrected in the subsequent operation)

nerve and skin flap was performed to repair the damaged MP joint of the thumb. During the follow-up of $1\frac{1}{2}$ years, active and passive ROM of the transplanted joint of the left thumb was 45°/70° and 35°/75°, and radiography showed the joint to be essentially normal.

Case 6

A 20-year-old female had sustained a severe injury to her right hand 1 year prior to admission. The initial injury consisted of contusion of the thumb, traumatic amputation of the index finger and the greater part of the second metacarpus, and comminuted fracture of the ring finger resulting in the bony ankylosis of the fourth MP joint. The transplantation of the free vascularized second left MTP joint with nerve was carried out to repair the damaged MP joint of the ring finger. During the follow-up of 6 months, the transplanted joint had active ROM 30°/40° and passive 25°/40°. Radiography showed no signs of degeneration.

DISCUSSION

It has been experimentally proved that an autogenous small joint transplantation with its nutrient vessels may be free from late degenerative changes[1,2]. The anatomically matched structure of MTP to MP joint rendered its vascularized replacement an ideal measure. In case of tendon and skin defect along with the stiffening joint, a composite MTP joint replacement may be done. The vascular pedicle of the transplant consists of the PDA, FDMA with its articular branch, a portion of the dorsal pedis vein arch, and a long saphenous vein. The calibers of DPA and saphenous vein are rather large for successful microsurgical anastomosis. The key to dissection of the joint is to protect from injury the articular branch of FDMA. It is, therefore, better done under magnification.

Having preserved the blood supply of epiphysis as well as metaphysis, vascularized MTP joint transplantation is quite suitable for infants without interference to finger growth.

In big joint transplantation, vasculonervous reestablishment of the transplant is indispensable in the avoidance of its late alteration. As to the small joint, is the vascularized graft without being reinnervated subject to late degeneration? This is still a question waiting for further discussion and answer. Experimentally[1,2], the vascularized small transplanted joints were exempt from degeneration in a follow-up study of more than 2 years. In our series, graft reinnervation plays no role in long-term survival. All survived without late degeneration in a follow-up of 6–30 months. Nevertheless, graft reinnervation is a physiological resource and was done in the last three cases.

The sclerotic bone of the metacarpus and phalanx should be removed completely in order to promote circulation. Any residual sclerotic bone tissue will cause nonhealing in the transplant. This complication occurred in one of our cases, for whom a secondary operation is needed to deal with the malunion of the graft.

REFERENCES

1. Buncke, H. J. *et al.* (1967). The fate of autogenous whole joint transplanted by microvascular anastomoses. *Plast. Reconstr. Surg.*, **39**, 333
2. Hurwitz, P. J. (1979). Experimental transplantation of small joints by microvascular anastomoses. *Plast. Reconstr. Surg.*, **64**, 221
3. Guo En-tan *et al.* (1980). Free vascularized small joint transplant, preliminary report of the second metatarsophalangeal joint transfer for the reconstruction of damaged metacarpophalangeal joint. *Acad. J. Second Military Med. Coll.* **1**(2), 12 (In Chinese)

17 Free Transfer of Fascia of the Scalp by Microvascular Technique Plus Skin Graft for the Repair of Postburn Clawhand Deformity

WEI LIAN-JUN, CHANG TI-SHENG, SHI YAO-MING and CHIA YUAN-ZRE
Department of Plastic and Reconstructive Surgery, Shanghai Second Medical College

Postburn clawhand deformity has long been a challenge to both plastic and hand surgeons because it involves not only the skin and subcutaneous tissue but also deep structures such as tendons, ligaments, bones and joints. A combination of all these factors makes reconstruction of the hand a difficult problem. The conventional reconstruction of clawhand deformity usually begins with the replacement of the scar tissue with a flap or tube transplantation which always requires several stages before deep structures can be handled safely. With the help of microvascular anastomosis technique, a one-stage free flap transfer can be substituted but, as we all know, the flap thus transferred is often too bulky in appearance. Since October 1980 we have been adopting a new surgical technique including a free scalp fascia transfer and a free skin graft on top of it. This new technique has been used in repairing seven cases of clawhand deformity with good results. The technique was first advocated by Smith in 1980 for repair of chronic leg ulcer.

CADAVER STUDIES

To verify the precise distribution of the vessels and their caliber as well as the maximum size of the scalp fascia available, we studied 52 specimens in 32 cadavers in October 1980, with the kind help of the Anatomy Department of the Shanghai Second Medical College. The results are as follows:

Distribution of vessels

The superficial temporal vessel has two branches, the posterior and the anterior. The posterior branch, together with its venae comitantes, anastomoses with the opposite counterpart at the top of the skull. Throughout its whole course one can see numerous collateral connections which have a different pattern of distribution even on both sides of the same cadaver. The anterior branch, which also has numerous connections along its course, traverses anteriorly and is anastomosed with the same vessel from the opposite side.

Caliber of the vessels

The vessels were dissected out and measured with a ruler. The caliber of the artery at the level of the tragus is 1.5–2.5 mm, and that of the vein 2.0–2.5 mm. At a level 5 cm above the tragus, the caliber of the artery is 1.5–2.0 mm and the vein 1.0–2.0 mm.

Location of bifurcation of superficial temporal artery

The superficial temporal artery bifurcates into an anterior branch and a posterior branch at various sites from the tragus. In 22 cadavers, the bifurcation is located at a spot 4.0–4.5 cm from the tragus, constituting 42.3% of 32 cadavers. This anatomic feature enables us to use the portion of the scalp fascia supplied by the anterior branch to repair the thumb, while that supplied by the posterior branch is used to repair the remaining four fingers. The portion in between the above two is used to repair the first web. To avoid compromise of blood supply to the fascia, the precise location of the vascular bifurcation should be defined as exactly as possible both preoperatively and intraoperatively.

Anatomical relationship between superficial temporal artery and vein

The superficial temporal artery takes a course anterior to the vein on 35 sides out of 52 sides in 32 cadavers, constituting 67.3%, while the artery is situated posterior to the vein on 17 sides, constituting 32.7%.

OPERATIVE PROCEDURES

The hair should be cut short enough preoperatively to permit identification of the course of the vessels and the location of the bifurcation either by a palpating finger or with the help of a Doppler's detector, and the courses of the vessels are marked with methylene blue. General anesthesia is used, and two surgical teams work simultaneously, one on the hand and the other on the scalp.

A T-mark is first made on the temporal region with its central limb lying directly over the course of the superficial temporal artery and its posterior branch, or lying along a line which bisects the angle formed by the bifurcation of the artery. The transverse limb is placed parallel to the sagittal suture of the cranium.

The dissection begins with a skin incision along this T-mark and care should be taken not to carry the incision too deep into the subcutaneous layer which is

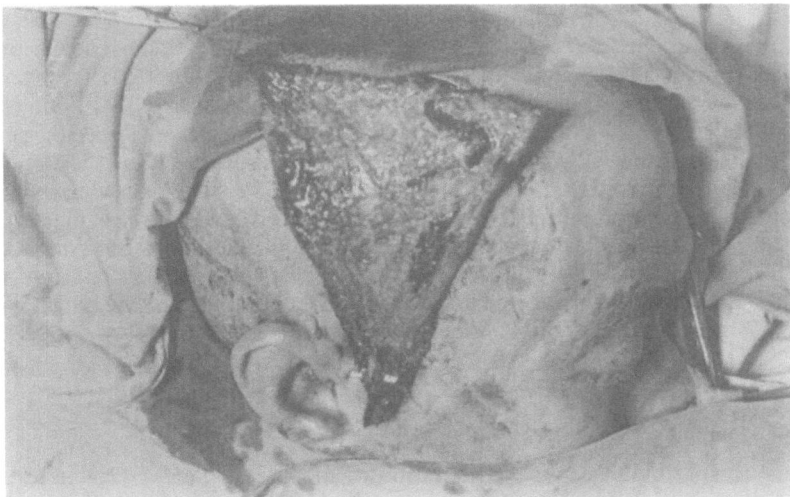

Figure 17.1 The temporal fascia has been lifted

usually very thin. Two scalp flaps are raised on both sides of the central limb. The plane of dissection is best placed just underneath the hair follicles in the superficial layer of the subcutaneous tissue to avoid damage to the hair follicles as well as the network of the superficial temporal vessels lying on the scalp fascia. When the required size of scalp fascia has been exposed, it is elevated from the pericranium (Figure 17.1), which should include the whole layer of the underlying areolar tissue in order to provide padding for the gliding tendons of the hand. After division of the vascular pedicle, the scalp fascia is transplanted to the dorsum of the clawhand and vascular anastomosis is performed between the superficial temporal vessels and the carpal branch of the radial artery and the cephalic vein. To complete the operation, a split thickness free skin graft is put on top of the revascularized scalp fascia. The donor wound in the temporal region can usually be closed primarily.

The maximum size of the scalp fascia in this series of patients is about 10×15 cm² and the caliber of the vessels is usually larger than 1.5 mm.

CASE REPORTS

Case 1

A male aged 18 years was admitted for both clawhands due to flame burn. Examination revealed hyperextension of the left thumb with dislocation of its MP joint due to scar contraction. In addition, the thumb was adducted resulting in contracture of the first web space (Figure 17.2).

The patient was placed under general anesthesia and two teams worked together. The scar tissue over the dorsum of the hand measuring 8×4 cm² was excised under the tourniquet. The dislocated MP joint was reduced after excision of its two accessory ligaments and elongation of the shortened extensor pollicis longus. The first web space was reopened by severance of the transverse head of the adductor pollicis, thus creating a wound measuring 8×10 cm^2. Both the radial artery (1.2 mm) and the cephalic vein (2.0 mm) were dissected out for vascular anastomosis. Another team harvested a scalp fascia of the same size which was transplanted to the wound in the hand. After revascularization by vascular anastomosis with 9/0 nylon suture, a split thickness free skin graft was put on the scalp fascia. Low molecular dextran was administered systemically for 5 days postoperatively. Both the skin graft and the scalp fascia took well. Follow-up examination showed good functional restoration of the hand (Figure 17.3). Angiography 2 months later revealed patency of the vessels.

Case 2

A 25-year-old male sustained thermal burn of his left hand 1 year before the operation; his hand had ultimately developed clawhand deformity. Physical

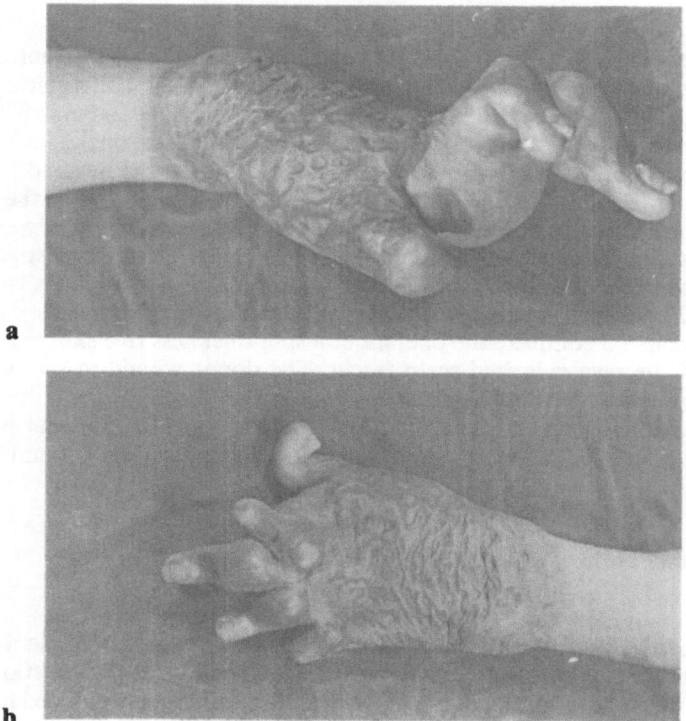

a

b

Figure 17.2 Clawhand after burn. **a,** Preoperative lateral view. **b,** Preoperative dorsal view

examination revealed that all the five MP joints, especially that of the already adducted thumb, were dorsally dislocated due to scar contraction over the dorsum of the hand. The operation was done by two teams working simultaneously. After excision of the scar, the transverse head of the adductor pollicis was severed to widen the first web space and all the five dislocated MP joints were reduced after resection of the accessory collateral ligaments. The shortened extensor pollicis longus was also lengthened. A piece of temporal scalpal fascia measuring 12×13 cm^2 was removed from the right temporal region and transplanted to the dorsum of the hand. Vascular anastomosis was performed between the superficial temporal vessels and carpal branch of the radial artery and the cephalic vein in the hand. A free split thickness skin graft was put on top of the revascularized scalpal fascia. Both the free skin graft and the scalpal fascia took well. Follow-up shortly after the operation showed good functional restoration, and patency of the vessels was confirmed by arteriography 2 months after the operation.

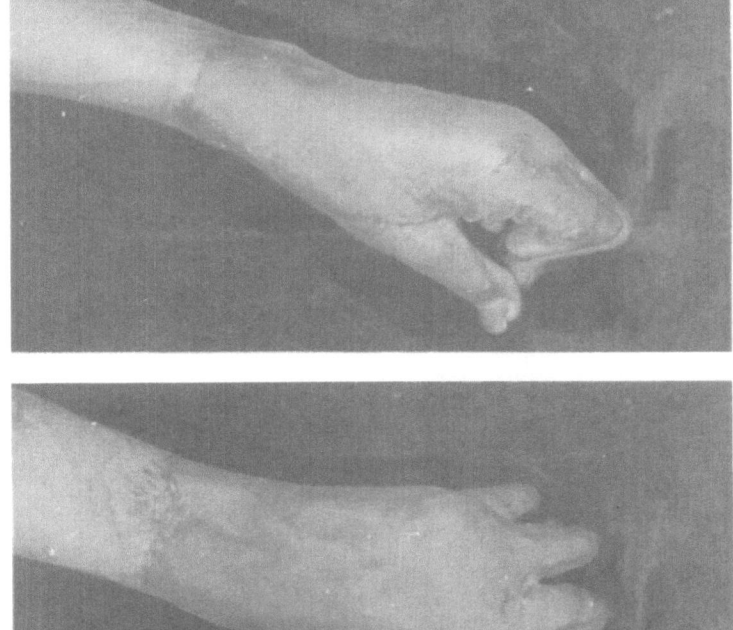

Figure 17.3 a, Postoperative lateral view. **b,** Postoperative dorsal view

DISCUSSION

The advantages of this operation are as follows.

(1) The operation can be completed in one stage, including the correction of deep structures. By making use of the bifurcation of the superficial temporal artery, it is possible to open the first web space and at the same time repair the thumb with the portion supplied by the posterior branch, and the other four fingers with that supplied by the posterior branch, and this procedure involves less risk to the blood supply of the transplant than that in a conventional free flap.

(2) The scalpal fascia is thin enough to fit the esthetic requirement of the dorsum of the hand.

(3) The caliber of the temporal vessels is large enough to ensure high rate of patency (larger than 1.5 mm) after microvascular anastomosis.

(4) The incisional scar of the donor site can be adequately hidden by the hair (Figure 17.4).

The only disadvantage of the scalpal fascia is that it seems to lack enough elasticity to meet the specific functional requirement of the hand. Therefore, its clinical use should be reevaluated after a long term follow-up.

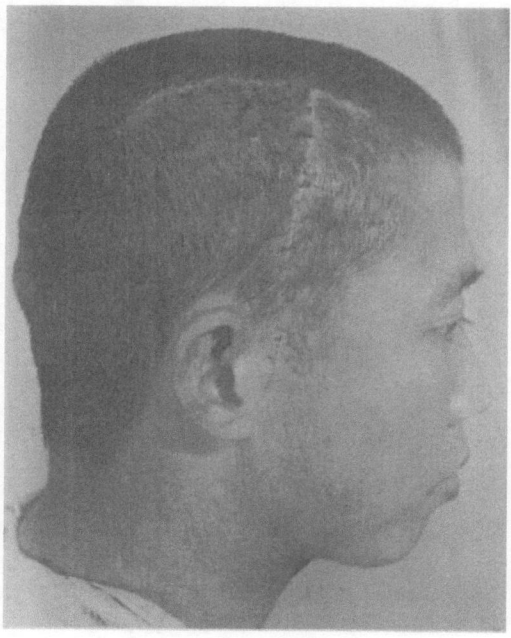

Figure 17.4 The scar line over the donor site

18 Sole to Palm Full Thickness Skin Graft

HAO ZHU-REN, CHEN WEI-ZHONG and CHEN PEI-YAN
Affiliated Hospital, North China Institute of Radiation Protection

For proper functioning of the hand, palmar skin, an integral part of the hand, plays an important role, and any defect in it, whether traumatic or pathologic, should be meticulously resurfaced. The conventional skin graft is far from satisfactory for the repair of a palmar skin defect. Consequently, sole to palm full thickness skin graft was proposed in 1955 by Webster[1], and used subsequently by Le Worthy (1963)[2] and Micks (1967)[3].

Nineteen sites in 13 patients with palmar skin defect were repaired by means of sole to palm full thickness skin graft in the past 4 years in our clinic. The technique is so rewarding that we should like to recommend it once again.

SURGICAL TECHNIQUE

Before operation, the donor site is examined to exclude any foot deformity, and at the same time to determine how much skin on the medial pedal region is available.

After the palmar scar has been excised and the cicatricial contracture released, a cloth pattern of the defect is taken and put on the sole to locate the proper donor site and the skin graft is obtained.

The sole skin is tightly bound to the deep fascia by tough fibrous bands which should be cut during graft removal. After removing the subcutaneous fat, the full thickness skin graft is transplanted to the palmar defect and maintained by tieover pressure dressing. Stitches are removed on the tenth to 14th postoperative day.

The donor site defect can be eliminated by direct approximation, in a small defect, or by split thickness skin graft, in a big one (Figures 18.1–18.3).

In finger pulp skin defect, ridged sole skin should be chosen, to mimic the new fingerprint (Figure 18.4).

143

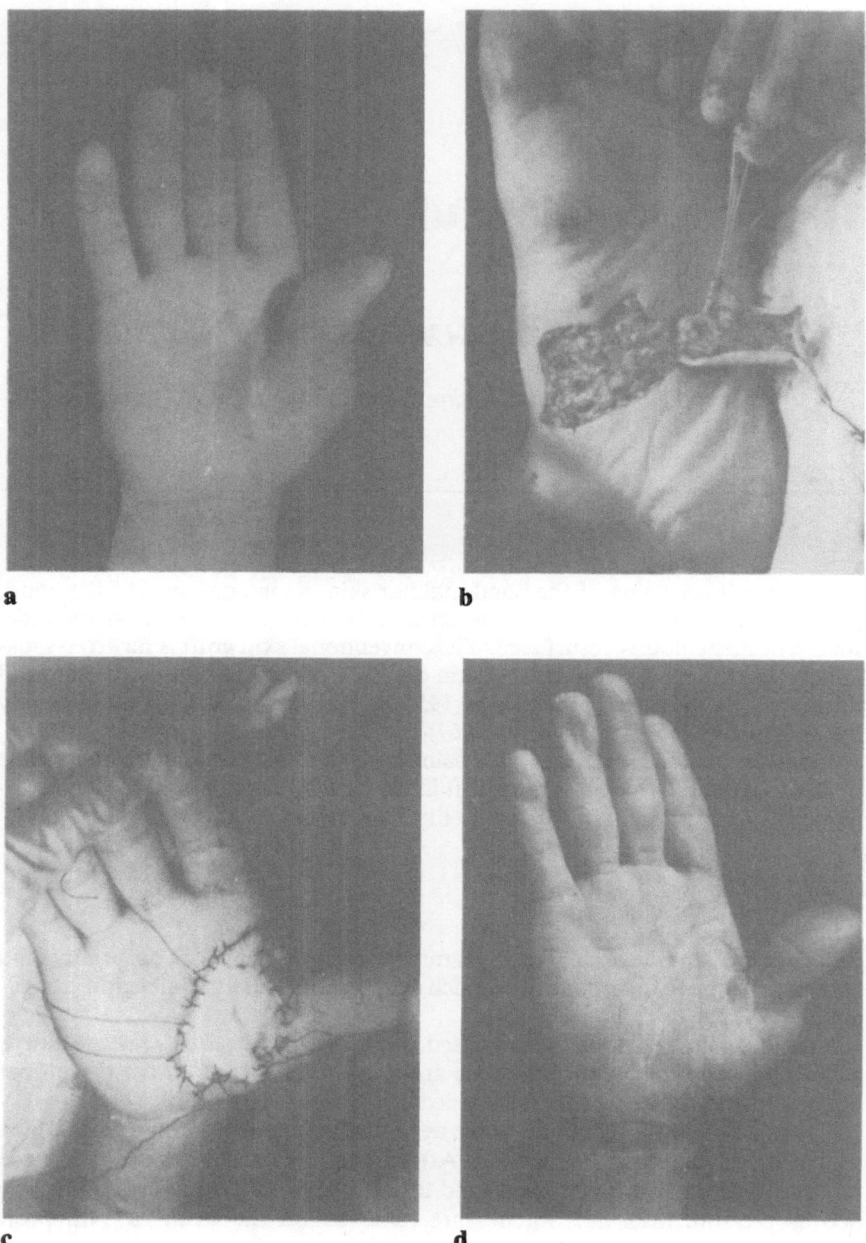

Figure 18.1 **a,** Cicatricial contracture of the right palm. **b,** Excision of the full thickness sole skin graft. **c,** Palmar skin defect covered with sole skin graft. **d,** Esthetic and functional results 26 months after operation

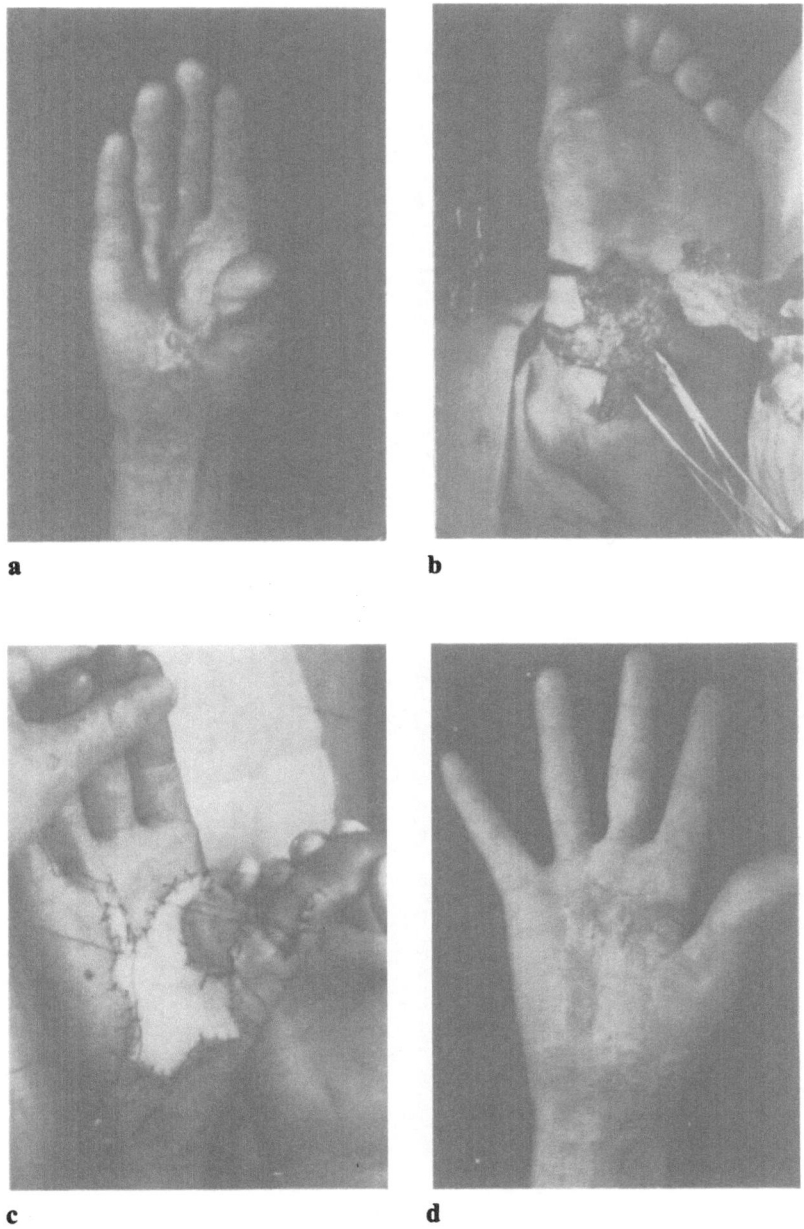

Figure 18.2 **a,** Severe cicatricial contracture of the right palm. **b,** Precise excision of the sole skin graft along the outline of the cloth pattern. **c,** The shape of the graft conforms exactly with the palmar defect. **d,** Esthetic and functional results 24 days after operation

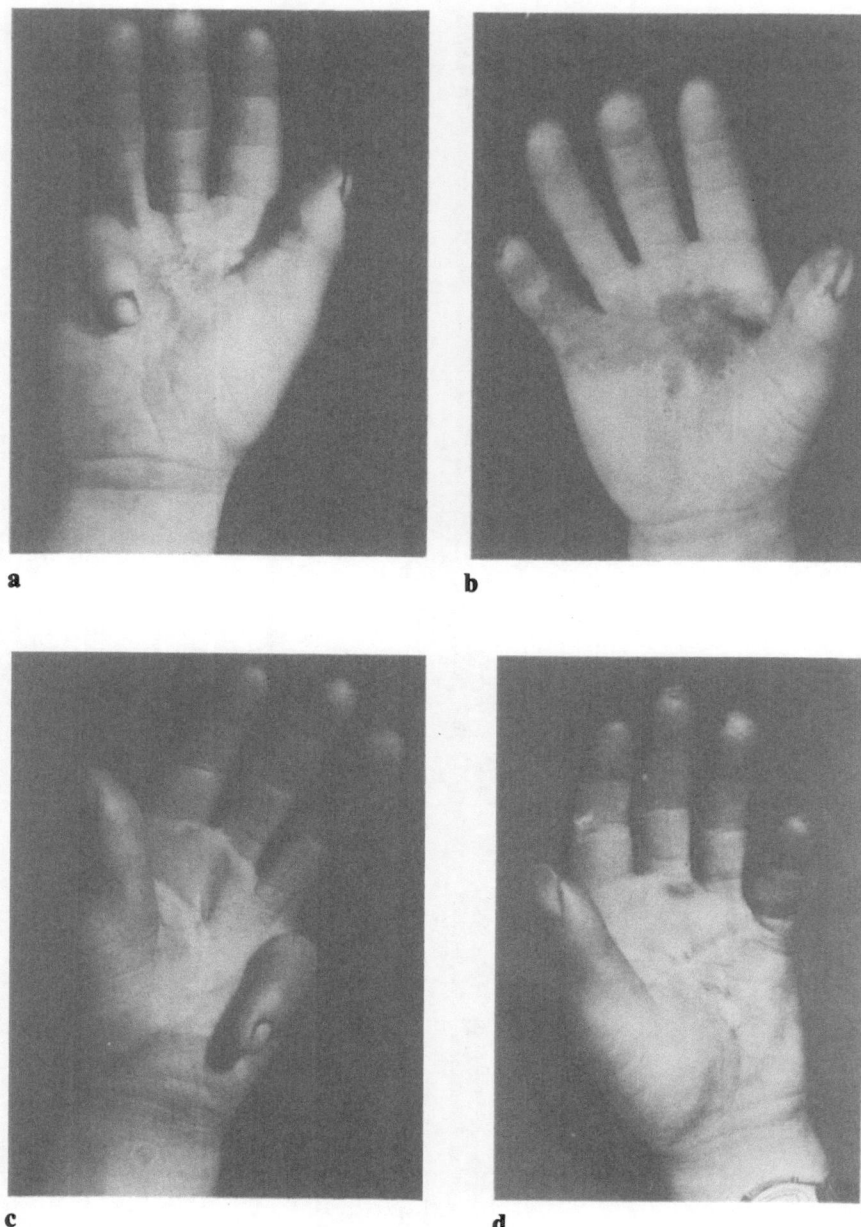

Figure 18.3   a, Right hand, before operation. **b**, Right hand palmar contracture repaired by conventional full thickness skin graft, seen 3 years after operation. **c**, Left hand, before operation. **d**, Left hand, 14 months after operation

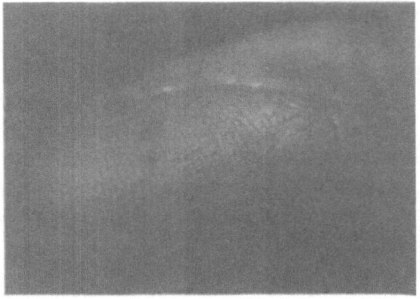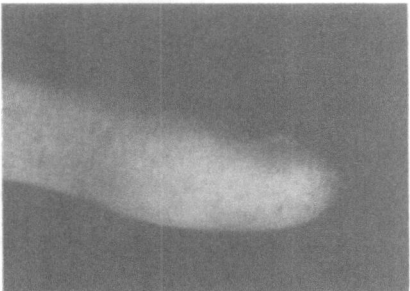

Figure 18.4 The thumb pulp, suffering from chronic radiation dermatitis, was repaired with a piece of sole skin graft, and has a new fingerprint

RESULTS

The age distribution of 13 patients (19 sites) ranges from 1.5 to 38 years. Of the 19 grafts, three were for fingertips, three for finger pulps, five for the palmar surface of the finger and the remaining eight for palmar skin defects.

In regard to the management of the wound on the donor site, split thickness skin grafts were used in 16 and direct suture in three.

Eighteen grafts took well but one was partially lost.

A follow-up study of 3–30 months was carried out on six patients. The grafts were firm and stable with good color match.

The repaired palms are capable of a great variety of complicated movements including heavy labor. The gross protective sensation and sweat function returned to the sole 4 months after operation.

DISCUSSION

Principal points for consideration are as follows.

(1) The sole of a foot consists of two different parts, the weight bearing and nonweight bearing regions. The keratic layer of the weight bearing sole skin is very thick and its function is too important for it to be used as a donor site. The skin of the nonweight bearing part, on the contrary, can be used without causing trouble when the patient walks.

(2) Generally speaking, the survival rate of a skin graft depends on its thickness; the thicker the graft, the more difficult its survival. In fact, the sole skin is not thicker than the conventional skin graft as one imagines. Microscopic measurement of the sole skin thickness revealed that the thickness of the sole dermis was equal to that of the arm skin dermis, except that the sole keratic layer is much thicker.

(3) The sole skin graft is of average thickness, but why is it far more resistant? The answer seems that its keratin layer is thicker, and its connection with

the deep tissues is very firm. For comparison, on two occasions, we tried skin grafts taken from the sole and upper arm on two hands of the same patient. Six and 16 months after operation respectively, grafts from the upper arm were rather dark, soft and fragile, but the color of the sole graft matched well with the recipient skin. The sensibility of the skin grafts taken from the upper arm is keener than that from the sole. So it seems to be the case that, for an ordinary worker, grafts taken from the conventional donor site may still be feasible, but for heavy manual workers or peasants the sole skin grafts would be more suitable.

(4) Under the microscope, we found that the epidermal basal layers of the palmar and sole skin contained many fewer pigment cells and no pigment granule could be seen, but those of the skin of the upper arm contained a lot of pigment granules and the content of pigment cells was nearly three times as much.

(5) A skin graft as large as 8×10 cm can be taken from the nonweight bearing area of the sole of a foot, so it is enough for resurfacing most palmar defects. When the palmar wound is too large to be covered, another skin graft from another site can be added at the same time.

(6) Since the sole skin graft practically does not contract after being removed, it can be cut precisely along the outline of the cloth pattern, and there is no need to cut more skin, unlike usual practice.

The sole skin graft lacks elasticity, so its form and size must fit the palmar raw surface exactly. The cloth pattern must be made as accurate as possible.

Certainly, this method has its drawbacks, such as being very detailed and complicated to perform, and the patient needs a longer stay in bed. But its good results, and noticeable improvement produced in hand functions, have encouraged us to introduce it again. And we are sure that this method is indicated at least for the manual laborers in the Northern provinces of our country whose donor feet can be protected by shoes when working.

REFERENCES

1. Webster, J. P. (1955). Skin grafts for hairless areas of the hands and feet. *Plast. Reconstr. Surg.*, **15**, 83
2. Le Worthy, G. W. (1963). Sole skin as a donor site to replace palmar skin. *Plast. Reconstr. Surg.*, **32**, 30
3. Micks, J. E. *et al.* (1967). Full-thickness sole skin grafts for resurfacing the hand. *J. Bone Jt. Surg. (Am).*, **49**, 1128

19 One-stage Surgical Treatment for Scar Contracture of Achilles Tendon following Burns and its Anatomic Basis

CHEN BI, WANG LIANG-NENG, QIU JIAN-GUANG and ZHAO DONG-SHENG

Department of Burns and Plastic Surgery, First Affiliated Hospital, The Fourth Military Medical College, Xi'an

Repair of the scar contracture of the Achilles tendon following severe burns of the lower extremities has presented a difficult problem. In the past, normal skin coverage was always required before the Achilles tendon could be lengthened. Thus the patient used to be under the heavy economic and emotional burdens of long hospitalization and multistage surgical procedures. To shorten the period of hospitalization, we designed a new method of Achilles tendon lengthening to correct the deformity in one stage, and good results have been obtained since 1976.

OPERATIVE PROCEDURE

Since 1976, in correcting this kind of deformity, we have designed a scar calcaneal tendon flap in rectangular form with a length–width ratio of about 4:1 or even 5:1. The tendon, together with the overlying scar, was incised longitudinally at its midline down to the alveolus fat tissue. On both sides of the incision, two flaps were thus designed with the pedicle of the medial one downward and that of the lateral one upward. The posterior portion of the ankle joint capsule was incised, and the Achilles tendon was lengthened and sutured side by side after the ankle joint had been corrected back to a right angle. Free skin grafts were applied to the secondary wounds. Pressure dressing and plaster of Paris casts were used to immobilize the ankle in a functional position. Four cases (altogether eight feet) were treated and the deformities were corrected with fairly good results with this procedure. Patients got out of bed 49–65 days after operation.

In these four cases, however, the flaps had been delayed in three feet prior to the tendon lengthening, and two of the medial flaps had circulatory embarrassment resulting in necrosis of about 2 cm at the distal ends; while in the five feet which did not have the 'delay' operation, three medial flaps also showed distal

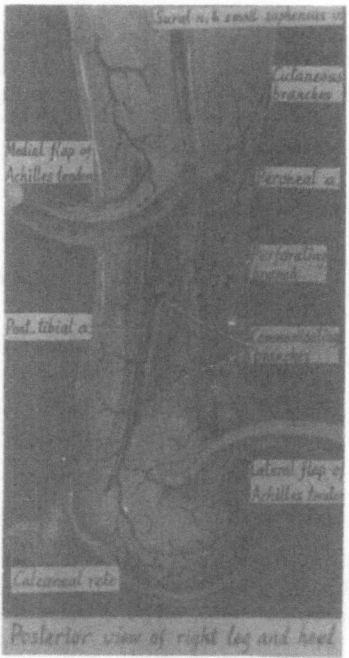

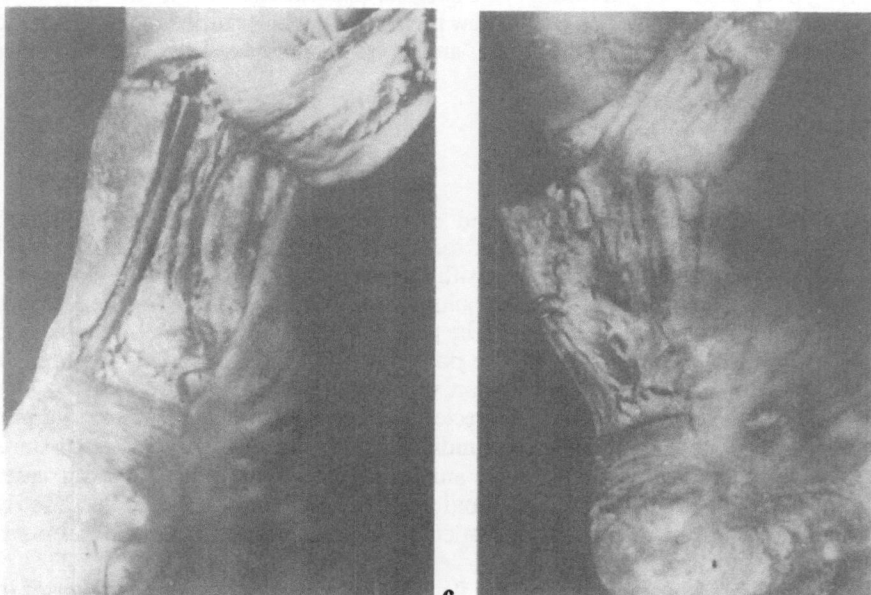

Figure 19.1   a, Vascular distribution of the lower half of the leg and calcaneus region. **b,** Medial flap and its vascular branches. **c,** Lateral flap and its vascular branches

necrosis, whereas all the eight lateral flaps, whether they were delayed or not, were in good condition without any circulatory embarrassment.

The details of skin blood supply near the Achilles tendon have been scarcely described in general anatomic textbooks[1,2]. For the investigation of the anatomic character of the flap circulation in this region, fresh cadavers were perfused with red latex in the arterial system and transparent specimens of infant and child cadavers were made. A total of seven cadavers was studied. It has been shown that the collateral circulation around the ankle is relatively abundant, since there are two or three communicating branches between the peroneal and posterior tibial arteries, and several arterial networks (calcaneus, lateral malleolar and medial malleolar networks), which are composed of the branches of the anterior tibial artery, posterior tibial artery and peroneal artery. Medial to the Achilles tendon, about 1 cm posterior to the medial border of the tibia, there are five or six branches of arteries arising from the posterior tibial artery to supply the tendon and its neighboring soft tissue. They anastomose with each other and also with the calcaneus network and medial malleolar network. The upper one or two branches are of greater caliber; they arise from the posterior tibial artery near the junction of the middle and the lower third of the leg. In the process of our operation, these main branches can be included in the medial flap when its base is slightly widened. Lateral to the tendon, five or six branches arise from the peroneal artery and supply the tendon and the skin lateral to it. These

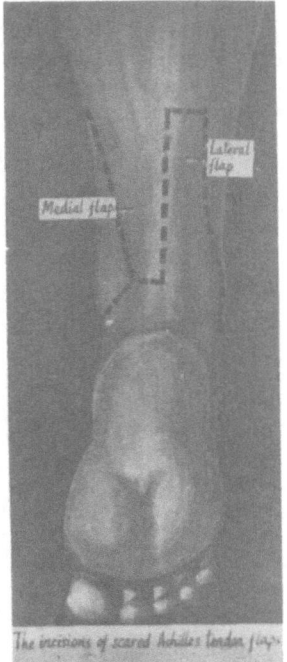

Figure 19.2 The incisions of the scarred Achilles tendon flaps

branches anastomose with each other, with the lateral malleolar and calcaneus networks and the nutrient vessel of the sural nerve (Figure 19.1) on which the branches posterosuperior to the lateral malleolar have several ascending twigs and contribute to the blood supply of the lateral flap.

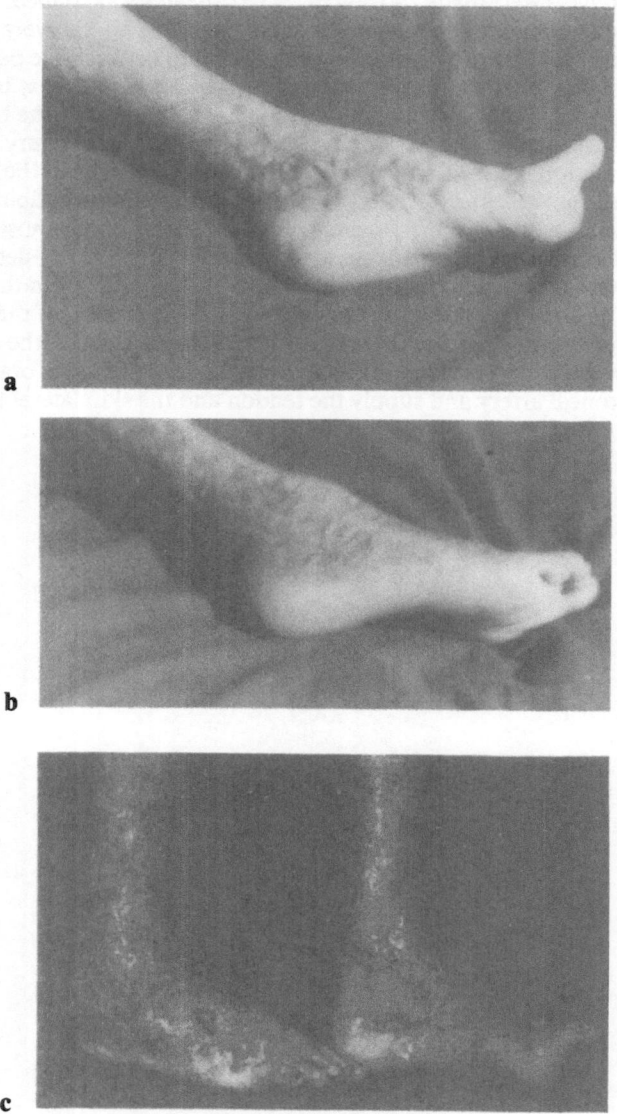

Figure 19.3 Case 1. **a,** Equinus deformity of left foot. **b,** Equinus deformity of right foot. **c,** Postoperative view of both feet

In accordance with the anatomic character of the flap circulation, the abundant collateral circulation of the medial flap, especially its distal portion, is easily damaged by ordinary incision or 'delay' operation unless the base of the flap is designed slightly wider than the distal end, as we have been doing recently. In this way, the main branches which arise from the posterior tibial artery supplying the medial flap can be preserved. Careful attention should, of course, be given to preserving the underlying vessels of the flaps and at the same time we should always keep an eye to the sural nerve during dissection. Over the past two years, five cases (seven feet) were treated by this modified technique without delaying of the flaps, and all the medial and lateral flaps healed per primam without any circulatory embarrassment. The patients got out of bed 23–55 days after operation.

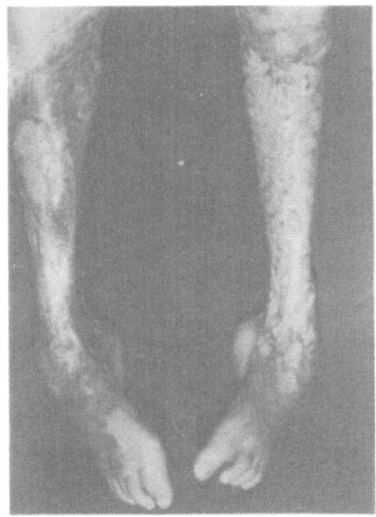

a

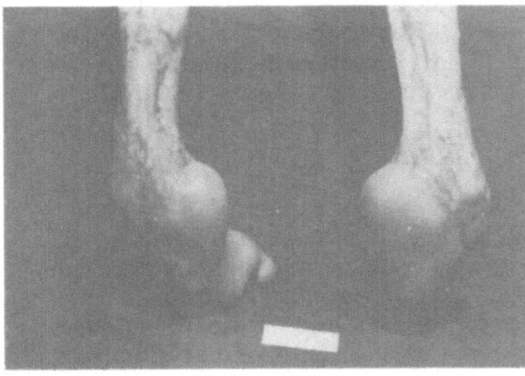

b

Figure 19.4   Case 2. Equinus deformity of both feet. **a**, Anterior view. **b**, Posterior view

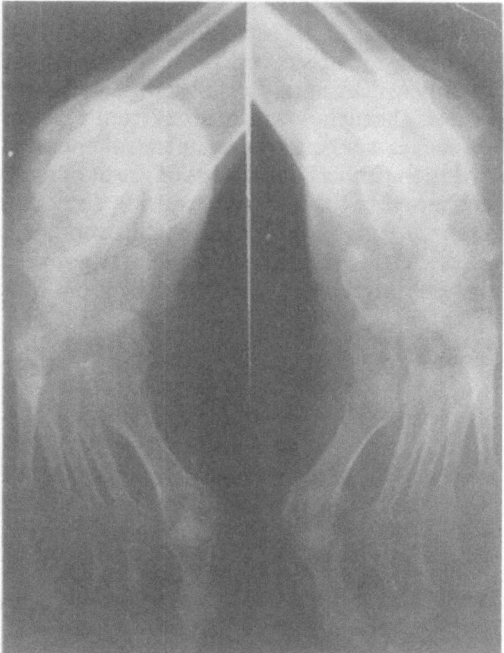

Figure 19.5   Case 2. X-ray film of both equinus feet demonstrates changes in bony structures

CASE REPORTS

Case 1

A female, 20, has a history of severe drop foot contracture after extensive burns of TBS 92% with third degree 74%. The feet or both ankle joints were corrected by lengthening the Achilles tendon and dividing the posterior capsule of the ankle joint in a one-stage operation. The wounds healed per primam. She got out of bed 25 days after operation (Figures 19.4–19.7).

Case 2

A female, 24, was admitted for severe talipes equinovarus and shortening of the Achilles tendon after severe burns of both lower extremities in 1982. The ankle joints were dropped 180° with inversion of 60° on the left side and of 30° on the right. The greater part of the triceps muscles of both sides was burned and the left Achilles tendon was almost destroyed. She had been confined to bed for 2½ years. The deformities were corrected by the modified procedure with an additional medial incision. Steinmann's pins were used to maintain the ankles in a functional position. The wounds healed per primam. She got out of bed 55 days

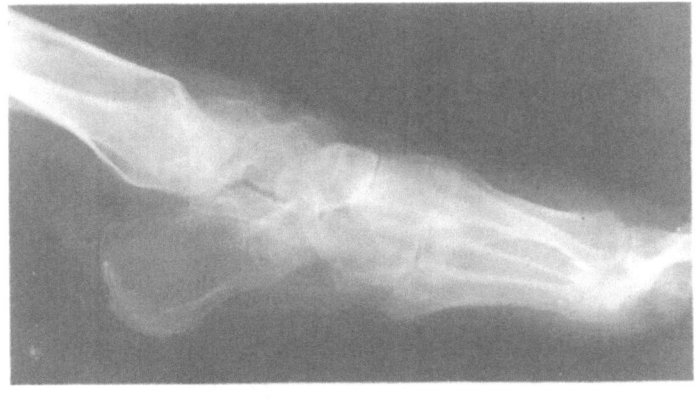

a

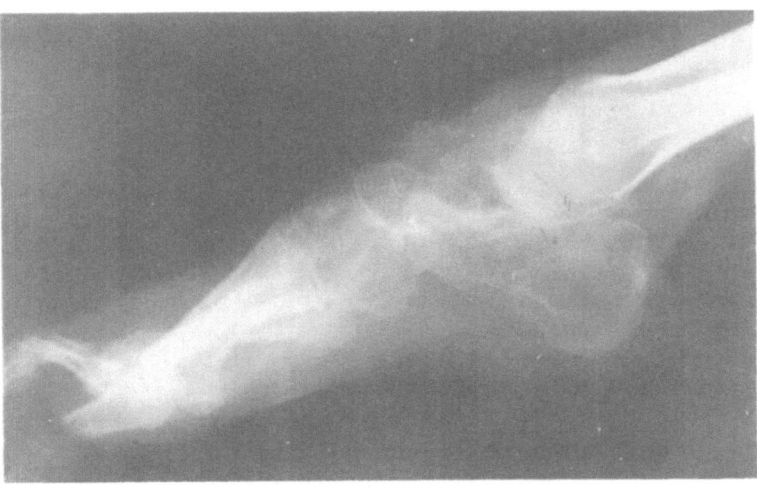

b

Figure 19.6   Case 2. **a**, X-ray film of the left foot. The tibia, fibula and metatarsals all lie in a straight line. **b**, X-ray film of the right foot

after the operation (Figures 19.2-19.7) and she enjoyed walking so much by herself (Figure 19.8).

DISCUSSION

As shown by anatomic investigation, the skin circulation on both sides of the Achilles tendon is relatively abundant. The communicating branches between the peroneal artery and posterior tibial artery, the calcaneus network, medial malleolar and lateral malleolar network all play an important role in the collateral circulation. That is the reason why the flap can survive even though its length–width ratio reaches 4:1 or 5:1. The lateral flap, though it is in reverse

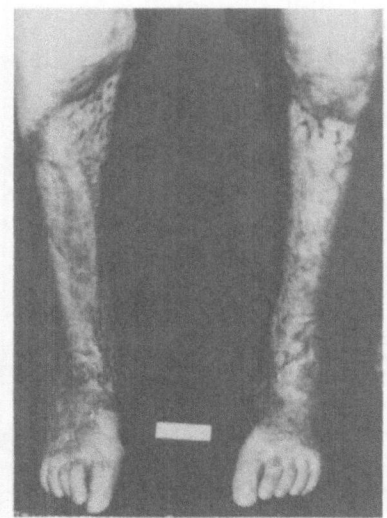

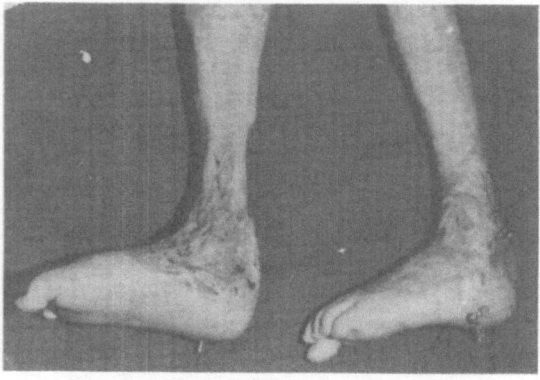

Figure 19.7   Case 2, 3 weeks after the operation. **a**, Anterior view of the feet. **b**, Posterior view

direction, always has a good blood supply, since its pedicle is supplied with abundant collateral circulation; while blood supply in the medial flap, in spite of the fact that it is in the same direction as the bloodstream, is not as good as that of the lateral one, since the small arterial networks from the surrounding area to the flap are cut off during operation. However, it can be sufficiently perfused by widening the base of the scarred Achilles tendon flap, thus the main branches arising from the posterior tibial artery are included in this medial flap.

In view of our clinical findings and anatomic investigation, we consider that the delaying of the flap is not necessary as it does not enhance its blood supply very much in this situation. The sural nerve which lies alongside the small

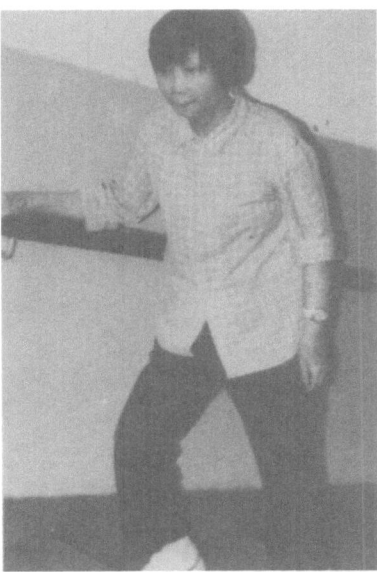

Figure 19.8   Case 2. The patient's walking gait 70 days after operation

saphenous vein should be preserved (assuming it had not been destroyed by burns). Neurolysis should be done of the posterior portion of the ankle joint capsule which often exists under this condition, so that it should be incised during the course of correcting the deformity by lengthening the Achilles tendon.

REFERENCES

1. Hollinshead, W. H. (1969). *Anatomy for Surgeons*. Vol. III, 2nd Edn., pp. 760–1, 805–8. (New York: Harper & Row)
2. Warwick, R. and Williams, P. L. (eds.) (1973) *Gray's Anatomy*. 35th Edn., pp. 681–4. (London: Longman)

20 Microvascular Transplantation of Prefabricated Free Thigh Flap

SHEN TZU-YAO

Department of Burns and Plastic Surgery, Beijing Ji Shui Tan Hospital, Beijing Institute of Traumatology & Orthopedics

In my previous paper entitled 'Vascular implantation into skin flap'[1], it was experimentally shown that a 'random-pattern' skin flap, with a transposed vascular bundle or an artery alone buried underneath, could be transformed to a 'secondary axial-pattern' skin flap (unpublished findings). The establishment of vascular communications between the flap and implanted vessels is constant after a period of time. This type of secondary, or prefabricated, axial-pattern skin flap can be successfully used in island transposition or microvascular transfer. In the light of this rationale, a prefabricated free thigh flap was designed and put into practice in 1981.

CASE REPORT

A 30-year-old male worker presented with a severe neck contracture and lip eversion following an extensive burn of 80% of TBSA and third degree 30% (Figure 20.1). Because of the extensive cutaneous scarring on his body surface, no conventional donor area was available for free flap transfer. A design of prefabricated axial-pattern skin flap on the relatively healthy area on his right thigh was proposed.

Preoperative markings

The upper anteriomedial aspect of the right thigh was used as a prefabricated axial-pattern skin flap with the long saphenous vein included in its medial portion. Two lines were drawn from the femoral artery pulsation to mark the imaginary courses of the transverse and descending branches of the lateral circumflex femoral artery (Figure 20.2).

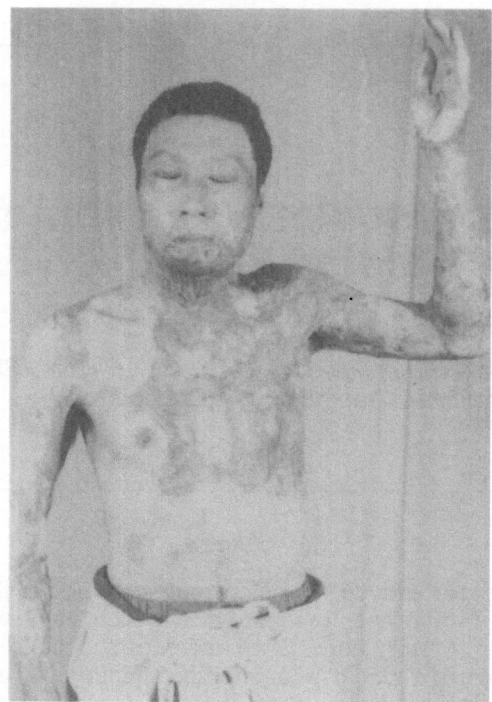

Figure 20.1   Severe neck contracture and lower lip eversion following extensive burn

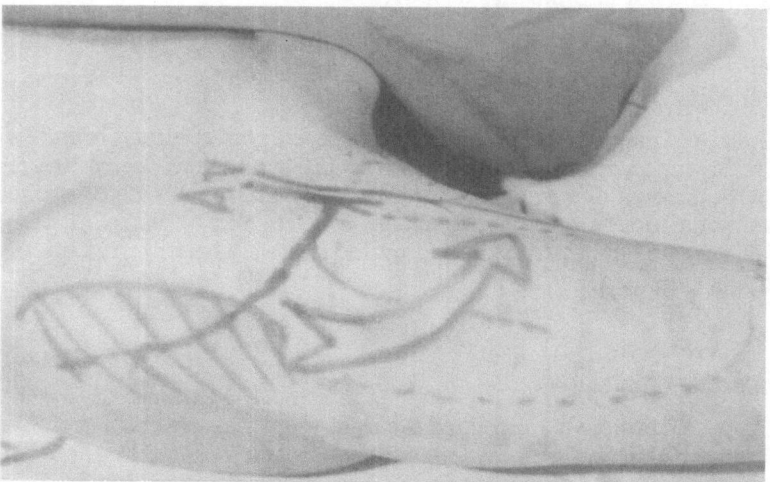

Figure 20.2   Right thigh donor site with dermographic drawing of the imaginary courses of the transverse and descending branches of the lateral circumflex femoral artery

First-stage operation

Under epidural anesthesia with the patient in a supine position, a curve incision was made from 10 cm below the anterior superior iliac spine to the anterolateral midthigh, and another curve incision made from the same point extending to the inguinal ligament to the femoral artery pulsation. A skin flap was raised to expose the upper portion of the quadriceps femoris and sartorius muscles. Having elevated the rectus femoris muscle and retracted medially the vastus intermedius muscle, the lateral circumflex femoral artery was isolated from its origin – the profunda femoris artery; its bifurcating branches – the transverse and descending branches, the latter travelling upside down in the space between the vastus lateralis and the vastus intermedius – were also located (Figure 20.3). The distal end of the vascular bundle was ligated and severed as far as possible just before it penetrated into the muscle belly. In order to increase the mobility of the descending branch, the transverse branch and other muscular rami were ligated and severed. The planned vessel was retrogradely isolated up to the bifurcation. Care should be taken not to jeopardize the motor nerve of the femoral nerve which lies along the vessels. Thus a vascular bundle of 14 cm long with its satellite vein was completely isolated for transposition and implantation purposes. The free bundle was pulled out of the superior border of the sartorius where the femoral artery met. A 5 cm segment of the distal bundle was buried in the skin flap through an incision made on its raw surface where its distal end was ligated and anchored to the subdermal plane (Figure 20.4). The flap was then sutured back into its original place. Postoperative Doppler monitoring of the buried artery revealed excellent pulsative 'swoosh'.

Second-stage operation

After a 5-week interval, through an incision made on the medial side to the femoral artery, the implanted artery was first dissected out and traced

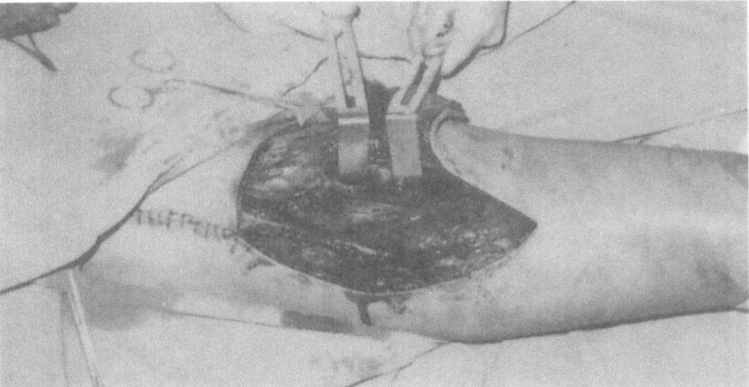

Figure 20.3 Rectus femoris muscle elevated and vascus intermedius retracted medially to expose the lateral circumflex femoral artery

proximally to its origin. The patency of the buried artery was evidenced by its naked-eye pulsation. The planned flap, sized 16×26 cm, was re-elevated with the transplanted branch of the lateral circumflex femoral artery and the long

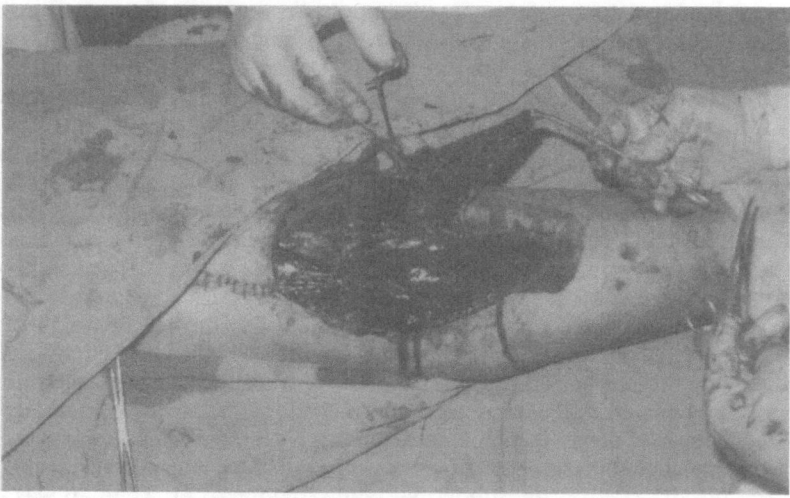

Figure 20.4 The descending branch of the lateral circumflex femoral artery was transposed and implanted into the thigh skin flap

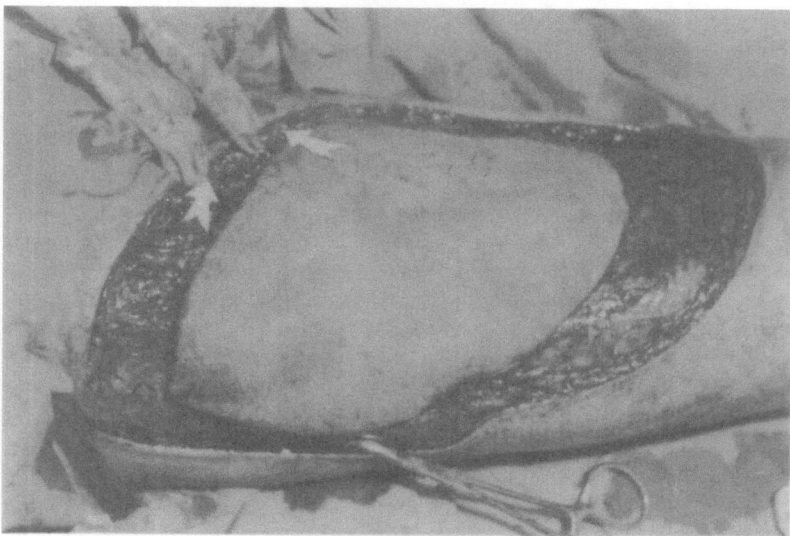

Figure 20.5 Five weeks after the first operation, the flap is raised. Medial arrow indicates the implanted arterial pedicle; lateral arrow indicates the greater saphenous vein

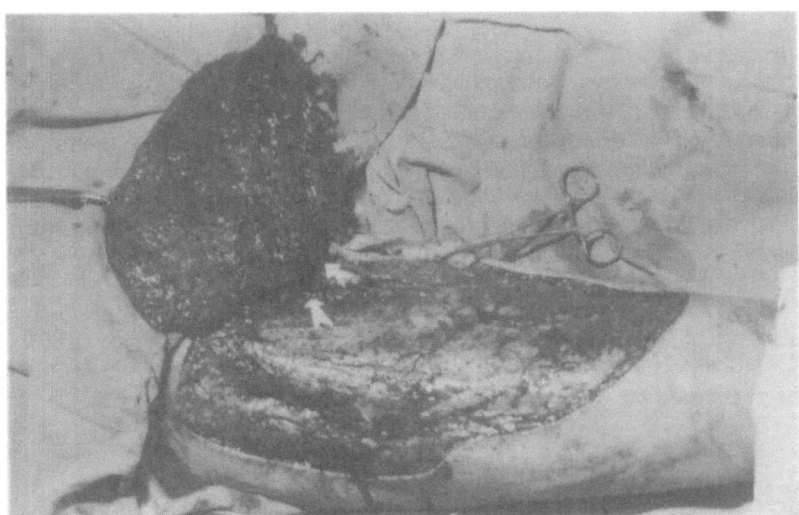

Figure 20.6 The prefabricated flap is completely mobilized with its vascular pedicle still attached

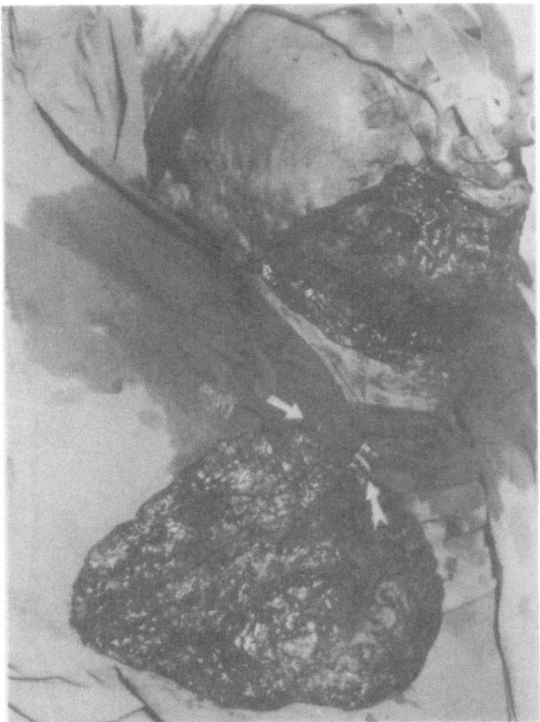

Figure 20.7 The skin flap is ready for transfer to the neck region

saphenous vein as the vascular pedicles. Pink and brisk bleeding on the cut edges of the skin flap was seen with rapid capillary refilling. After the recipient bed was prepared, the flap was completely isolated with detaching vascular pedicles (Figure 20.5). The donor long saphenous vein and a subcutaneous vein, 5 mm and 2.5 mm in diameter respectively, were anastomosed in end-to-end fashion to the external jugular and superficial facial veins, 5 mm and 3 mm in diameter respectively. The former implanted artery, 3 mm in diameter, was sutured in end-to-end fashion to the superficial facial artery of the recipient with 9/0 monofilament nylon (Figures 20.6–20.8).

The flap survived uneventfully after the reestablishment of the blood circulation with excellent color match and satisfactory contour (Figure 20.9). The donor site defect was resurfaced with a split thickness skin graft. No functional embarrassment was noted on the donor limb afterwards.

DISCUSSION

The advantages of this technique are evident: (1) anatomic constancy of the sufficiently large vascular bundle permitting easy dissection, the vascular calibers

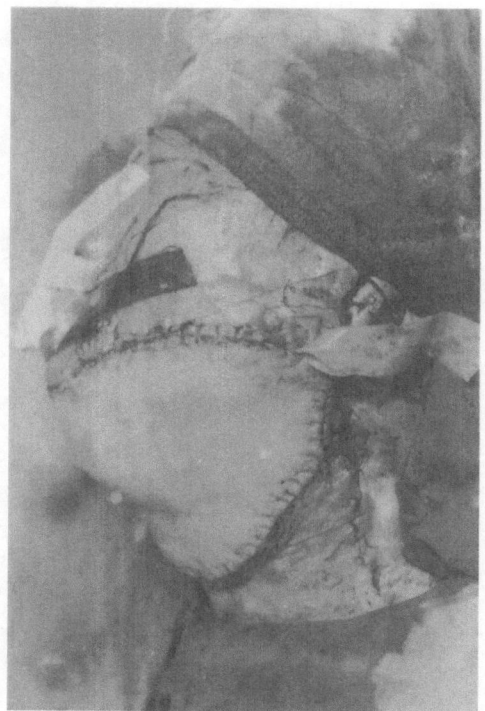

Figure 20.8   View immediately after the free prefabricated flap transplantation

yielding a high patency rate after anastomosis, (2) a skin flap of the best quality in dimension, thickness and color match and (3) unobtrusive donor site without functional sequelae, quite acceptable to the patient. Among the flaps currently used, no flap of such quality has ever been found. Its clinical use merits consideration.

The skin flap has a noticeable cutaneous nerve branch available for skin flap reinnervation. In this case, the flap had not necessarily been reinnervated.

The feasibility of transforming a 'random-pattern' skin flap into an 'axial-pattern' by means of transplanting a vascular bundle and the rapidity of arborization budding into the recipient skin flap are beyond one's imagination. The prefabricated axial-pattern skin flap on rabbits could be safely transferred as early as 8 days after vascular implantation. In this case, we did not perform the second-stage operation until 5 weeks later, for various reasons. Depending on the circulatory status of the flap during operation, it seems that the interval between two operations could be shortened, say, to 3 or 4 weeks. In spite of the two-stage operations, we believe this kind of secondary axial-pattern skin flap has its particular indication in those patients who have no conventional free flap donor area for microvascular transfer.

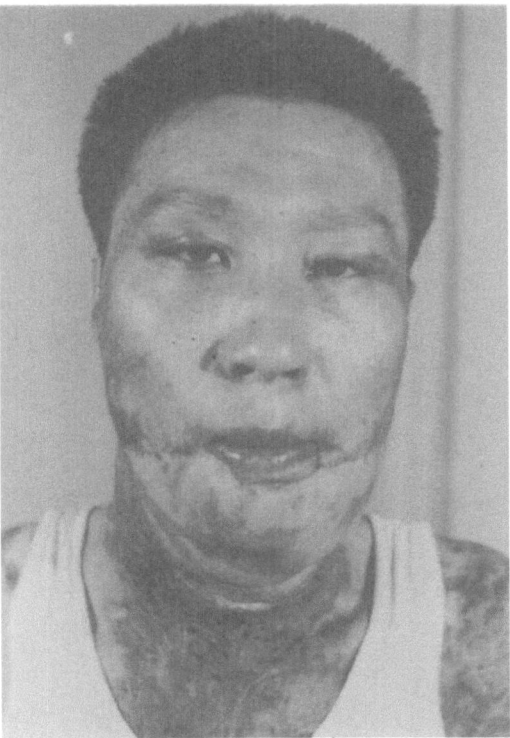

Figure 20.9   Complete survival of the flap 1 year after operation

SUMMARY

A 'random-pattern' skin flap can be transformed into an 'axial-pattern' by means of vascular implantation. The descending branch of the lateral circumflex femoral artery was used to prefabricate the axial thigh flap. After a 5-week interval, the prefabricated or secondary free flap was successfully transferred to the neck with microvascular anastomosis.

REFERENCE

1. Shen Tzu-yao (1981). Vascular implantation into skin flap. Experimental study and clinical application: A preliminary report. *Plast. Reconstr. Surg.*, **68**, 404

21 Surgical Treatment of Lymphedema of the Extremities (A Study on Lymphaticovenous Anastomosis in Comparison with the Method of Excision and Skin Graft)

YU GUO-ZHONG, ZHU JIA-KAI, PANG SHUI-FA and LIU JUN-CHI

Division of Microsurgery, First Affiliated Hospital, Zhongshan Medical College

Lymphedema of the extremity is a chronic and obstinate disease which causes much distress to the patient. In the past 50 years various methods of surgical treatment have been tried, but none of them is satisfactory. However, the method of excising diseased tissues and skin graft has still been widely accepted. Under the influence of the development of microsurgery in recent years, lymphaticovenous anastomosis (LVA) in an attempt to bypass lymphatic blockage has been employed. This operation seems to be a more rational method for the reestablishment of lymphatic drainage.[1]

CLINICAL MATERIALS

Since 1962, excision of pathologic tissues and skin graft for the treatment of limb lymphedema has been practised in our hospital in a number of cases. Of these, 18 had complete records available for clinical analysis. Thirteen were males and five females. The total number of limbs involved was 21. In all cases the disease was in the lower extremity with marked thickening and swelling of the skin and subcutaneous tissues. After the operation, there was improvement in all, but three of them developed postoperatively ulcers in the dorsum of the foot or ankle which required adjunctive reoperation. Another patient who underwent the same operation at another hospital and who developed recurrent lymphedema was submitted to reoperation at our clinic.

Since May 1979, 17 cases (18 limbs) had been selected for LVA. Four were males and 13 females. The youngest patient was 13 years and the oldest 58 years of age. The lower limb was involved in 14 cases and the upper limb in three. They have been followed-up for 6–22 months. Among the seven cases of lymphedema secondary to irradiation, radical mastectomy or filariasis, it was definitely relieved in six (86%). There were only three cases (30%) showing improvement among the remaining ten cases of primary lymphedema. Five patients have had frequent exacerbations of lymphangitis, including one whose lymphedema was not relieved by LVA. Their postoperative lymphangitis attacks were remarkably lessened.

SURGICAL TECHNIQUE

Since the limb lymphatic trunks lie along both sides of the major superficial veins (long saphenous in the lower limb and basilic as well as cephalic veins in the upper extremity), the surgical approach to the lymphatic trunks should be made through skin incisions in the vicinity of these superficial veins. In the case of leg LVA, skin incisions should be placed in the upper and lower fourth of the anteromedial aspect of the leg; in the thigh lymphedema, incisions are put on its proximal and distal parts. An alternative is to make the incision near the site of obstruction based on the lymphangiography. The same principle is applied to the choice of skin incisions on the upper limbs. If it is planned to make four incisions on one limb, it is desirable to make two incisions at one time. For direct visualization of the lymph vessels, Evans' blue solution (10 mg/2 ml in 4 ml of 1% procaine) must be injected beforehand. Injections at several intradermal points are given along a horizontal line 6–10 cm below the planned site of incision. Light massage is then applied to facilitate the flow of stained lymphatic fluid. A transverse incision 6–9 cm long is subsequently made. Traction sutures are inserted into the wound edges on both sides to keep the wound well exposed. Using a small curved hemostat, globule fat tissues are carefully cleared away while searching for venules and lymphatic vessels. At this moment the operating microscope is of great help. Due attention should be paid to the differentiation of venules, small nerves, fibrous bands, lymph vessels and arterioles, so as to avoid the mistake of anastomosis afterwards. Venules and lymph vessels should be well protected from injury, the fibrous bands cut and cleared away, and small nerves preserved or severed according to whether they hinder the operative exposure. Arterioles are rarely seen in the field. They may exist, in which case they may be identified by observing their pulsation.

It must be realized that the subcutaneous venules lie superficially, but the lymph vessels suitable for anastomosis are situated in the deep layer of the wound. Be sure not to sacrifice or to injure the superficial veins while searching for the lymph vessels. After the venules and lymph vessels have been found, they must be carefully isolated under a surgical microscope. The venule is tied, a microsurgical clamp applied proximally, and the venule is then cut between the ligature and clamp. The proximal end of the cut venule is irrigated with heparin in normal saline. The distal end of the vessel is then anastomosed to the proximal end of the venule with four to six interrupted sutures of 11/0 nylon and on an atraumatic needle. After anastomosis the clamp is released and finger pressure is applied to facilitate the lymphatic flow. If the bluish-stained lymph can easily be seen to pass through the site of anastomosis, it indicates that the opening is adequately patent. When many venules and lymphatics are found, LVAs have to be made as many as possible for better bypass of the lymphatic blockage. Finally, the wound is thoroughly irrigated and closed with special care for the underlying LVAs.

DISCUSSION

Excision of diseased tissues and skin graft

Radical excision of pathologic tissues followed by skin graft, although being an operation which is purely esthetic rather than therapeutic (lymphatic obstruction relief), does correct elephantoid limb to a quasinormal appearance. However, being traumatic and hemorrhagic (average blood loss of 600 ml) with scarring graft skin liable to ulcer formation, this operation is now only reserved for those of the advanced cases of elephantiasis with sclero-crescentic skin. For those with a mild degree of lymphedema, and limb skin not much thickened, the results of such a radical operation are disappointing to most plastic surgeons.[2]

LVA is designed to establish a new lymphatic pathway for the obstructed lymph flow and thus to relieve the lymphedema. The operation is less traumatic and blood transfusion is seldom necessary. There is no postoperative skin problem. It is indicated for mild limb lymphedema, the skin of which is still mobile and resilient. The operation is quite effective in reducing the limb swelling, the postoperative lymphangitis becomes less frequent and the disease is controlled if not eradicated. However, the LVA is less effective in patients with primary lymphedema which is most probably due to lymphatic maldevelopment or agenesis. In case of LVA failure, excision of the diseased tissues followed by skin graft is an alternative.

In summary, as regards the choice of operative procedures, the following points may be considered.

(1) Early mild secondary lymphedema is best treated by LVA especially for those patients with frequent attacks of lymphangitis.

(2) In relatively severe secondary lymphedema with the involved limb elephantiasis, the skin being thickened but not very coarse, LVA may be considered. In case of LVA failure, alternative surgical excision procedure may still be carried out.

(3) In very severe lymphedema with greatly swollen extremities and coarse skin, excision of the diseased tissues and skin graft should be considered.

(4) In our series of patients, primary lymphedema of uncertain etiology responded poorly to LVA. Therefore, its indication should be seriously questioned.

Some keypoints to LVA

Lack of sufficient venules for LVAs

This is rather a technical error. An inexperienced surgeon is too anxious to approach lymph vessels without due attention to the superficial layer in such a way that many venules are accidentally destroyed. The lymph vessels of appropriate size lie deeper in the incision. If the superficial venules hinder their exposure, they may be cut distally, their ends flushed with heparin solution and well protected for anastomosis. In case there is only one superficial venule available, it may be traced down to find out its bifurcation and utilize the branches to be anastomosed with two lymph vessels[3].

Insufficient number of lymph vessels

In such a case, the vessel should be carefully inspected to see if the size is distinctly increased and if there is a reversed lymph flow. If these developments have actually happened, both the distal and proximal cut ends may be anastomosed to the proximal ends of two venules.

Retraction of the cut end of lymphatic vessels

Sometimes this happens and makes it difficult to find its opening for anastomosis. To avoid this, a thin layer of perilymphatic fat should be left intact during dissection. Furthermore, the wall of the lymph vessel may be cut to half circumference; stitches are inserted through the edges of the lymphatic vessel and venule first and the same stitches are put for another half circumference.

Proper techniques in the method of excision and skin graft

The chance of recurrent lymphedema and development of ulcers at the ankle and the dorsum of foot are rather great. To avoid these, the surgeon should do the following: (1) widely excise the diseased tissue, (2) carefully stop the bleeding, (3) thick split or full thickness skin graft[4] and (4) full contact to the recipient area.

SUMMARY

In conclusion, although LVA is a newly developed technique and sounds more rational, yet it cannot replace the old method of excision and skin graft. Certainly, many problems are involved in the method of LVA. However, there is great hope of having them solved by further studies on the pathophysiology of the lymph vessels as well as the microsurgical techniques so as to obtain better results.

REFERENCES

1. O'Brien, B. M. *et al.* (1977). Microlymphatic-venous anastomosis for obstructive lymphedema *Plast. Reconstr. Surg.*, **60**, 197

2. Chang Ti-sheng *et al.* (1958). The surgical treatment of lymphedema of the lower extremities: A preliminary report. *Chinese J. Surg.*, **6,** 139
3. Zhu Jia-kai *et al.* (1980). Lymphedema of the limbs treated by lymphaticovenous anastomosis. *Chinese J. Surg.*, **18,** 416
4. Miller, T. A. (1980). Charles procedure for lymphedema: A warning. *Am. J. Surg.*, **139,** 290

22 Free Omentum Transplantation – Report of 30 Cases

JIANG SHU-YING, YING RU-QIN, SONG, WEN-SHEN, QIAN JUN-SHAN and WANG RUI-LONG
Department of Plastic Surgery, 202 Hospital of the PLA

YANG GUO-FAN, CHEN BAO-JU, GAO YU-ZHI and LIU XIAO-YAN
Department of Plastic Surgery, General Hospital of Shenyang Military Arrondissement

Being rich in vascularization, resistant to infection, and having great capacity for absorbing and repairing, omentum has been used for many years in efforts to repair tissue defects of organs inside or outside of the abdominal cavity, especially for the enhancement of blood supply of ischemic tissues. The introduction of microsurgery has enlarged the scope of omentum transplantation. Since 1978, 30 cases of free omentum transplantation have been done by us, and we report the results here.

CLINICAL DATA

Among the 30 cases (24 male, and their ages ranging from 16 to 35 years) nine were of Buerger's disease; seven hemifacial atrophy; one cerebral artery stenosis; three postburn scalp defect; three postburn clawhand; one chronic leg ulcer; two traumatic leg soft tissue defect; one degloving injury of the hand; one chronic leg osteomyelitis; one postburn soft tissue defect of the jaw and neck; and one case of ischemic necrotic contracture of the forearm. Total omentum transplantations were done in 15 patients and partial in the other 15. No abdominal complications were observed during a follow-up study of 1–3.6 years. End-to-side microvascular arterial anastomoses were done in eight cases of Buerger's disease, and end-to-end in another 22 cases. All venous anastomoses were done in end-to-end fashion. Vascular anastomoses were done under the microscope in 12 cases.

SURGICAL TECHNIQUE

Under general or epidural anesthesia, the operation was carried out by two surgical teams.

Preparation of the omentum

Laparotomy was done through an upper midline abdominal incision. The vasculature and thickness of the omentum and the extent of the recipient area determined the size of the omentum to be removed (total or partial omentectomy). The gastroepiploic vascular arch was freed by dividing the right and left gastroepiploic vessels along the greater curvature of the stomach, and the omentum freed from the transverse colon. For the convenience of vascular anastomosis, the left gastroepiploic vessels were severed deep to the junction of the gastroduodenal artery, as the caliber of the vessels was greater there. In cases of Buerger's disease, the gastroepiploic artery was cut near its opening to the gastroduodenal artery, and a portion of the gastroduodenal arterial wall was included to form a dish-shaped cut end where the anastomotic lumen is fairly enlarged. The omentum was then immersed in a solution containing heparin and lidocaine. The abdomen was closed in layers.

Preparation of the recipient site

In cases of Buerger's disease, or hemifacial atrophy, the recipient area should be explored first to assure the patency of the recipient vessels before laparotomy. The recipient vessels of choice are arteria (a.) and vena (v.) temporalis superficialis, a. facialis, v. facialis anterior, a. thyroidea superior and v. jugularis externa in the scalpofacial region; a. radialis and v. cephalica in the upper extremities and a. femoralis and v. saphena magna, a. tibialis anterior, a. tibialis posterior and its accompanying branches in the lower extremities. In postburn clawhand, release of contracture by complete scar excision is mandatory. In Bell's palsy, a subcutaneous 'pocket' is to be created in the atrophic side. In Buerger's disease, a tunnel under the deep fascia of the leg is created to permit free passage of the omentum flap. In unilateral cerebrovascular stenosis, a retro-auricular subcutaneous tunnel should be made for the passage of the omentum. Adequate debridement of the fresh or chronic wounds is indispensable.

Free omentum transplantation

Reestablishment of circulation of the omentum was completed by venous anastomosis prior to arterial. In patients with Buerger's disease, the omentum could be lengthened along the course of the blood vessels of the flap. In hemifacial atrophy, the omentum should be securely suspended in the 'pocket'. In cerebrovascular stenosis, the omentum was to be attached to the arachnoid membrane via the subcutaneous tunnel. In case of coexistent skin defect, after tamponade of the defect by vascularized omentum, a split thickness skin graft was put on top of it.

RESULTS

All omentum flaps survived. Satisfactory results were obtained in 29 cases, i.e.

all except one. Detailed results are as follows.

(1) In eight of the patients with Buerger's disease, the results were encouraging. Pain at rest and intermittent claudication disappeared. Skin temperature and colour improved and toe ulcers healed. In the one case regarded as failure, the pain at rest recurred after a 3-month subsidence. Leg amputation became obligatory owing to the superinfection of the ischemic necrosis.

(2) In seven patients with hemifacial atrophy, postoperative esthetic appearance was satisfactory.

(3) In three patients with postburn scalp defect, operative results were good. In particular, in one of them, in addition to repair of the scalp defect, an ethmoid sinus fistula was surgically closed, followed by an immediate total nose reconstruction.

(4) Lower leg lesions, including chronic ulcer, post-traumatic soft tissue defect and chronic osteomyelitis, were satisfactorily repaired in four patients. In these cases, the recipient vessels were often buried deep in the scar tissues and thus a longer donor vascular pedicle was necessary for the success of flap transplantation. The omentum flap has the advantage of providing a longer vascular pedicle.

(5) In one patient with a total degloving injury of the hand, the whole hand was wrapped with the omentum which was then overgrafted with a piece of split thickness skin graft. During operation, the avulsed fifth fingertip was transplanted to the stump of the amputated thumb, the avulsed ring finger was reconstructed and finally the thumb and index, middle and ring fingers were all wrapped with the omentum flap covered with a piece of split skin graft. The transplanted omentum and skin graft on the hand, as well as the fingers, all survived. Though the omentum flap and skin graft on the index, middle and ring fingers survived, however, the distal digital segments of these three fingers were amputated because of infection of the DIP joints. The function of the hand was partially restored. Though being a solitary case treated by this method, the functional result achieved is far superior to that achieved by the conventional method.

(6) In three patients with postburn clawhand, postoperative functional results were significantly improved, but MP joint contracture and tendon adhesions need to be tackled further.

(7) In each of the three patients with traumatic complex soft tissue defect comprising one case of scalp-facial defect, one of forearm defect and one of maxillocervical defect, double (omentum and forearm skin flap) flap transfer was successfully carried out in a one stage operation.

(8) A patient with unilateral cerebrovascular stenosis suffered from hemiplegia for 4 years. Three months after omentum transplantation, the anesthesia on the hemiplegic extremities disappeared, terminal blood circulation improved and flexion deformity of the right hand was alleviated. But no further improvement was noted even 1 year after operation.

DISCUSSION

In the light of our experience in 30 patients, free omentum transplantation may be employed in the following five conditions.

Filling up depression deformity

Being soft, elastic and plastic, the omentum is esthetically superior to other tissues in achieving good morphology. In cases of bone defect such as seen in chronic oesteomyelitis, free omentum transplantation improves the vascularization of the ischemic bone significantly.

Enhancement of blood circulation to recipient site

In Buerger's disease, the circulation of the lower extremity can be improved considerably by omental graft. This method is superior to the pedicle omentum flap in that it can be extended as far as the dorsum of the foot.

Providing rich vascularized tissue bed for split skin grafts

The vascular omentum covered by split skin graft constitutes an ideal composite skin flap of the best quality. It is far better than the split thickness skin graft in elasticity, plasticity and friction resistance. For example, in a case of chronic leg ulcer of 17 years' duration, after a mere split skin graft, the ulcer healed temporarily only to break down many times. The patient was finally admitted to our hospital with two big leg ulcers. After debridement, a 26×20 cm^2 wound was created with a poorly vascularized bed, obviously inadequate for a split thickness skin graft. A vascularized omentum graft covered above by a skin graft was therefore adopted. The vascularization of the leg was improved after healing. In a patient with a big scalp defect, use of omentum covered above by a skin graft achieved a smooth contour of the reconstructed scalp with no recurrence of ulcer.

Providing well-vascularized tissue cover for exposed tendons, bones and joints

In degloving injury of the hand, or in clawhand, the tendons, ligaments, bones and joints were usually involved and a split skin graft could not take. In this case, the vascularized omentum can be utilized to wrap around the exposed joints and ligaments and thus provide an adequate vascular bed for the skin graft.

Vascularized omentum as interpositional flap in double flap transplantation

The gastroepiploic arch of the omentum can be anastomosed on both ends to permit the transplantation of a double flap in this series, i.e., the omentum was transplanted by anastomosing one end of the gastroepiploic arch to the recipients to be anastomosed with the vessels of a skin flap. This makes possible the repair of extensive soft tissue loss in a one-stage operation. In one case reported here with multiple craniofacial injury deformity, after debridement, a $28 \times 12 \, cm^2$ fresh wound was created with exposure of the cranium. The omentum transplantation was carried out by anastomosing the right gastro-epiploic vessels to the left superficial temporal vessels and a split skin graft was put onto the omentum. The ethmoid fistula was repaired with a piece of omentum. The radial artery and the cephalic vein of the forearm flap were anastomosed to the left gastroepiploic vessels of the transplanted omentum, and total nose reconstruction by forearm flap was simultaneously performed. The results of reconstruction in a one-stage operation on multiple deformities were excellent.

REFERENCES

1. Mclean, D. H. and Buncke, H. J. Jr. (1972). Autotransplant of omentum to a large scalp defect with microsurgical revascularization. *Plast. Reconstr. Surg.,* **49**, 268
2. O'Brien, B. McC. (1977). *Microvascular Reconstructive Surgery,* pp. 235–6. (Edinburgh: Livingstone)
3. Nishimura, A. (1979). Omentum transplantation in Buerger's disease. *Operation,* **33**, 297

23 Homologous Vascularized Ovary Transplantation: A Case Report

ZHU JIA-KAI, YU GUO-ZHONG and LIU JUN-CHI
Division of Microsurgery
HUANG CHENG-DA
Division of Orthopedics
ZHANG ZHI-YING, FANG YUE-XING and ZHUANG GUANG-LUN
Department of Obstetrics and Gynecology, The First Affiliated Hospital, Zhongshan Medical College, Canton

Bilateral oophorectomies, an integral part of en bloc excision of malignant ovarian tumor, acceptable to elderly women, can hardly be tolerated by young women for whom prolonged estrogen substitution therapy is necessary to overcome endocrine disturbance. Subcutaneous ovary allograft was advocated by some, but ischemia and rejection of the transplant made the positive result only temporary. Following the introduction of microsurgery, vascularized autograft of the fallopian tube and ovary succeeded in animal experiments. No successful case of ovary homograft has ever been reported clinically. A case of homologous vascularized ovary transplantation succeeded perfectly in 1979 in our clinic.

CASE REPORT

A 35-year-old woman had sustained menorrhagia. A total hysterectomy and bilateral oophorectomies were performed in 1976, because both ovaries showed cystic changes and were thought to be malignant, even though the pathologic diagnosis indicated myxocystic tumor of the right ovary and a follicular cyst of the left one after operation. Ten days after the operation she suffered from symptoms including severe dizziness, lassitude, masculinized voice and dryness of the vagina – a serious endocrine disturbance. However, after administration of stilbestrol, these symptoms improved, although not completely.

On November 7 1977, a free implantation of an allo-ovary gave her some improvement, but this only lasted 6 months. The symptoms appeared again, and worsened. She lost her appetite, had anorexia, vomiting, marked loss of subcutaneous fat and secondary sexual characteristics. Furthermore, she did not respond to treatment with stilbestrol, and she was not able to work at all. She was then brought to the Microsurgical Department for a homologous vascularized ovary transplantation on September 7 1979.

A vascular ovary was carefully dissected from a 44-year-old donor who underwent total hysterectomy for a uterine myoma. After perfusing the graft with 4 °C heparinized Ringer's lactate solution, we implanted it subcutaneously in the groin and anastomosed the vessels of the graft to the deep femoral artery and great saphenous vein. Diameters of the artery and vein were 1.5 mm and 2.5 mm respectively. A 9/0 monofilament nylon microsuture was used. The ischemic time of the graft was 2 h 50 min. We used 100 mg azathioprine (Imuran) before the operation and 1000 mg hydrocortisone at the beginning of the operation for immunosuppression and both were continued for 3 days. Afterward, prednisone 60 mg was given once a day. There were three episodes of rejection postoperatively, and large doses of hydrocortisone were used to control them. After 3 months, a daily dosage of prednisone 25 mg and Imuran 25 mg or cyclophosphamide (Endoxin) 100 mg once a day alternatively every 10 days were maintained.

After the transplantation, her symptoms subsided, a female voice and sexual activity were recovered. The vaginal smear showed evidence of a slight decrease in the estrogen level, the follicle-stimulating hormone in the urine decreased from 100–150 mouse uterine units, the estrogen increased from 1 μg to 10 μg, and pregnanediol increased from 0 mg to 0.8 mg. She has been followed up for 2 years. The patient takes the immunosuppressive drugs less regularly. She only notices some hoarseness in her voice, and the estrogen level in her urine is lower than before, but she can now work as usual.

CONCLUSION

A homologous vascularized ovary transplantation was performed in a young woman suffering from a severe endocrine disturbance with satisfactory results for 2 years following the transplantation.

24 Microsurgical Replantation of an Amputated Penis: A Case Report

YU GUO-ZHONG, PANG SHUI-FA, LI FO-BAO and ZHU JIA-KAI

Department of Surgery, The First Affiliated Hospital, Zhongshan Medical College, Guangzhou

With progress in microsurgery, successful microsurgical replantation of the penis has been reported in the literature[1-3]. Here we report a successful replantation of an amputated penis by use of microsurgical technique.

CASE REPORT

A 35-year-old patient had his penis amputated with scissors by his wife on August 22, 1980. Three hours after the incident, the patient came to us with the amputated penis 5 cm long without any refrigeration treatment. The penis stump was about 4 cm long (Figure 24.1).

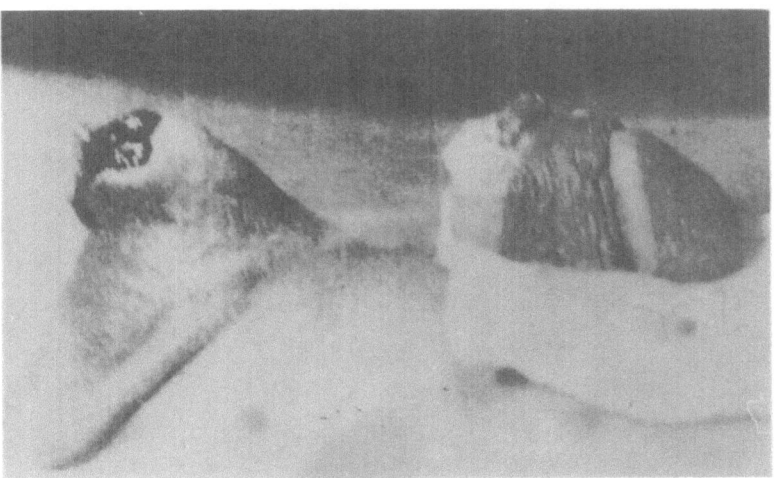

Figure 24.1 Completely amputated penis

The replantation was done under continuous caudal anesthesia. A No. 16 urethral catheter was introduced via the amputated penis and stump penis urethra into the bladder as a temporary stent. Urethral anastomosis was made with interrupted 3/0 catgut sutures. The tunica albuginea was joined with continuous 3/0 catgut sutures. The repair of vessels and nerves was done under the operating microscope. Two dorsal arteries both 0.5 mm in diameter and one dorsal vein 3 mm in diameter were anastomosed with interrupted 9/0 nylon sutures. Immediately after the reestablishment of the circulation, the glans became pink in colour. The amputated penis was ischemic for 10 hours. The skin was closed with interrupted sutures after two dorsal nerves had been stitched together. After a suprapubic cystostomy, the urethral catheter was removed.

Intraoperative and postoperative intravenous infusion of low molecular weight dextran, postoperative intramuscular injections of tolazoline, stilbestrol and antibiotics as well as oral aspirin were given. The glans remained pink colored after operation. Two weeks after operation, the suprapubic catheter was removed without there being any complaint of voiding difficulty. A hematoma complicating a small area of skin necrosis in the proximal part of the replanted penis was discovered, and split thickness skin grafting was all that was necessary. The patient was discharged with perfect healing of the wound (Figure 24.2).

Nine months after operation, the sensation and erection of the replanted penis were completely recovered. The patient can urinate without any difficulty of urethral stricture.

The urinary diversion by suprapubic cystostomy eliminated the urethral catheter, which is a foreign body liable to cause irritation and infection of the urethral anastomosis. The risk of urethral stricture is thus largely obviated.

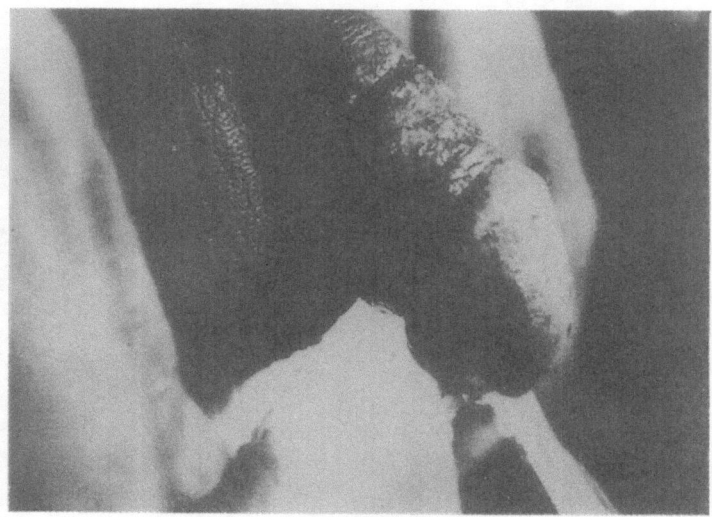

Figure 24.2   Replanted penis before discharge, with free passage of urine

REFERENCES

1. Cohen, B. E. *et al*. (1977). Successful clinical replantation of an amputated penis by microneurovascular repair: Case report. *Plast. Reconstr. Surg.*, **59**, 276
2. Tamai, S. *et al*. (1977). Microsurgical replantation of a completely amputated penis and scrotum: Case report. *Plast. Reconstr. Surg.*, **60**, 287
3. Henriksson, T. G. *et al*. (1980). Microsurgical replantation of an amputated penis. *Scand. J. Urol. Nephrol.*, **14**, 111

25 Observation on Morphologic Changes in Blood Vessels in Experimental Random Pattern Skin Tubes

NIU XING-TAO, QU HONG-YE, SUN YU-LIANG and LIU XIN
Department of Plastic Surgery, The Third Teaching Hospital, Beijing Medical College

LI XUE-YU, SHEN GUI-MING and LIU JI-HENG
Department of Anatomy, Beijing Medical College

Skin tubes are widely used for tissue defect repair and organ reconstruction in plastic surgery. It has long been proved that a random pattern skin tube, scarcely vascularized by innominate vessels immediately after its reconstruction, exhibits a very rich vascularization after a couple of weeks, that its subcutaneous fat can be liberally trimmed off and its cut distal end during transfer can be folded without any risk of blood supply disturbance. The sequence of events in morphologic changes in blood vessels in random skin tubes and the mechanism of the revascularization are two unresolved problems in the realm of plastic surgery.

The angiographic study of skin tube revascularization in rabbits by Conway[1] was rather simple in design. Besides the demonstration of the formation of axial-pattern vessels in the skin tube, the anatomic and morphologic changes in blood vessels had not been observed in detail. The works on blood vessels in the skin tubes and flap by Hynes[2] and Braithwaite[3] were limited to clinical observations without morphologic consideration. In order to elucidate the sequence of events on morphologic changes in blood vessels in the skin tubes, we undertook an angiographic study in rabbits, by means of abdominal aorta infusion of Chinese ink at fixed intervals after the creation of skin tubes. Having been dehydrated and treated with wintergreen oil, the skin tube preparations became transparent and were examined under the dissection microscope.

MATERIALS AND METHODS

Thirty adult rabbits weighing 2.5–3.5 kg were used for experimentation. Each animal had two tubed flaps ($2 \times 5 \, cm^2$ each) created on either side of its back. The skin flaps were perpendicularly arranged to the long axis of the body in

185

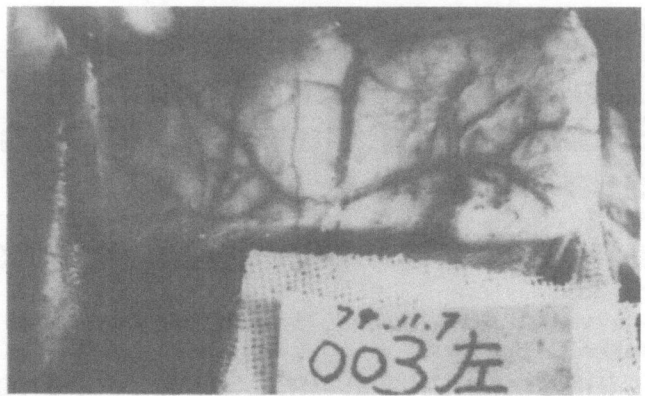

Figure 25.1   Type 1, skin tube vascular distribution

order to exclude any possible inclusion of axial vessels which are longitudinally located. Anesthesia was by intravenous infusion of 5% sodium pentobarbital solution (0.5 ml/kg). Three types of skin tubes were recognized according to the vascular pattern of collaterals of the main longitudinal vessels: type 1 having a couple of collaterals in the whole length of two skin tubes, the distance between the origins of the two collaterals being < 5 mm (Figure 25.1); type 2, the same as type 1 except for the distance being > 5 mm (Figure 25.2); and type 3 having no complete collaterals (Figure 25.3). There were 25 skin tubes each of type 1 and type 2 and ten of type 3. Five fixed intervals immediately after the construction of skin tubes, namely, 30 minutes, 3 days, 1, 2 and 4 weeks after operation, were used for the angiographic study of the skin tubes. Under general anesthesia, the abdomen was opened and Chinese ink solution infused directly into the

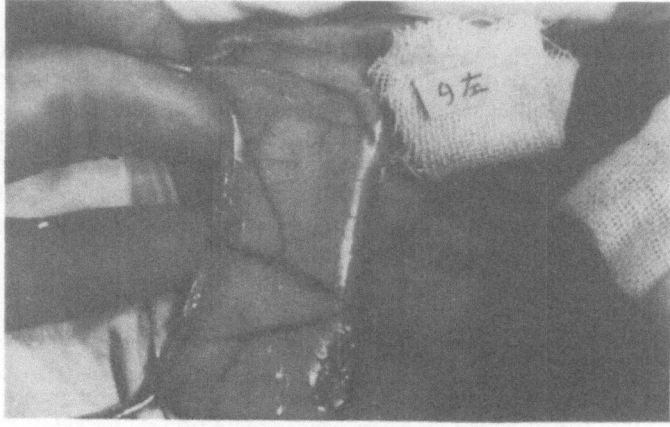

Figure 25.2   Type 2, skin tube vascular distribution

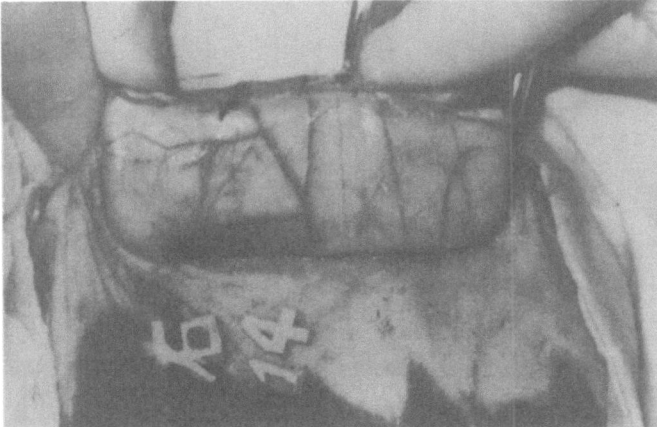

Figure 25.3   Type 3, skin tube vascular distribution

abdominal aorta at a rate of 40 drops per minute, the total volume of infused solution being 150 ml/kg. Each animal was kept in a freezer at 0 °C for 24 h after death. Each skin tube was opened along its suture line, unfolded and soaked in 5% formalin solution for 24 h. The specimen was dehydrated with alcohol and made transparent by immersion in wintergreen oil. A 25 × microscope was used for angiographic examination.

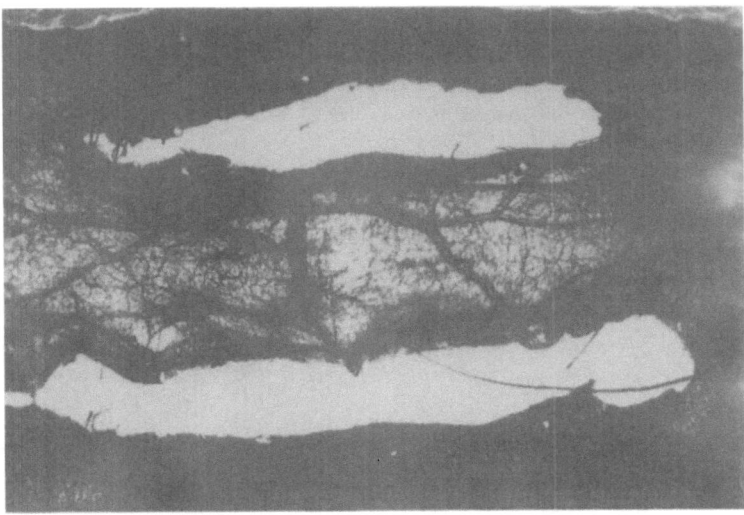

Figure 25.4   Vascular pattern of Type 1, 3 days after operation. Marked dilatation of vessels whose courses were rearranged into one parallel to the axis of the tube. (Translucent specimen under dissection microscopy)

RESULTS

Macroscopic examination

Edematous congestion of various degrees had occurred in all skin tubes immediately after their construction; it disappeared 3–4 days after operation in type 1 and 2 skin tubes. Two weeks after operation, hair growth began to appear in the skin tubes. The edematous congestion was more pronounced in type 3 skin tubes; here the midportion dried up gradually and eventually the whole tube was lost.

Microscopic features of transparent specimens

Five fixed interval groups were examined.

(1) Thirty minute group. Skin tube vasodilation occurred in all these types, especially pronounced in anastomotic branches of remnant collaterals.

(2) Three day group. In type 1 skin tubes, vasodilation was prominent in such a way that collateral branches were engorged or even tortuous and tended to arrange themselves parallel to the long axis of the skin tube (Figure 25.4). Morphologic changes in anastomotic branches were less prominent in type 2 skin tubes (Figure 25.5). In type 3 skin flaps, no vasodilation could be seen among anastomotic branches (Figure 25.6).

(3) One week group. From the original collateral branch, a tortuous axial vessels pattern along the length of the skin tube was formed in type 1 skin

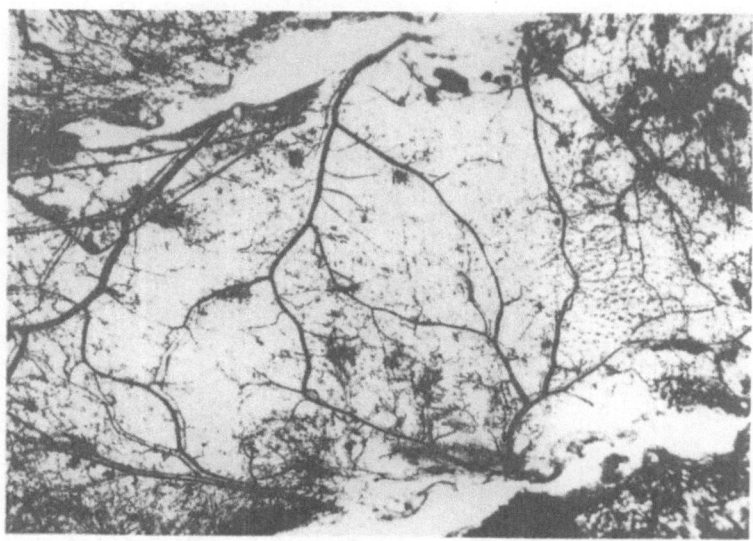

Figure 25.5 Vascular pattern of Type 2, 3 days after operation. (Translucent specimen under dissection microscopy)

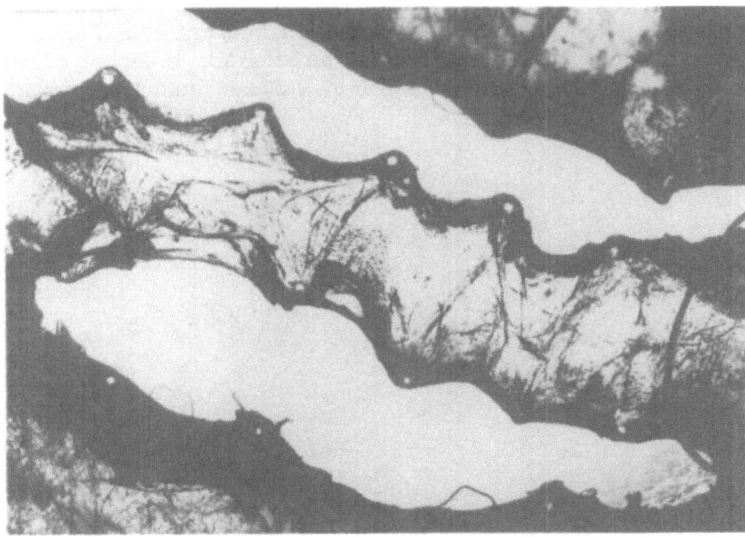

Figure 25.6   Vascular pattern of Type 3, 3 days after operation. (Translucent specimen under dissection microscopy)

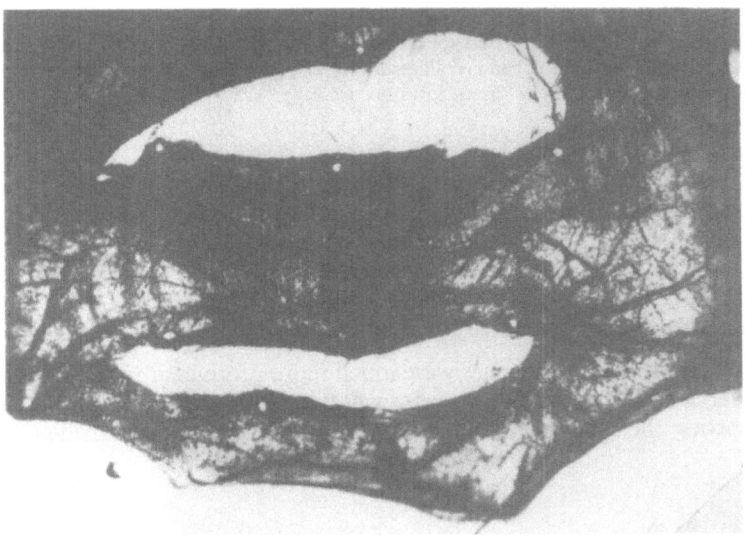

Figure 25.7   Vascular pattern of Type 1, 1 week after operation. Transformation into an axial-type vascular system was noted. (Translucent specimen under dissection microscopy)

tubes (Figure 25.7). In type 2 skin tubes, patent and convoluted anastomoses were observed among the collateral branches (Figure 25.8). In type 3, filling defect occurred in anastomotic branches of remnant collaterals. Degeneration changes in vascular branches precluded the formation of vascular axis.

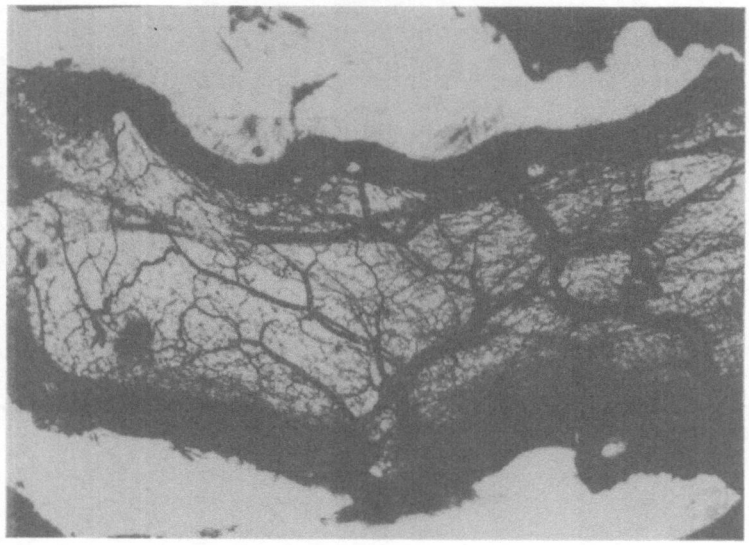

Figure 25.8   Vascular pattern of Type 2, 1 week after operation, with patent anastomoses between vascular branches and collateral vessels, but there was marked tortuosity. (Translucent specimen under dissection microscopy)

(4)   Two to four week groups. Establishment of an 'axial-pattern' vascular system was completed in type 1 skin tubes; it is almost parallel to the long axis of the skin tube. In type 2 flaps, the establishment of this pattern was somewhat delayed; it took place in the fourth week. In type 3, most of the skin flaps dried up before the 2–4 week intervals, so that no satisfactory specimens were available for examination.

All these morphologic changes were much more prominent in the veins than in the arteries and the lumen of the veins was two to three times bigger than that of the arteries; the same phenomena were seen in anastomotic branches.

DISCUSSION

Early morphologic changes in the skin tubes are hyperemia and edema. Microscopically, vasodilation is seen, being more prominent in the venous system. This is in complete accord with the opinion of Kilner, Debakey and Ochsner –

free back flow of the tissue fluid and venous flow are essential to skin tube survival. Venous congestion is the main factor in the loss of a skin tube.

In type 1 skin tubes, a preexisting complete collateral with short anastomotic branches makes the tube circulation more easily established. In type 2 tubes, which have long anastomotic branches, the establishment of an 'axial-pattern like' vascular system seemed more difficult. However, it was achieved eventually, though delayed a little. In type 3 tubes, the preexisting vasculature is too poor to establish an 'axial-pattern like' vascular system and skin tubes accordingly died.

This experiment showed blood vessels in random skin tubes can gradually convert themselves from a random arrangement to an 'axial-pattern like' system. It should be emphasized that the preexisting blood vessels for canalization and remolding are indispensable for vascularization of the skin tube. Some virtually collapsed vessels reopened, others widened in caliber and some of the main vessels gradually narrowed down and became obliterated. These changes may probably be the consequence of alteration in the direction of blood flow, and no newly formed vascular bud was found. It is suggested that the establishment of an 'axial-pattern like' vessel system in a tubed flap is based on its preexisting blood vessels.

CONCLUSION

The skin flaps, 60 in number in 20 rabbits, were made on either side of the back. Based on the original vascular patterns, skin flaps were divided into three types. Morphologic changes in vasculature and skin tube survival were determined. It is postulated that a preexisting original vasculature is indispensable to the establishment of a satisfactory 'axial-pattern like' vascular system within a skin tube. Canalization and remolding of preexisting vessels are essential to the revascularization. No newly formed vascular buds were seen. The vasculature changes were more prominent in the venous side than the arterial. Therefore, in the designing of a skin tube, efficient vasculature of the donor site should be emphasized. Free venous return of the skin tube is indispensable to its survival.

REFERENCES

1. Conway, H. *et al.* (1949). Vascularization of tubed pedicle. *Plast. Reconstr. Surg.*, **4**, 133
2. Hynes, W. (1950). The blood-vessels in skin tubes and flaps. *Br. J. Plast. Surg.*, **3**, 165
3. Braithwaite, F. (1950). Preliminary observations on the vascular channels in tube pedicles. *Br. J. Plast. Surg.*, **3**, 40

26 Medullary Cavity – A Substitute for Venous Return in Vascularized Bone Transplantation – An Experimental Study

GAO JING-HENG, XU ZHEN-KUAN, ZHENG HUA-XIANG, WANG YU-MING and HOW ZAIN
Department of Surgery, Zunyi Medical College
WANG WEI-MIN
Department of Pathology, Zunyi Medical College, Guizhou

Being a complex process, bone union has been an important subject of research for many years. Experimental island bone transplantation with both arterial and venous pedicles was performed by Strauch[1] (1971) and Ostrüp[2] (1974) and clinical application was successfully carried out in 1975 by Taylor[3]. In regard to the venous return of the bone graft, many authors considered that its interruption plays a role of promoting bone growth. This chapter reports the results of experimental arterial bone graft of which the venous return was interrupted.

MATERIAL AND METHODS

Twenty-five dogs, weighing 10–24 kg, were divided into two groups: (1) control group of ten dogs without vascular pedicle of the bone graft and (2) experimental group of 15 dogs, with arterial bone grafts.

Experimental group

Under intraperitoneal pentobarbital anesthesia, a midline incision on the inner side of the foreleg was made down through deep fascia (Figure 26.1a). Flexor muscles were retracted to expose the median artery and its branches (radial artery and ulnar artery). Right after its dividing into radial artery, and on its way down anteromedially along the middle and lower segments of the radius, it gives off nutrient branches to the lower third of the radius (Figure 26.1b). The distal ends of the radial artery with its accompanying veins were cut and ligated, the radius was transected with a wire saw at the levels of upper third (corresponding

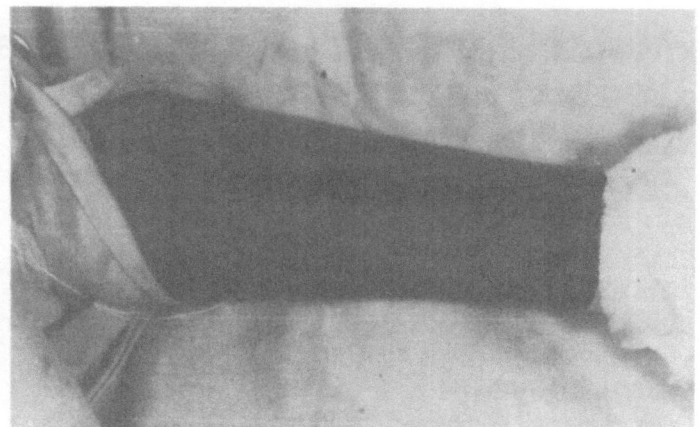

a

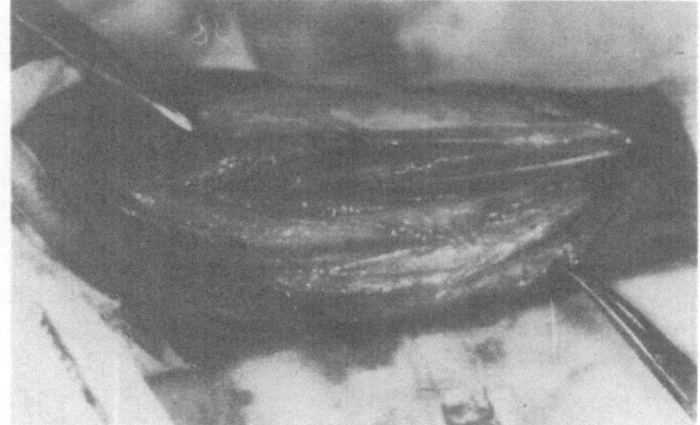

b

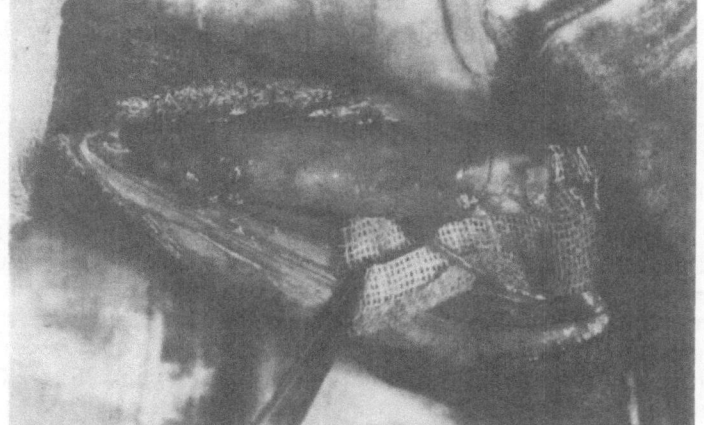

c

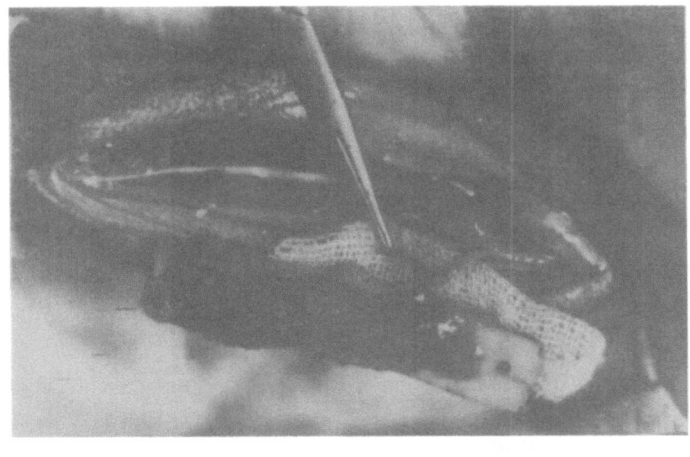

d

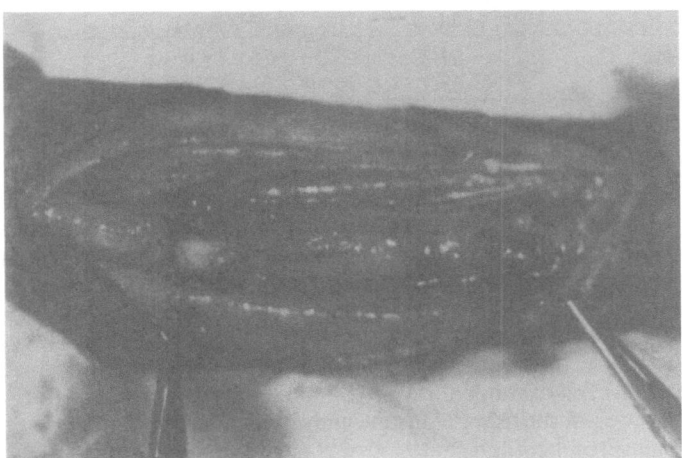

e

Figure 26.1 **a,** Midline incision on the inner side of the foreleg. **b,** The radius and the median artery with its branches are exposed. **c,** Anterior view of the bone graft. **d,** Lateral view of the bone graft. The graft is completely isolated except being connected with the radial artery. **e,** *In situ* replacement of the bone graft

to where the radial artery parts from the median artery) and the lower third, and the accompanying veins were cut and ligated at the same level. Nearly all the soft tissues were dissected away so that the transected bone is isolated completely, excepting only its connection with the radial artery (Figure 26.1c,d). Bleeding from the medullary cavity of the free bone graft was noted. The isolated bone graft was then replaced *in situ* (Figure 26.1e) by transfixing both ends with stainless wire, and so were the soft tissues. Finally the incision was closed and dressed routinely. Postoperatively, observation of the bone graft for its survival and healing was carried out by radiography, angiography and pathologic section.

Control group

Operative procedure was the same as described above, but the arterial pedicle was not preserved.

RESULTS

Experimental group

The available results of observation in 11 of the 15 dogs are listed in Table 26.1. The time interval lapse of observation ranged from 2 to 18 months.

Table 26.1   Results of *in situ* bone grafts in the experimental and control groups

Group	Callus formation (days)	Bone bridge formation (days)	Marrow cavity communication (days)
Experimental	27.8	55.9	378
Control	33.7	90.5	570

Roentagenogram (11 cases)

Healing of both ends of the graft occurred in ten cases, a total number of 20 bone ends. The earliest periosteal response is demonstrated on the ninth postoperative day. The average time for the external callus to develop and surround the bone graft is 27.8 days. In ten bone ends aligned snugly, time lapse for the bone bridge formed from external periosteal callus is 38–73 days (average 55.9) (Figure 26.2) and for transition from the blur of the fracture line to the reestablishment of communication of the medullary cavities is 378 days (Figure 26.3). However, in the other ten bone ends, which were not in good apposition, delayed union resulted and nine out of the ten were distal bone ends.

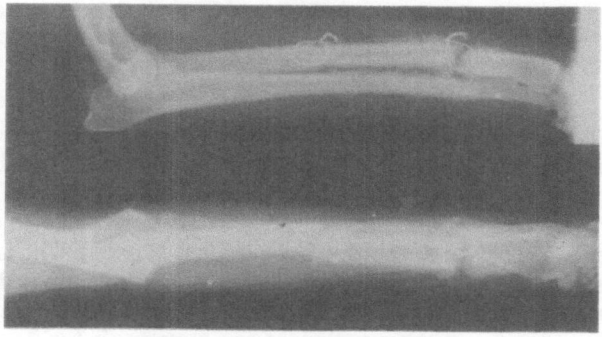

Figure 26.2   Bone bridge formation

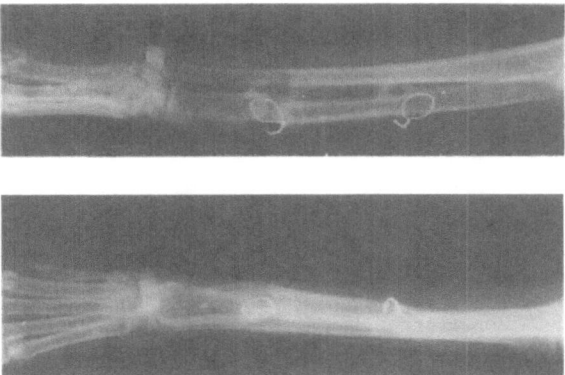

Figure 26.3   Bone marrow cavity communication

One case failed to heal because the periosteum on the proximal end of the graft has been excised, resulting in no periosteal response in the early stage, low density on the angiogram and bone absorption in the late stage (Figure 26.4).

Angiogram

The vascular network was demonstrated in seven cases. Density of the bone graft in the angiogram was increased as compared with that in the plain film, indicating the existence of vascularity (Figure 26.5).

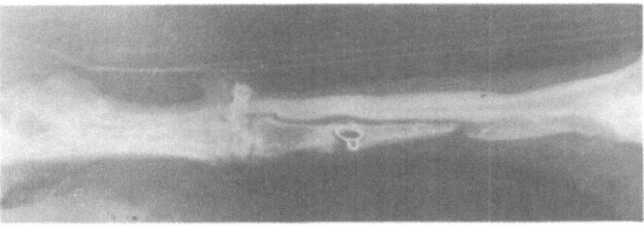

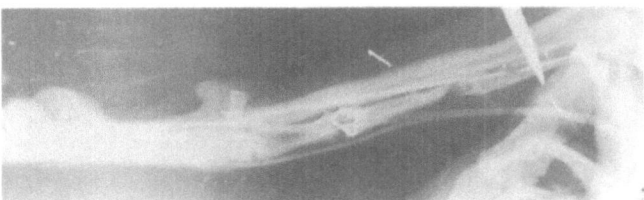

Figure 26.4   Late bone absorption and nonunion of the graft resulted from periosteal excision during operation

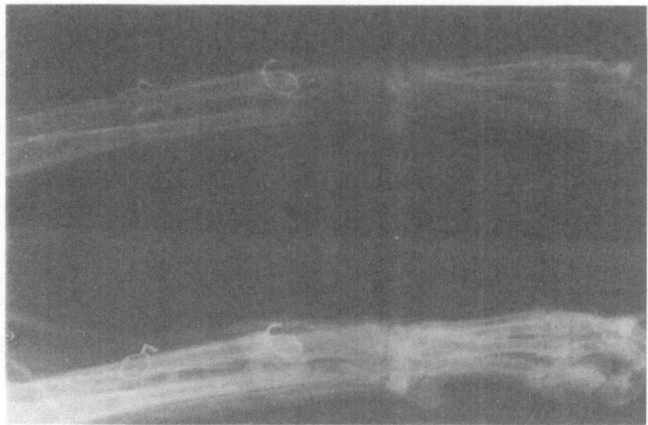

Figure 26.5 Plain film (*above*), angiograph film (*below*). Density of the bone graft is increased in comparison with that in the plain film, suggesting existence of vascularity

Pathology

Bony healing as well as completion of the trabecular remodelling are shown 12 months postoperatively in dog No. 4 in the proximal end of the transplanted bone segment. But there is only periosteal proliferative fibrous tissue in the distal bony junction. Not many trabeculae are shown in the normal bone near the distal end of the graft (Figures 26.6, 26.7).

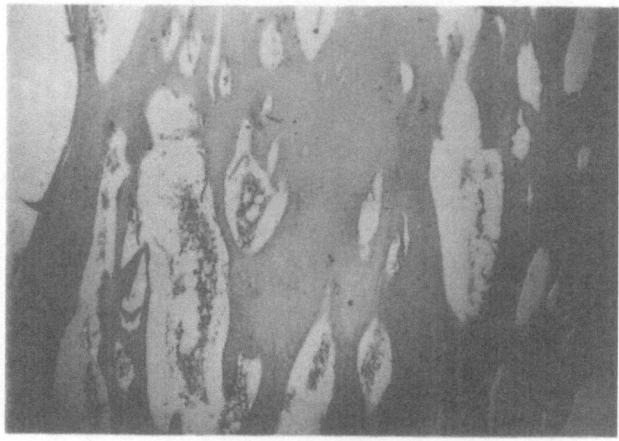

Figure 26.6 Bone union and completion of trabecular remodeling in the proximal end of the graft 12 months after operation

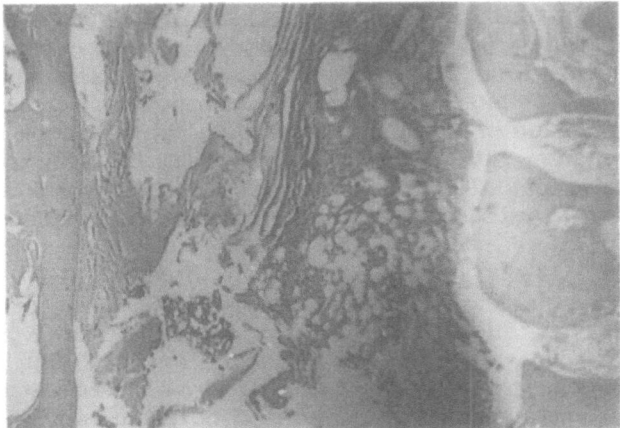

Figure 26.7   Small amount of trabeculae was found in the normal bone near the distal end of the graft

Control group

Part of the observation result was obtained from four of the ten dogs. The time of observation covered a period of 34–570 days. On the 16th postoperative day, only a small amount of periosteal reaction could be seen radiologically. Encircling of the transplanted bony segment by external callus is completed after 337 days on an average. It took an average of 90.5 days for the formation of a bony bridge from the blur of the fracture line. Communication through the medullary cavities was resumed after 570 days.

DISCUSSION

In this experiment, a free radius graft model with radial arterial pedicle only was set up for autogenic orthotopic bony transplantation. The course of the radial artery was operatively confirmed to be constant in 25 dogs. There were two or three nutrient arteries entering the medullary cavity in the middle and lower segments of the radius. Experimental results can be observed postoperatively by X-ray film, isotopic scanning, angiogram or even by pathologic section. Considering its simplicity in manipulation and certainty in index observation, it seems to be a relatively good model for the study of bony transplantation with vascular pedicle.

Of the 11 experimental dogs, ten showed good healing and callus formation, which encircled the segment completely. It took 27.8 days on average (10–45 days) for the transplanted bone segment to heal. And on average (38–73 days), 55.9 days were needed to show blur of the fracture line and formation of a bony bridge, and an average of 378 days (360–420 days) for the resumption of communication through the medullary cavity. However, in four dogs of the control group, it took 33.7 days (16–45 days) for the formation of callus, and 90.5 days on average (80–101 days) for the blur of the fractured line and bony bridge formation. Kruse[4] (1974) reported that occlusion of venous return with a tourniquet could promote the union of fracture in dogs. In two of his 12 experimental dogs, union of fracture, distal to the tourniquet, took place within 41–269 days (average 103 days), while no union was seen in his control group. This result is in conformity with our experiment. Therefore, it seems that bone flap with arterial pedicle alone (without venous pedicle) can enhance fracture healing.

Keck[5] (1965), Kelly[6] (1968), Singh[7] (1971), Brookes[8,9] (1972) and Kruse[4] (1974), based on further investigation, using a tourniquet or tying off the main vein, proposed as reasons that (1) increase in medullary cavity pressure after occlusion of venous return will stimulate bone growth, (2) supply of growth material will be increased for the venous return-occluded bone and (3) on account of temporary venous return blockage, the resulting decrease in local pH and increase in P_aCo_2 can accelerate the production of bone cell. Brookes[9] (1972) pointed out that by blockage of venous return of bone, a part of the venous blood will drain into the epiphyseal vein, and a part will permeate through the bony tissue into the collateral veins of the surrounding soft tissues. As the bone cells are in an environment of low pH and high P_aCo_2, bone union will be accelerated.

Kruse and colleagues observed that increasing venous pressure distal to the blockage is only temporary. Three weeks after the blockage, pressure will drop down to nearly normal level. In this experiment, the venous return of the bone flap is blocked by ligating the radial vein, and venous return of the graft will drain through the marrow cavity into the epiphyseal veins and through the permeation of the bony segment into the collateral veins formed in the surrounding soft tissues. Though the medullary cavity pressure is not measured in this experiment, it is most probable that it would be increased temporarily with lowering of pH and increase in P_aCo_2. This experiment serves to explain the mechanism of bone union acceleration.

Kruse *et al.* proved experimentally that the important function of blocking the venous return is to produce more periosteal callus by early stimulation of fracture periosteum and to accelerate new bone growth, shown mainly in the phase of periosteal reaction.

The results of this experiment also prove the fact that acceleration of healing of the bone flap is made possible by enhancing the periosteal callus formation. Mckibbin[10] reported that the external periosteum is the leading factor in the whole process of bone union. At present, most authors argue that if the subperiosteal bone was resected leaving the periosteal tube intact, the subperiosteal callus ring can still be evolved, enhancing the production of a new bone. This has been proved in clinical practice; therefore, the importance of a periosteum in the bone union should by no means be denied.

This experimental model may be used to study the mechanism of bone union. It proves preliminarily that bone flap with intact arterial supply alone in the vascular pedicle type is able to accelerate the bone healing by enhancing the formation of periosteal callus. This experimental result affords a working base for using arterial pedicle bone flap in clinical practice.

REFERENCES

1. Strauch, B. *et al.* (1971). Graft of island bone. *Br. J. Plast. Surg.*, **24**, 334
2. Ostrüp, L. T. *et al.* (1974). Distant transfer of a free, living bone graft by micro-vascular anastomosis. An experimental study. *Plast. Reconstr. Surg.*, **54**, 374
3. Taylor, G. I. *et al.* (1975). The free vascularized bone graft. A clinical extension of microvascular techniques. *Plast. Reconstr. Surg.*, **55**, 533
4. Kruse, R. L. *et al.* (1974). Acceleration of fracture healing distal to a venous tourniquet. *J. Bone Jt. Surg.*, **56**, 730
5. Keck, S. W. *et al.* (1965). The effect of venous stasis on intraosseous pressure and longitudinal bone growth in the dog. *J. Bone Jt. Surg.*, **47**, 539
6. Kelly, P. J. *et al.* (1968). Effect of unilateral increased venous pressure on bone remodeling in canine tibia. *J. Lab. Clin. Med.*, **72**, 410
7. Singh, M. *et al.* (1971). Bone growth and blood flow after experimental venous ligation. *J. Anat.*, **108**, 315
8. Brookes, M. *et al.* (1972). Venous shunt in bone after ligation of the femoral vein. *Surg. Gynecol. Obstet.*, **135**, 85
9. Brookes, M. *et al.* (1972). Bone blood pH and gas tensions after femoral vein ligation. *Surg. Gynecol. Obstet.*, **135**, 873
10. Mckibbin, B. (1978). The biology of fracture healing in long bone. *J. Bone Jt. Surg.*, **60B**, 150

Part II

Recent Advances in Burns Surgery in China

27 Clinical Significance of Changes in Excreted Fraction of Filtered Sodium (FE$_{Na}$) in Severe Burn Patients

CHEN YU-LIN, FANG ZHI-YANG and XU FENG-XUN

Burn Unit, Changhai Hospital, the Second Military Medical College, Shanghai

Correct and timely monitoring of renal function in severe burns is helpful and closely related to prognosis. Some investigators have recently described how diagnosis and differential diagnosis of acute renal insufficiency can be made by observing the changes in FE$_{Na}$ (the excreted fraction of the filtered sodium)[1,2], which is a relatively simple, sensitive and accurate monitoring measure. Changes in FE$_{Na}$ in the whole course of 31 severe burn cases have been observed by the present authors and are analysed in this chapter.

CLINICAL MATERIAL

The FE$_{Na}$ test was performed in patients with severe burns from 1978 to 1981. Patients were divided into two groups, survivors and nonsurvivors. The survivors group was further categorized into a subgroup of ten, with 80–100% TBSA burnt, and a subgroup of nine with 40–79% TBSA burnt. The group of nonsurvivors comprised 12 cases (Table 27.1). FE$_{Na}$ of both survivors and nonsurvivors was observed.

Table 27.1 General Data

Group	Subgroup	Patients cases	Age (M ± SD)	Sex (M : F)	TBSA burnt (%) (M ± SD)
Survivors	1	10	20–56 (28.7 ± 10.5)	9 : 1	80–100 (89.60 ± 7.12)
	2	9	21–59 (32.8 ± 13.5)	8 : 1	40–79 (60.11 ± 13.96)
Non-survivors		12	21–51 (33.0 ± 9.1)	5 : 1	60–100 (86.42 ± 3.75)

Table 27.2 Changes in FE$_{Na}$ in survivors

Group	Patients	3rd post-burn day	Week postburn						
			1	2	3	4	5	6	7
Survivors	19	3.65±2.32	4.50 ±3.05	3.68 ±1.40	3.03 ±1.43	4.34 ±2.34	3.24 ±1.30	3.31 ±1.46	2.32 ±1.53
Subgroup 1	10	3.32±2.41	3.84 ±1.31	3.59 ±0.67	3.18 ±1.61	4.40 ±2.45	3.71 ±0.68	4.27 ±1.09	2.11 ±1.78
Subgroup 2	9	4.06±2.29	5.23 ±4.22	3.89 ±2.27	2.80 ±1.20	4.25 ±2.38	2.67 ±1.70	2.03 ±0.58	2.52 ±1.60

Table 27.3 Relationship between FE$_{Na}$ and escharectomy

Group	Patients (cases)	Shock phase	Week postburn						
			1	2	3	4	5	6	7
Escharectomy operation within week 1	12	4.05 ±2.36	4.99 ±3.63	3.72 ±1.75	2.63 ±1.10	4.36 ±1.93	2.98 ±1.29	3.18 ±1.56	2.67 ±1.42
Escharectomy operation thereafter	3	2.65 ±0.97	3.89 ±1.22	3.76 ±0.88	4.61 ±1.62	4.04 ±2.31	4.37 ±0.64	—	—
No escharectomy	4	3.26 ±2.04	3.47 ±1.88	3.55 ±0.73	2.67 ±1.71	4.64 ±5.64	—	—	—

Relationship between FE$_{Na}$ and burns

The FE$_{Na}$ of the survivors was tested on the third postburn day and for the rest of the course up to the end of 7 weeks. The results are outlined in Table 27.2.

Table 27.2 indicates that the FE$_{Na}$ values of the survivors on the third post-burn day increased (> 3). This high level persisted and reached a first peak by the end of the first postburn week. The second peak appeared by the end of the fourth postburn week and values were then gradually brought down to normal (< 3) by the end of the seventh postburn week.

No obvious differences in FE$_{Na}$ values were found between the two subgroups shown in Table 27.2. This implies that the extent of TBSA burnt was not a decisive factor influencing the postburn value of FE$_{Na}$.

As is shown in Table 27.2, most of the patients presented high values of FE$_{Na}$ in the first postburn week. Since most of the escharectomy operations were done during the first postburn week, it was imperative to make clear the relationship between FE$_{Na}$ and escharectomy. Comparisons of FE$_{Na}$ values were thus made between operated-on groups and nonoperated-on groups and between those with escharectomy performed within the first postburn week and those where it was performed later (Table 27.3).

Table 27.3 shows that although there was an elevation of FE$_{Na}$ in the non-operated-on group and in the group of patients who received their operation after the first postburn week, neither group reached the peak value of 4.99, while the FE$_{Na}$ values of the group operated on within the first postburn week reached their peak at the end of the first postburn week. Escharectomy plus the after-math of burn shock might be the contributing factors which caused the elevation of FE$_{Na}$ resulting, so to speak, from the damaged renal tubules.

Relationship between FE$_{Na}$ and administration of antibiotics

It was shown in Table 27.2 that FE$_{Na}$ reached a second peak in the fourth post-burn week. This was presumed to be the adverse reaction to long term use of aminoglycosides.

Table 27.4 indicates that the administration of aminoglycosides was another contributing factor of elevation of FE$_{Na}$ which seemed most prominent during the fourth postburn week.

Changes in FE$_{Na}$ in patients who died

Changes in FE$_{Na}$ within a few days prior to death were observed. A comparison

Table 27.4 Relationship between FE$_{Na}$ and antibotics used in the fourth week postburn

Group	Cases	TBSA burnt	III degree burns	FE$_{Na}$ in 4th week
Aminoglycosides	9	81.44 ± 14.13	50.89 ± 25.79	5.43 ± 2.01
Other antibiotics	6	6.217 ± 11.94	47.17 ± 25.44	2.69 ± 1.85
p Value				< 0.05

Table 27.5 Change in FE_{Na} value in nonsurvivor group

| Group | Patients | Days prior to death | | | | |
		5	4	3	2	1
ARF	2	—	—	41.70 ± 34.74	59.77 ± 42.94	51.83 ± 43.28
NonARF	10	4.03 ± 1.99	4.44 ± 2.54	5.20 ± 4.56	8.55 ± 10.05	4.17 ± 3.35
p Value		—	<0.01	<0.01	<0.01	<0.01

was made between those patients suffering the complication of acute renal failure (ARF) and those not suffering ARF. A significant difference in FE_{Na} value was observed between the ARF group and the nonARF group ($p < 0.01$) (Table 27.5).

Significance of FE_{Na} in early diagnosis of acute renal insufficiency

One case was selected for an attempt to work out whether FE_{Na} was a more sensitive parameter for the early diagnosis of ARF in comparison with the conventional method adopted (Table 27.6).

No conclusion could be drawn, however, since the marked elevation of FE_{Na} 5 days prior to death was accompanied by concomitant alteration in other laboratory determinations (Table 27.6).

DISCUSSION

The capability of tubular reabsorption of glomerular filtered sodium markedly decreased during renal tubular damage or obstruction of the urinary tract. Therefore, by calculating the sodium excreted, the quality and degree of renal functional derangement can be judged:

$$
\begin{aligned}
FE_{Na} &= \frac{\text{Sodium excreted}}{\text{Sodium filtered}} \times 100 \\
&= \frac{U\,Na \times V}{p\,Na \times GFR} \times 100 \\
&= \frac{U\,Na \times V}{p\,Na \times C\,Cr} \times 100 \\
&= \frac{U\,Na \times V}{p\,Na \times \dfrac{U\,Cr \times V}{p\,Cr}} \times 100 \\
&= \frac{U\,Na \times p\,Cr}{p\,Na \times U\,Cr} \times 100
\end{aligned}
$$

Note that U Na = urine sodium (mmol/l); V = urine output (l); p Na = plasma sodium (mmol/l); GFR = glomerular filtration rate; C Cr = Creatinine clearance rate; U Cr = urine creatinine (mg/dl); p Cr = plasma creatinine (mg/dl).

Espinel and his colleagues[1] postulated that FE$_{Na}$<1 implied prerenal azotemia; FE$_{Na}$>3 represented acute tubular necrosis or obstruction of the urinary tract. The normal value was set at 1–3. In the present study we observed that the FE$_{Na}$ values of critical burns appeared to be elevated on the third postburn day. The average figure was 3. This figure persisted till the end of the first postburn week and then gradually sloped down. A second peak of elevation was found in the fourth postburn week. Final restoration to normal range (>1,<3) was expected at the seventh postburn week. We propose that the elevation of FE$_{Na}$ on the third postburn day may be due to ischemic and hypoxic damage to the renal tubules and intraluminal aggregation of red blood cells, hemoglobin, and may occur during the shock stage[2]. The high level of FE$_{Na}$ in the first post-burn week was related to escharectomy. The second peak of FE$_{Na}$ value, which was found during the fourth postburn week, was probably due to tubular damage from infection and inappropriate use of antibiotics. It is worth drawing attention to the fact that the administration of antibiotics of the aminoglycoside group brought about obvious elevation of FE$_{Na}$ value[3-5].

Table 27.6 Comparisons between FE$_{Na}$ and other determinations of a nonsurvivor, with ARF (TBSA burnt 60%, IIΓ 51% BSA)

Criteria of chemical determinations	Days prior to death				
	5	4	3	2	1
FE$_{Na}$	24.31	17.52	66.27	90.14	82.44
24 h urine output (ml)	820	520	92	57	6
Urine creatinine (mg/dl)	31.2	21.2	22.5	15.0	10.7
Plasma creatinine (mg/dl)	8.25	7.5	9.25	11.6	10.35
U/p creatinine	3.78	2.83	2.43	1.29	1.03
UUN (mg/dl)	104.0	148.0	41.5	118.0	130.0
BUN (mg/dl)	52.5	61.75	68.0	70.33	55.45
U/p UN	1.98	2.40	0.61	1.68	2.34
Urine osmolality (mmol/kg H$_2$O)	316	346	328	331	329
Plasma osmolality (mmol/kg H$_2$O)	313	337	351	373	360
U/p osmolality	1.01	1.03	0.94	0.89	0.91
Urine Na (mmol/l)	92	114	88	144	140
Free water clearance rate (ml/h)	−0.32	−5.78	0.23	0.27	0.34

FE$_{Na}$, urine osmolality, urine sodium, and the ratio of urine creatinine to plasma creatinine were used in monitoring acute renal insufficiency in 87 cases by Greco and his colleagues[2]. They found that the diagnostic accuracy of the four criteria appeared to be 86/87, 46/87, and 65/87 respectively. Hence, the criteria including FE$_{Na}$ were proved to be effective and accurate. Nevertheless, the clinical evaluation of FE$_{Na}$ in the early diagnosis of ARF cannot be made in the present study.

Generally speaking, appropriate early fluid resuscitation, maintenance of hemodynamic stability during escharectomy, and judicious use of antibiotics are the key links in maintaining renal function in burn patients and FE$_{Na}$ is a simple and reliable criterion monitoring renal function.

REFERENCES

1 Espinel, C. H. *et al.* (1976). The FE$_{Na}$ test use in the differential diagnosis of acute renal failure. *J. Am. Med. Assoc.*, **236**, 579
2 Greco, F. D. *et al.* (1981). Role of the laboratory in management of acute and chronic renal failure. *Ann. Clin. Lab. Sci.*, **11**, 283
3 Emmerson, A. M. *et al.* (1980). Nephrotoxicity with gentamicin or tobramycin. *Lancet*, **12**, 96
4 Simmons, C. F. *et al.* (1980). Inhibitory effects of gentamicin on renal mitochondrial oxidative phosphorylation. *J. Pharmacol. Exp. Ther.*, **214**, 709
5 Lerner, S. A. *et al.* (1979). Suggestion for monitoring patients during treatment with aminoglycoside antibiotic. *OHNS*, **87**, 222

28 Pathomorphologic Study of the Kidneys of Severe Burn Patients and its Relationship to Renal Dysfunction

SHI JINQUAN, YANG ZONGCHENG, LI AO, CHEN CONGLAIN and SHI TONGZHOU

Department of Pathology, Burn Center and Laboratory of Electron Microscopy, Third Military Medical College, Chongqing

Renal dysfunction not infrequently complicates severe burns, but its exact nature and pathogenesis remain not yet clearly understood. Opinions have been diverse. In the middle years of this century, it was claimed by many authors that the pathological basis of acute renal failure was mainly attributable to degeneration or/and necrosis of the renal tubules. Terms such as 'lower nephron nephrosis' or 'acute tubular necrosis' were applied[1-3]. Later, Sevitt[4] of Birmingham proposed that glomerular changes also played an important role in the pathogenesis of acute renal failure. In 1960, Dr Yan of our department, after a pathologic study of the kidneys of 24 severe burn patients, found that in most cases the glomeruli exhibited consistent morphologic changes, characterized by widening of the intercapillary space of tufts due to accumulation of eosinophilic material and monocytic infiltration resulting in glomerular ischemia[5]. He postulated that glomerular abnormalities might be the main cause of renal dysfunction in severe burn patients.

The purpose of the present study is to investigate both the histologic and ultrastructural alterations in the kidney, especially the glomeruli, and explore the correlation between the morphologic changes and functional disturbances in severe burn patients.

MATERIALS AND METHODS

From July 1979 to May 1982, the left kidneys of 17 severely burned patients who died in our Burn Center were obtained immediately after death. As soon as the kidney was exposed, a piece of the renal tissue was excised and readily fixed in 4% phosphate buffered glutaraldehyde solution for electron microscopy examination. The whole left kidney was then removed and fixed in 10% formalin for histologic study[6,7].

Electron microscopy

Samples of 16 kidneys were studied. After preliminary fixation with 4%
glutaraldehyde, the renal tissue was transferred to 1% OsO_4 solution for 2 h, and
then embedded in Epon 812 (seven samples) or epoxy resin 618 (nine samples).
Semithin sections (1 μm thick) were used for orientation. Ultrathin sections
(40–60 nm), cut with an LKB 8800 ultramicrotome and stained with lead cortrate
and uranyl acetate, were examined under DXA_4-10 and DXB_2-12 EM.

Light microscopy

Two or more tissue blocks were examined for each kidney. Conventional
paraffin sections and hematoxylin–eosin staining were done. Special stains
including periodic acid–Schiff (PAS), Jones methenamine silver and Dunn
Thompson hemoglobin stain were also performed when indicated.

Patient groups

Seventeen patients are divided into two groups: Group I, with apparent renal

Table 28.1 Main clinical data of 17 patients

Group*	Case no.	Sex & age (y)	TBSA burned %	Time of death (postburn days)	BUN (mg%)	p Cr (mg%)	Creatinine clearance rate (l/d)
I	1	M 45	82	6	93	4.2	25
	2	M 31	70	7	142	8.3	7
	3	M 59	90	7	80	5.2	54.3
	4	M 28	91	7	86	6.2	35.7
	5	M 30	60	8	156	10.2	8.4
	6	M 37	70	8	106	3.4	43
	7	F 45	97	8	92.3	6.3	54
	8	M 31	90	10	135	7.0	
	9	M 59	96	15	115	3.1	52
	10	M 46	92	22	61	2.8	34
II	11	M 5	40	9	20	2.5	
	12	F 34	65	11	49.2	3.4	
	13	F 50	98	14	38	4.0	54
	14	M 4	54	22	13		
	15	M 19	95	23	60	3.8	
	16	M 6	40	65	12.5	0.9	15.8
	17	M 26	97	103	43	2.5	72

* Group I with apparent renal insufficiency; Group II without apparent renal insufficiency

insufficiency, ten cases; and Group II, without apparent renal insufficiency,
seven cases. Their main clinical data are summarized in Table 28.1.

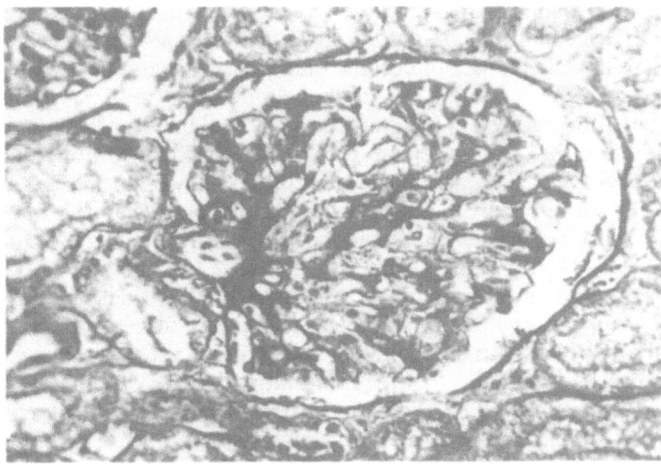

Figure 28.1   Glomerular ischemia, widening of mesangial area with increased amount of PAS-positive eosinophilic material. Case No. 4, PAS × 250

RESULTS

Light microscopic findings

A. Glomeruli

Endothelial cells of glomerular capillary loops appeared swollen, and capillary lumina were frequently occupied by polymorphonuclear leukocytes and/or

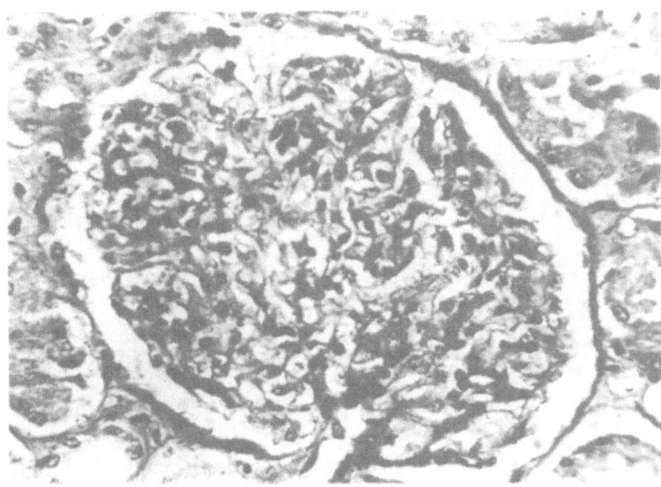

Figure 28.2   Glomerular ischemia, widening of mesangial area, increased number of glomerular cells. Case No. 9, PAS × 250

monocytes. Mesangial areas became widened and usually filled with increased PAS-positive eosinophilic materials. In some cases glomerular cells increased in number so that the glomeruli became enlarged, with narrowing of the capsular spaces. The above changes led to the glomerular capillary loops becoming ischemic in various degrees (Figures 28.1, 28.2). The glomerular capsular space as a rule contained many coarse or fine eosinophilic granules. The parietal epithelial cells of Bowman's capsule became swollen and cuboidal, and occasionally they appeared columnar, simulating epithelial cells of the proximal convoluted tubule. Glomerular capillary hyaline thrombi were found only in one case.

In this chapter, swelling and/or hyperplasia of glomerular cells (including capillary endothelial cells, mesangial cells, and visceral epithelial cells of Bowman's capsule) and widening of mensangial area as well as glomerular ischemia are referred to as 'acute glomerulopathy'.

In order to evaluate the degree and extent of acute glomerulopathy, a semi-quantitative histopathologic method was employed. One hundred glomeruli from the superficial to the deep portions of the renal cortex were counted at random and each glomerulus was graded on a scale of 0–3. The final score of acute glomerulopathy was reached by adding up the scores of 100 glomeruli as shown in Table 28.2.

Table 28.2   Final score of glomerulopathy

Case no.	Final score
1	150
2	160
3	75
4	86
5	214
6	144
7	118
8	166
9	190
10	83
11	44
12	144
13	112
14	25
15	122
16	30
17	88

Renal tubules

The histologic findings in renal tubules are summarized in Table 28.3. Cloudy swelling of the proximal convoluted tubules and dilatation of tubular lumen, especially the distal tubules, were rather common. Hydropic change was encountered in about half of the cases. Casts in the distal convoluted tubules,

Table 28.3 Histologic findings in tubules

Case no.	Proximal convoluted tubules				Distal convoluted tubules			Casts in Henle's loops & collecting tubules
	Cloudy swelling	Hydropic changes	Dilatation tubular lumen	Necrosis	Dilatation tubular lumen	Casts	Necrosis	
1	+	−	++	+	++	+	−	+
2	++	−	−	+	++	+	−	++
3	+	+	−	−	+	+	−	+
4	−	+++	−	−	+	+	+	+
5	++	++	+	+	+++	+	+	++
6	++	++	+	+	+++	+	−	−
7	++	−	−	−	+	+	−	+
8	++	−	−	+++	+	++	+	+
9	−	−	+	+	+	++	+	+
10	+	−	−	+	++	++	++	++
11	++	+	++	−	++	++	−	+
12	++	++	+	+	+	+	−	+
13	+	−	−	−	−	−	−	+
14	+	+++	++	+	+	+	+	−
15	−	+++	++	−	−	−	++	++
16	−	−	+	−	+	+	+	+
17	−	−	+	−	+	+	−	+

Henle's loops and collecting tubules were outstanding and often distended or/and blocked the tubules. There were two types of casts: (1) pigmented casts – brownish in color, coarsely or finely granular, and hemoglobin stain positive – and (2) hyaline casts. Tubular necroses occurring in both proximal and distal convoluted tubules were mild in degree and focal in distribution in most cases, but in a few cases they were rather severe and widespread.

Interstitium

Focal infiltration with lymphocytes, plasma cells and mononuclear cells were found in about half of the cases.

Electron microscopic findings

Glomeruli

The glomerular findings demonstrated under the light microscope were confirmed by electron microscopy. Enlarged capillary endothelial cells with increased amount of cytoplasm were found frequently. The number of organelles, especially rough endoplasmic reticulum (RER), increased in the enlarged endothelial cells. RER was arranged in whorled or fingerprint fashion

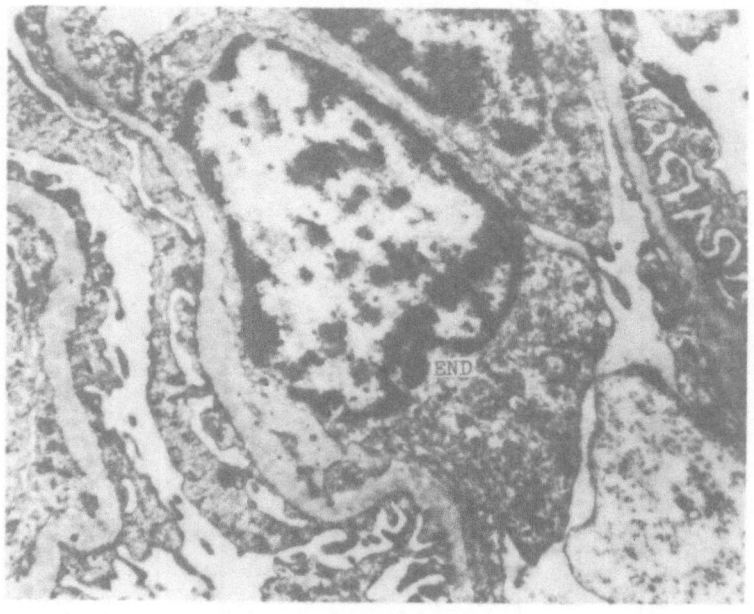

Figure 28.3 Glomerular capillary endothelial cell (END) becomes enlarged with increased amount of cytoplasm. Case No. 7, ×7000

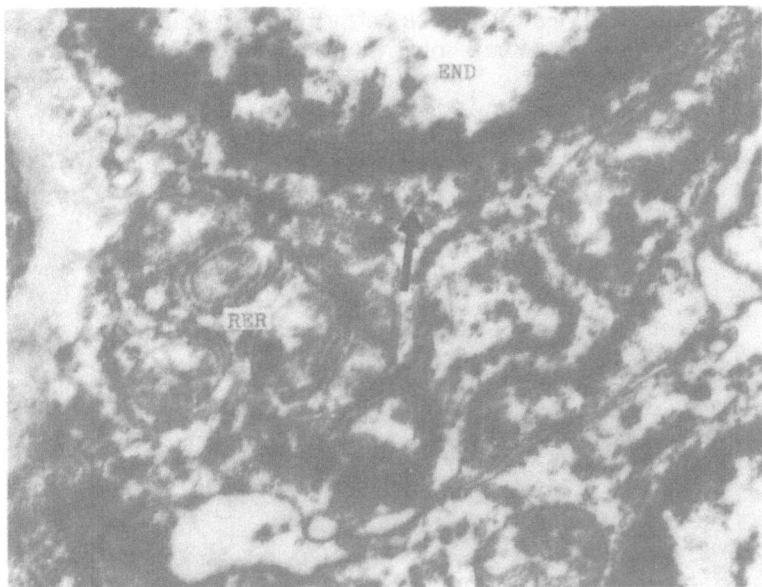

Figure 28.4 There occur hypertrophy of rough endoplasmic reticulum (RER), in whorled fashion, beneath the nucleus of endothelial cell. Free polysomes (arrow) probably increased. Figure 28.3 magnified × 21 000

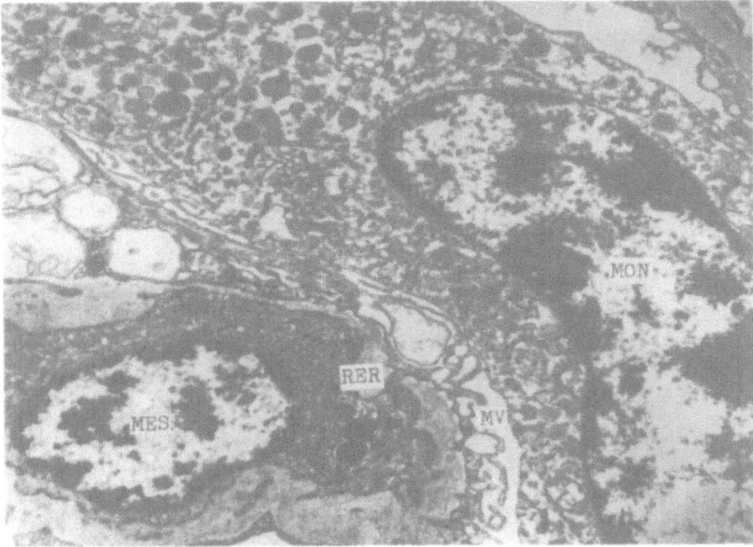

Figure 28.5 A monocyte (MON) is located in the capillary lumen, plasma membrane of endothelial cell shows microvilli formation (MV), mesangial cell (MES) endowed with well-developed RER. Case No. 15, × 7000

around the nucleus (Figures 28.3, 28.4). In some cases there were increases in free polyribosomes. Sometimes microvilli formed from plasma membrane of endothelial cells were found protruding into the capillary lumina which were usually already occupied by polymorphonuclear leukocytes or monocytes (Figure 28.5), and thus made the capillar lumina become narrowed or obliterated. In some cases endothelial cells revealed mitochondrial swelling and dilatation of RER. Occasionally, they became highly swollen, with formation of numerous vacuoles due to intracellular edema.

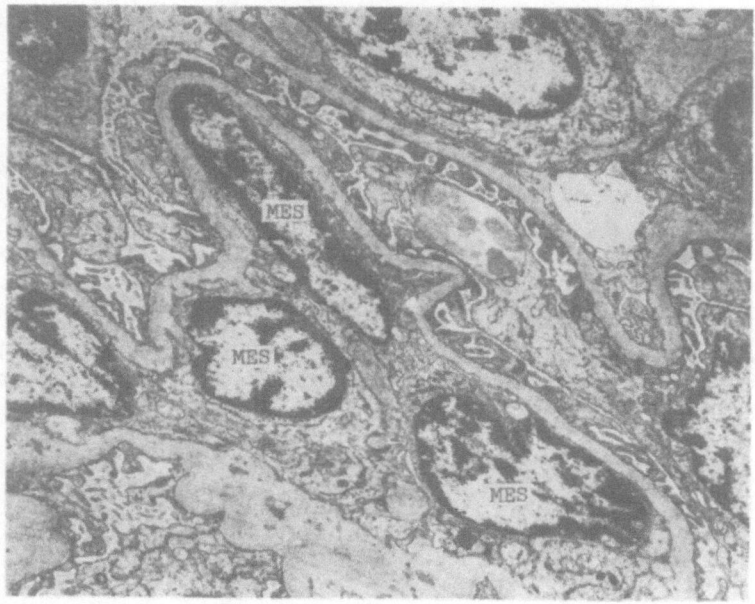

Figure 28.6   This electron micrograph shows hyperplasia of mesangial cells (MES). Case No. 5, ×4200

Mesangial areas were widened and associated with increased numbers of mesangial cells which also became hypertrophied with increased amounts of cytoplasm and well developed RER (Figures 28.6, 28.7). However, in some cases degenerative changes in mesangial cells such as mitochondrial swelling and dilatation of endoplasmic reticulum were revealed.

With the exception of two cases, the podocytes were essentially normal in this group of patients. In one case they showed high amplitude of swelling, manifesting mitochondrial swelling, dilatation of endoplasmic reticulum and formation of numerous vacuoles. In another case they were packed with numerous laminated membranous structures, i.e. myelin figures (Figure 28.8).

The parietal epithelial cells of Bowman's capsule revealed mitochondrial swelling, vacuole formation and distortion of nuclei due to compression of vacuoles.

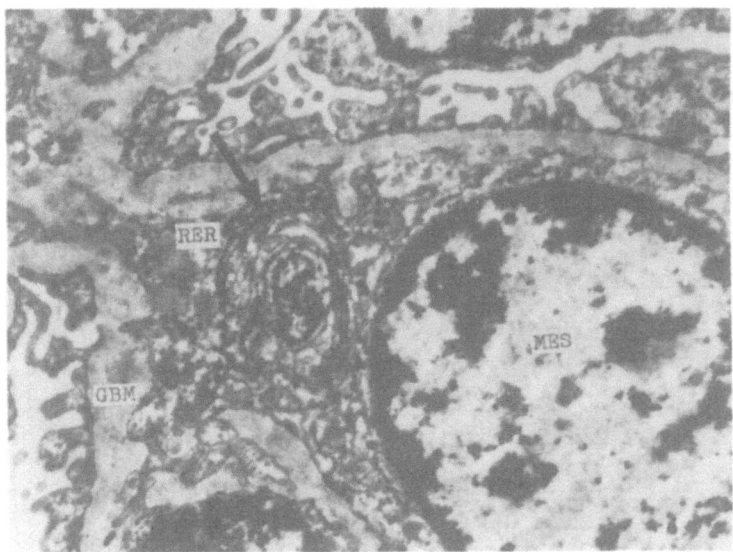

Figure 28.7 Mesangial cell (MES) exhibiting hypertrophy of RER, arranged in finger-print fashion (arrow). Case No. 7, × 14 000

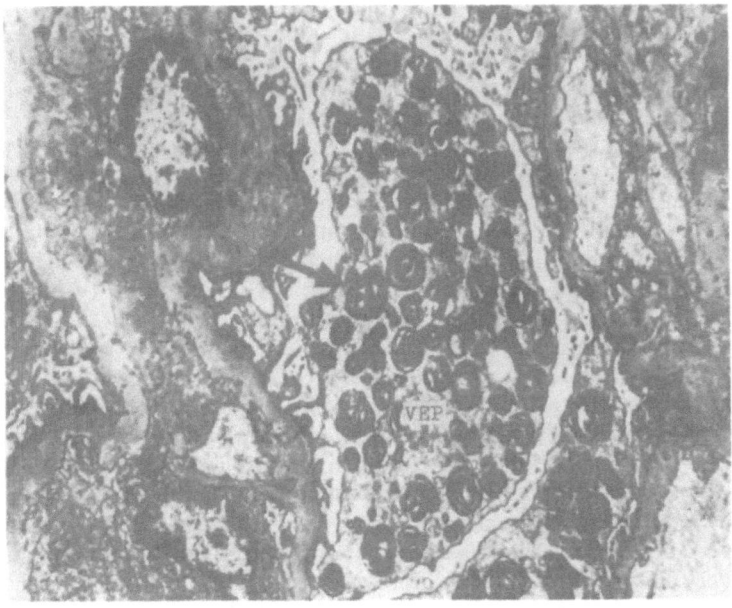

Figure 28.8 The cytoplasm of a podocyte is packed with numerous myelin figures. Case No. 6, × 5600

Renal tubules

The epithelial cells of the proximal convoluted tubules showed mitochondrial swelling and vacuolation. In most cases there were marked increases in lysosomes located just beneath the microvilli. In some cases hypertrophy of RER was demonstrated in the proximal tubules.

The epithelial cells of distal tubules also showed vacuolar degeneration, and in some cases revealed hypertrophy of RER.

DISCUSSION

In our present study, it is obvious that damage to the kidneys of severe burn patients involves not only the renal tubules but also the glomeruli, which further confirms our previous conceptions proposed by Dr Yan[5]. The glomeruli exhibited conspicuous and consistent morphologic changes characterized by (1) enlargement of capillary endothelial cells with increased amount of cytoplasm and hypertrophy of RER, (2) hyperplasia and hypertrophy of mesangial cells and (3) presence of polymorphonuclear leukocytes in the capillary lumina. Thus, capillary loops became narrowed or obliterated, resulting in glomerular ischemia. These changes are referred to as 'acute glomerulopathy'. The morphologic features of acute glomerulopathy are somewhat similar to those of acute proliferative glomerulonephritis. Acute proliferative glomerulonephritis is considered to be an immune complex disease and electron dense deposits could be found at the epithelial side of the glomerular basement membrane. Nevertheless, in the series in the present study, no such deposit was ever found.

The pathogenesis of postburn acute glomerulopathy is deferred. As postulated by one of the present authors[8], it might be a result of composite effects due to various factors, such as hypoxia, ischemia, or toxic materials, especially bacterial toxins; or the renal tissue might first be made attenuated by hypoxia or ischemia during the shock stage, then worsen or be damaged by bacterial toxins and toxic materials liberated from severe infection. Although immune complex deposit was not found in the pathologic sections of the present series, we are still not quite sure that an immunologic factor could be safely ruled out in the pathogenesis. This deserves further investigation. In the light of our morphologic study it is probable that cellular swelling[9,10] might be induced by hypoxia or ischemia; and mesangial cell proliferation, and hypertrophy of both mesangial and endothelial cells, especially hypertrophy of RER, might be looked upon as increased functional activity reacting to various noxious agents.

In order to explore the relationship between the histopathologic changes and renal dysfunction, and the actual role of glomerulopathy in the development of azotemia, we have correlated acute glomerulopathy and tubular necrosis with the occurrence of azotemia, as shown in Table 28.4.

There were ten cases revealing apparent acute glomerulopathy and tubular necrosis of various degrees simultaneously, and all of them developed azotemia. There were four cases with acute glomerulopathy of mild to moderate degree without tubular necrosis, and three of these developed azotemia. There were two cases with moderate tubular but mild glomerular lesions, and one case with mild acute glomerulopathy only, and none of these had azotemia. It seems probable

Table 28.4 Correlations of glomerular and tubular lesions with occurrence of azotemia

Total no. cases	Acute glomerulopathy	Tubular necrosis	Azotemia (cases)	No azotemia (cases)
10	+-+++	+-+++	10	0
4	+-++	-	3	1
2	±	+-++	0	2
1	±	-	0	1

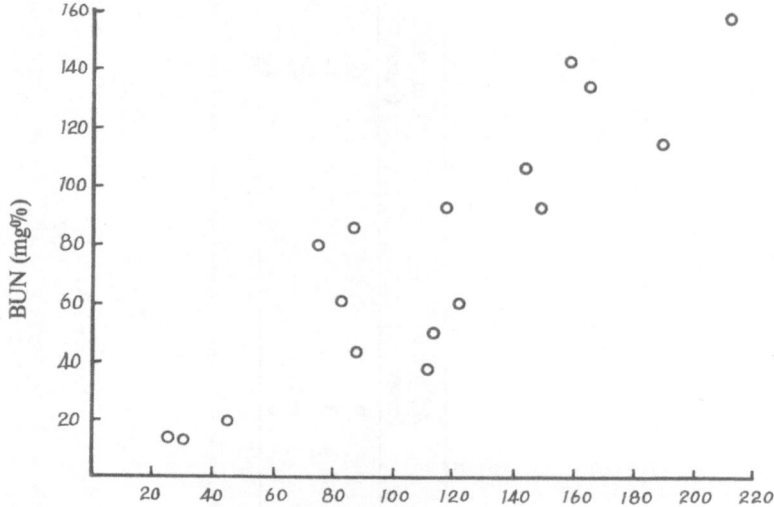

Figure 28.9 Scatter diagram of glomerulopathy scores vs BUN level

that acute glomerulopathy plays a more important role than tubular necrosis in the development of azotemia or renal insufficiency.

Furthermore, for the purpose of ascertaining the relationship between the degree of acute glomerulopathy and severity of azotemia, scatter diagrams were made by using final scores of glomerulopathy as abscissa and blood urea or plasma creatinine (p Cr) level as ordinate.

With the aid of rank correlation method it was found that a positive correlation exists between glomerulopathy and BUN or p Cr level, that is to say, increase in either BUN or p Cr level is parallel to the degree of acute

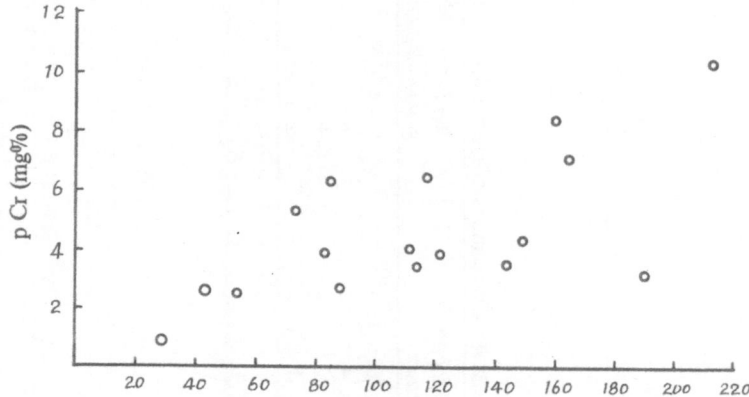

Figure 28.10 Scatter diagram of glomerulopathy scores vs plasma creatinine (p Cr) level

glomerulopathy (Figures 28.9, 28.10). It was further clarified that the occurrence of azotemia is mainly caused by glomerulopathy resulting in a fall in the glomerular filtration rate.

It must be pointed out that the renal lesions, especially tubular lesions, as shown in Table 28.3, are frequent findings in severely burned patients. However, the development of renal dysfunction depends upon the degree and extent of glomerular lesions. If the glomerular lesions are rather mild or focal, renal functional derangement may not occur because of the kidney's high compensatory power.

REFERENCES

1. Lucké, C. B. (1946). Lower nephron nephrosis. *Mil. Surg.*, **99**, 371
2. Oliver, J. (1953). Correlation of structure and function and mechanism of recovery in acute tubular necrosis. *Am. J. Med.*, **15**, 535
3. Sevitt, S. (1956). Distal tubular and proximal tubular necrosis in the kidneys of burned patients. *J. Clin. Pathol.*, **9**, 279
4. Graber, I. G. and Sevitt, S. (1959). Renal function in burned patients and its relationships to morphological changes. *J. Clin. Pathol.*, **12**, 25
5. Yan, S. N. *et al.* (1960). Patho-morphological study of the kidneys and its relationship to renal dysfunction in 24 burned patients. Paper presented at *Symposion on Burns, The 7th Military Medical College, Chongqing*
6. Artz, C. T. *et al.* (1979). *Burns.* p. 48. (Philadelphia: Saunders)
7. Trump, B. F. *et al.* (1973). Cellular change in human disease. *Hum. Pathol.*, **4**, 89
8. Li Ao *et al.* (1974). Acute nephropathy following burn sepsis – A restudy. In *Proceedings of the National Military Burns Seminar, the Treatment and Research in Burns.* p. 173
9. Summers, W. K. *et al.* (1971). The no reflow phenomenon in renal ischemia. *Lab. Invest.*, **25**, 635
10. Johnston, W. H. *et al.* (1977). Glomerular mesangial and endothelial cell swelling following temporary renal ischemia and its role in the no-reflow phenomenon. *Am. J. Pathol.*, **89**, 153

29 Changes in Cardiac Contractility in Burn Shock

CHEN ZHOUDAO, FU WIJUN, YANG YUMING, CHEN JIANGUO and LU ZHENDONG
Department of Physiology
YU KEDA
Department of Bioelectronics, Second Military Medical College, Shanghai

Based on the evidence obtained from experiments on myocardial mechanics, some investigators[1] have proposed taking the following indices as measures for the contractility of the intact heart, since these may be relatively less influenced by the factors before and after load on the heart: (1) the maximum rate of change in the left intraventricular pressure (expressed as dp/dt max.), (2) the ratio of dp/dt to the value of the instantaneous left intraventricular pressure (as $(dp/dt)/p$) and (3) the left intraventricular pressure–rate of pressure change loop ($p - (dp/dt)$ loop, or simply 'cardiac force loop'). These indices have been used widely in the investigation of hemorrhagic, toxic as well as traumatic, shock[2] and also in acute hypoxic tolerance of the heart[3] to measure the condition of cardiac involvement. But in burn shock, most of the investigators evaluated the functional condition of the heart by determining the cardiac output and calculating the heart work[4-6], and few of them approached this problem through direct measurement of the cardiac contractility on the basis of myocardial mechanics. In the work reported in this chapter, the cardiac contractility of dogs during the course of their burn shock was estimated by measuring and calculating their first derivatives of the left intraventricular pressure, the velocity of shortening of the contractile elements of the myocardium (VCE) and the left intraventricular pressure – the rate of pressure change loop ($p - (dp/dt)$ loop).

METHODS

Experiments were performed on 15 mongrel dogs of both sexes, weighing 9.3–14.7 kg. Under intravenous anesthesia (sodium pentobarbital 30 mg/kg), the dog was intubated and artificial ventilation was instituted by a Starling respirator. Left thoracotomy was done through the fifth intercostal space, the heart was partially exposed and an F6 lucite catheter was introduced into the left ventricle by punching the apex of the heart. The intracardiac catheter was connected to an arterial transducer (Mpu 0.5, Nihon Kohden). Parameters were measured and processed by a polygraph (RM 46 Nihon Kohden). In the meantime, the signals from the carrier amplifier and from the processor (time constant 1.0 ms, high frequency filter 50 Hz) were connected respectively to the X and Y terminals to display the $p - (dp/dt)$ loop. After these procedures, the pericardium was sutured in place and the chest wall closed. Thirty minutes after the withdrawal of the artificial respiration, the animal regained its spontaneous respiration with normal amplitude and rhythm. Experiments started.

Eight animals were grouped as the experimental group and the other seven as controls. The shoulder girdle, the back and the gluteal regions were shaved and were burned with a 5000 W bromotungsten lamp. A third degree burn wound of 40% of the BSA was thus produced. Records were taken just after the burn and every 30 min afterward, until the death of the animal. The animals of the control group were treated similarly except no burn was inflicted; records for controls were taken every 30 min through a period of 12 h. The data were treated statistically.

RESULTS

The animals of the experimental group died within 4–5 h after the burn, and all those of the control group survived within 12 h. The cardiac involvements of the animals were as follows.

(1)   The peak values of the left intraventricular pressure (LVSP) of the control animals were maintained at the level of 125–150 mmHg with mild drift.

The LVSP of the experimental animals showed an initial slight elevation followed by a sharp drop. At the end of the second postburn hour it fell to about 80% of the preburn level. At the end of the fourth postburn hour it fell to about 59%. The LVSP of the experimental animals was read as 84 mmHg when the animal showed the signs of shock. However, at the same instant, the LVSP of the control animals remained high, at 145 mmHg. The difference in LVSP value of the controls and the experimental animals, at the end of the second postburn hour, was very significant ($p < 0.01$) (Figure 29.1).

(2)   The maximum rate of change in the left intraventricular pressure (dp/dt max.) of the control group dropped from 4100 mmHg/s to 3100 mmHg/s, through the entire course of observation of 12 h. The average rate of reduction in dp/dt max. value was approximately 80 mmHg/s.

In contrast to the control group, the rate of reduction in the value of dp/dt max. in the experimental animals was prominent, showing an average of 500 mmHg/s. The values of dp/dt max. at the end of the second and fifth postburn hours had been reduced to about 67% and 35% of the preburn level. The difference between the experimental animals and controls was very significant ($p < 0.01$). The dp/dt max. of the experimental animals dropped to 1332 mmHg/s, while that of the controls was maintained at 3757 mmHg/s at the fifth postburn hour, which was about twice the former level (Figures 29.2, 29.3).

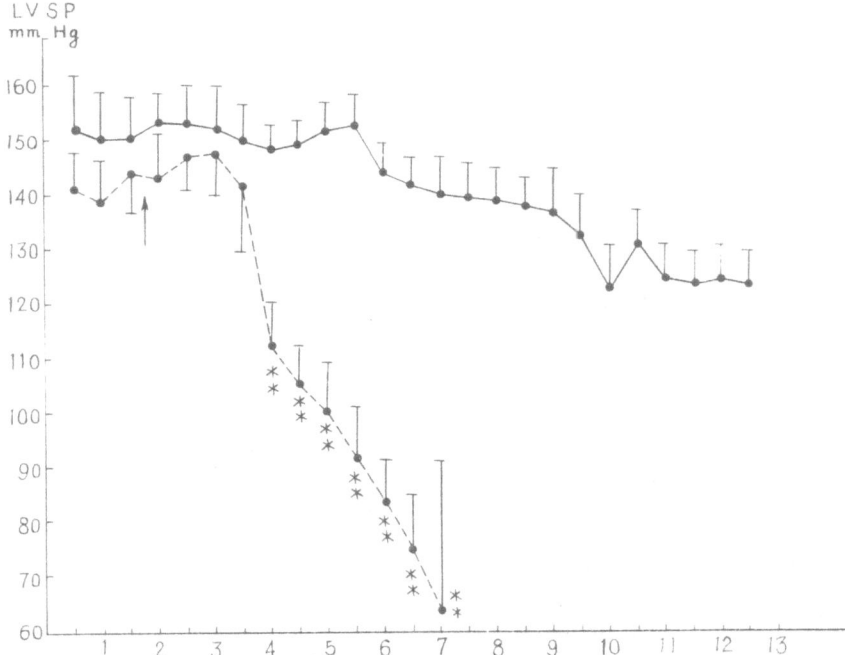

Figure 29.1 Changes of the left ventricular systolic pressure of the experimental dogs.
_____ = Control (mean ± SEM); - - - -= burn (mean ± SEM); * = p<0.05; ** = p<0.01

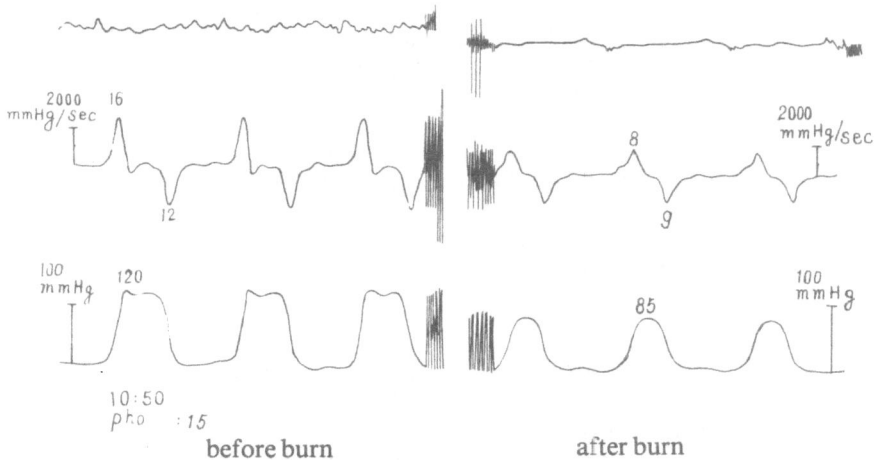

Figure 29.2 Left ventricular pressure recorded and *dp/dt* max. change during pre- and
postburn periods. Top: ECG tracings; middle: *dp/dt* ; bottom: left ventricular pressure

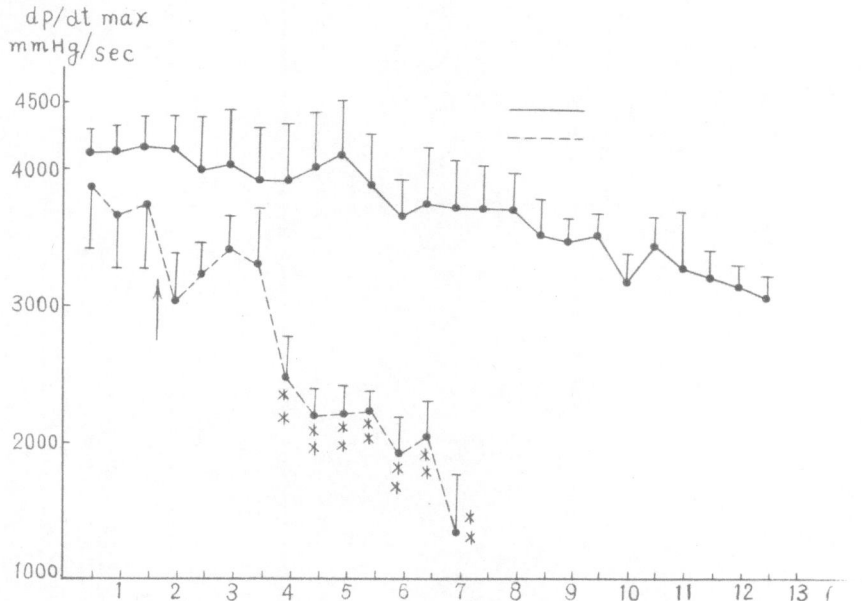

Figure 29.3 Changes of *dp/dt* max. of the experimental dogs. _____ = Control (mean ± SEM): - - - - = burn (mean ± SEM); * = $p<0.05$; ** = $p<0.01$

(3) The third item we observed was the ratio of maximum rate of change in the left intraventricular pressure to the instantaneous left intraventricular pressure, or the isovolumic instantaneous pressure (IP) (*dp/dt* max./IP). It was believed that the value of *dp/dt* max./IP is less influenced by the factors before and after loads on the contractility of myocardium. So it was taken as a better index to express the actual contractility of the heart, also known as VCE or the index of contractility.

In the control group, the *dp/dt* max./IP value was maintained at approximately 40/s during the period of the first 8 h and was relatively stable. In the experimental group, on the other hand, the *dp/dt* max./IP value varied markedly in the initial stage after burn. It quickly dropped within 2½ h to about 30/s, which was approximately 80% of its preburn value, and maintained this low level. The difference between these two groups was marked ($p<0.05$) (Figure 29.4).

(4) By the expression of the cardiac force loop (*p* - (*dp/dt*) loop), the strength (*p*) and the velocity of force development (*dp/dt*) of the heart during the cardiac cycle was displayed graphically as a loop to reflect the characteristics of the pumping efficiency of the heart. The areas within the extent of the loop (L_0) and of the different phases (L_1–L_4) were measured and calculated. They were expressed arbitrarily in units.

In the control group, the L_0 values were relatively stable, being maintained within the range of 80–90 units in the initial stage of the experi-

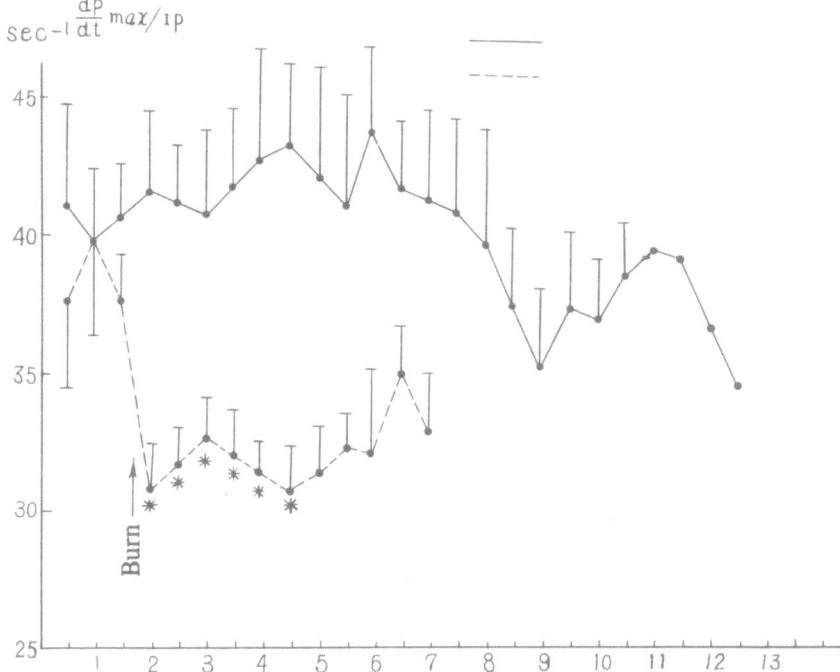

Figure 29.4 Changes of *dp/dt* max./IP of the burned dogs. _____ = Control (mean ± SEM): - - - - = burn (mean ± SEM); * = $p < 0.05$; ** = $p < 0.01$

ment, then fell gradually. In the experimental group, the value of L_0 showed an initial elevation of 10 units and then followed by a depression, appearing as a diphasic curve. The elevation stage lasted about $1\frac{1}{2}$ h and the depression stage about 3 h. During the depression stage, L_0 dropped

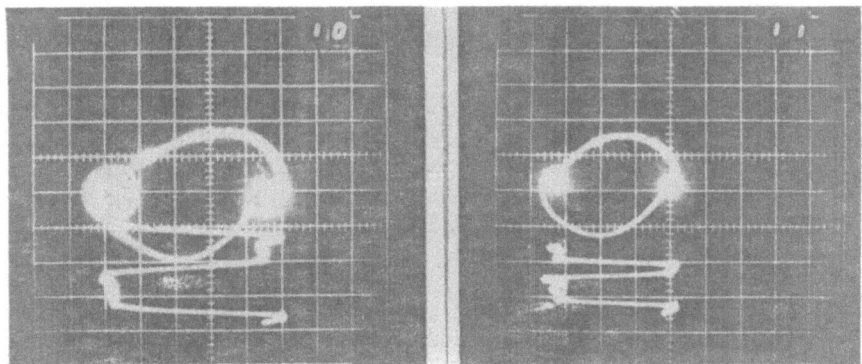

Figure 29.5 Recorded $p - (dp/dt)$ loop change before and after burn

sharply to the values of 30–40 units, which correspond to 45–84% of the
original. However, in the control group, the L_0 value dropped to 79–84%
of the original only. Beginning from the second hour postburn, the area
measured of the cardiac force loop (L_0) decreased significantly ($p < 0.01$)
(Figures 29.5, 29.6).

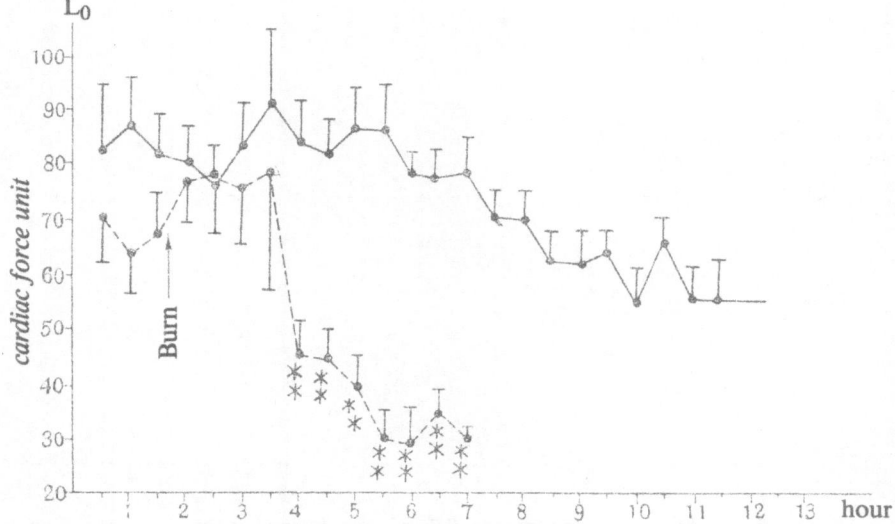

Figure 29.6 Changes of $p - dp/dt$ loop (L_0) of burned dogs. _____ = Control
(mean ± SEM); – – – – – = burn (mean ± SEM); ** = $p < 0.01$

The areas of L_1–L_4 showed corresponding changes. The changes in the
areas L_1, L_2 and L_4 were parallel to L_0. Moreover, they showed a diphasic
pattern (elevation followed by depression). The elevation was most
prominent in L_4, in which it elevated to the extent of 10 units.

L_1 corresponded to the isovolumic contraction of the ventricle (Figure
29.7).

(5) There was usually increase in heart rate after burn. During the first
30 min–1½ h after the burn, the heart rate increased from the original value
of 190/min to 220/min, which differed markedly from the control group
($p < 0.05$). The rapid heart rate continued throughout the whole course of
the experiment till the animal died.

DISCUSSION

Extensive burns usually induce multiple organ systems to fail, including the
cardiovascular system. A study on this problem was carried out by measuring

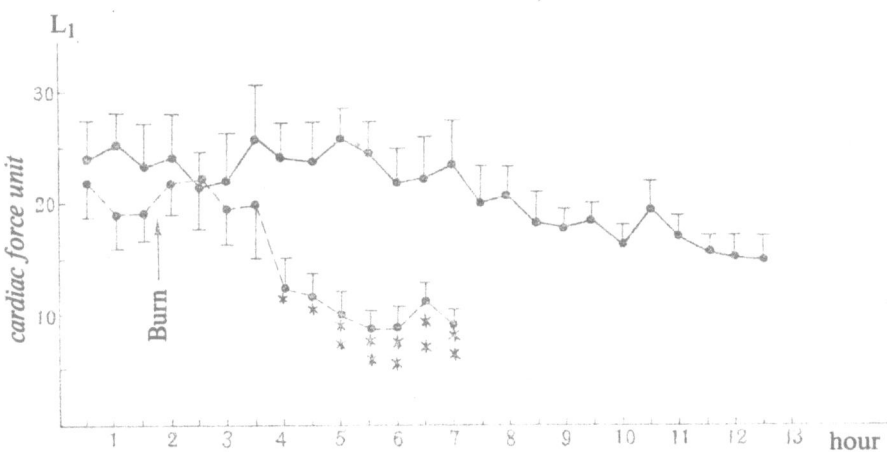

Figure 29.7 Changes of p - dp/dt loop (L_1) of burned dogs. _____ = Control (mean ± SEM);- - - - - burn (mean ± SEM); * = $p < 0.05$; ** = $p < 0.01$

and calculating the postburn myocardial contractility directly. We have found that at the first hour postburn, all the indices of myocardial contractility such as LVSP, dp/dt max., L_0 and L_1–L_4 exhibited a transient elevation. Probably, all of the changes in these indices were produced by an overall action of the sympathetic nervous system, after which a period of depression ensued. The reduction in value of dp/dt max., L_1 and L_0 implied that there happened to be a reduction in myocardial contractility during the isovolumic phase of the cardiac cycle. In 1973, Shtykhno et al.[7] measured the dp/dt of the left intraventricular pressure of a burned rabbit. However, they determined the changes of the first hour and the 24th hour only. We suppose they might not have caught the right time to reflect the actual cardiac involvement following severe burns.

Since the change in dp/dt max./IP preceded the decrease in LVSP and the signs of shock, taking this parameter as an index may exclude the influences before and after loads on the function of the myocardium. Probably, in addition to the peripheral resistance and the circulatory blood volume, the changes in myocardial contractility might play an important role in the development of burn shock, but also reflect a more sensitive index of the early myocardial change in burn shock. During the late stage of burn shock, the value of dp/dt max./IP rose slightly. The mechanism of this paradoxical result seemed to be that the magnitude of drops of intraventricular pressure during the isovolumic stage exceeded that of dp/dt max.

The pumping action of the heart was affected by the blood volume, the right heart filling, the peripheral resistance and the contractility of the myocardium. The last factor was reevaluated in the present study. Our work together with Vornovitsky's performance[8] on isolated papillary muscle of the rabbit heart showed that the cardiac contractility in burn shock was markedly impaired.

We also found that the reduction in dp/dt max. and L_4 might be considered as the early signs of burn shock. In the early stage of cardiac involvement, both the contractility of the heart and the nature of diastole were affected to a certain degree.

According to some investigators[9], there is evidence that the value of dp/dt max. is influenced by the heart rate. The faster the heart rates the larger the magnitudes of dp/dt max. and vice versa. Thus the inotropic factor might be overshadowed by a chronotropic one. In the present work, with the increase in heart rate, we did find the appearance of negative inotropic effects such as lowering of the dp/dt max. and the dwindling of force loop, which implied that the reduction in contractility of the heart was not due to the influence of negative chronotropic effect of the heart.

REFERENCES

1. Mason, D. T., Spann, J. F. Jr. and Zelis, R. (1970). Quantification of the contractile state of the intact human heart. *Am. J. Cardiol.*, **26**, 248–57
2. Brückner, J. B. *Kreislaufschock*. pp. 275–84, 359–72. (Berlin, Heidelberg, New York: Springer)
3. Hu Xu-chu, Ning Xue-han *et al.* (1978). Studies on acute hypoxic tolerance of the heart. *Acta Physiol.*, **30**(1), 29–39. (In Chinese)
4. Birke, G., Liljedahl, S.-O. and Linderholm, H. (1959). Studies on burns. V. Clinical and patho-physiological aspects on circulation and respiration. *Acta. Chir. Scand.*, **116**, 370–94
5. Fang Zhi-yang, Ge Sheng-de *et al.* (1979). Hemodynamics, hemorrheologic changes and disseminated intravascular coagulation at the shock stage in burned dogs. In *The Treatment and Research in Burns. Proceedings of The National Burns Seminar.* pp. 227–31. (In Chinese)
6. Yuan Shu-nan, Jiang Kun-yuan, Li Ao *et al.* Effects of some drugs on hemodynamics in severely burned patients at the early stage. *Symposium on Burns. The Third Military Medical College of the PLA, Chongqing.* pp. 178–88. (In Chinese)
7. Shtykhno, Y. M. and Markovskaya, G. I. (1973). Effect of thermal injury on the contractile function of rabbit heart. *Patho-Physiol. Exp. Ther.*, **3**, 64–6
8. Vornovitsky, E. G., Lenkova, N. A. and Vasilets, L. A. (1979). Changes in the contractile activity of the rabbit myocardium during burn shock. *Bull. Exp. Biol. Med.*, **87**(1), 6–8
9. Andrew, G., Wallace, N., Skinner, S. Jr. and Mitchell, J. H. (1963). Hemodynamic determinants of the max.dp/dt of the left ventricular pressure. *Am. J. Physiol.*, **205**, 30–6

30 Successful Treatment for Two Extensive Third Degree Burn Patients

XU FENGXUN
Burn Unit, Changhai Hospital, The Second Military Medical College, Shanghai

MA YUANZHANG
Juzhou Chemical Industry Hospital, Zhejiang

PU SUSONG
Burn Unit, The Second Teaching Hospital, Zhejiang Medical College

---

Treatment for third degree burns exceeding 90% of the BSA remains a very difficult problem. Only a few papers concerning the successful treatment of such patients have been published and only eight survivors have been reported. They are documented exclusively in the Chinese medical literature[1-5]. In the present chapter, we report two more cases. They were injured by the explosion of a boiler in May 1981.

HISTORY AND TREATMENT

Case 1

A male, 19 years old, weighing 60 kg, sustained an extensive burn of 100% of the TBSA including 92% third degree (Figure 30.1). He was complicated by moderate inhalation injury and a brain contusion with coma and hemiplegia of the right side (Figure 30.2). At admission, the patient was in a state of shock with a blood pressure of 76/44 mmHg and a pulse rate of 56/min. Cathetered urine revealed hemoglobinuria. Fluid resuscitation was instituted immediately. The blood pressure was soon brought up after a rapid infusion of 1000 ml of balanced electrolyte solution. Hemoglobinuria was gradually cleared up 24 h after the burn. The patient had experienced an uneventful shock stage (Table 30.1). Severe diarrhea occurred on the ninth postburn day, and continued for 7 days with an average of ten bowel movements daily. Bacterial culture of the mucous watery stool showed a growth of *Staphylococcus albus*; no *Escherichia coli* was found. The diarrhea gradually reduced after several retention enemas with *E. coli* isolated from normal children's stool. Except on the lower extremities, the third degree burned eschar of the trunk was excised and the wounds were covered with intermingled allo/autografts. Both arms were

233

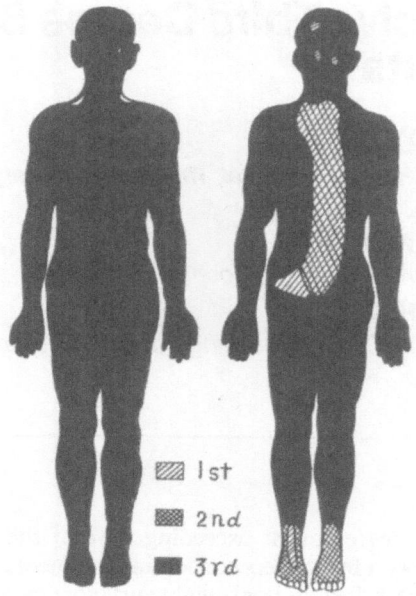

Figure 30.1   Diagram of BSA burned in Case 1

amputated because of dry gangrene. The patient gradually regained consciousness on the 21st postburn day. Intravenous fluid administration and antibiotic therapy were withdrawn on the 36th postburn day.

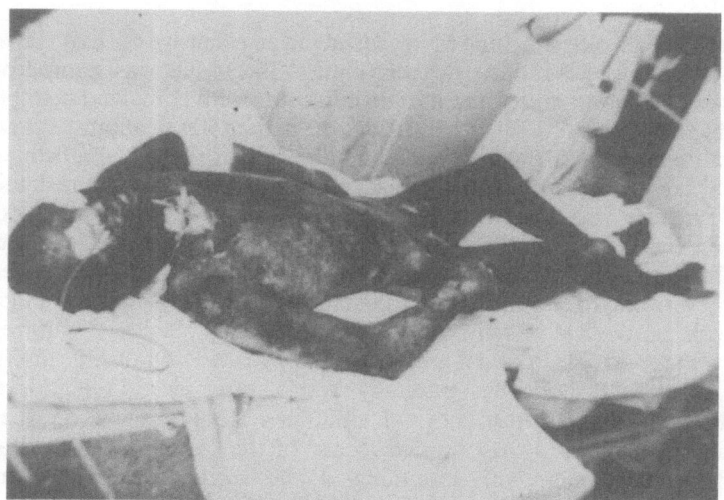

Figure 30.2   Case 1

Table 30.1 Fluid therapy and urine output of the first 72 hours

		Colloid					Electrolyte									Fluid intake/ urine output
Case	Time	Blood	Plasma	Dextran	Human albumin	Ringer's solution	5% Glucose in normal saline	Balanced electrolyte solution	5% Sodium bicarbonate	Water per os	20% Mannitol	Total	Colloid/ electrolyte	Urine	Urine/h	
1	1st 24 h	1610	400	1000			1600	1000	720	2870	750	9950	1:110	1985	83	5:1
	2nd 24 h	800	800				2250		600	1680	1000	7105	1:176	4610	192	1.5:1
	3rd 24 h	800	400		20		1600		200	2750		5770	1:148	4795	200	1.2:1
2	1st 24 h	1220	400	1000			1350	1000	920	1780	750	8570	1:12	2135	88.9	4:1
	2nd 24 h	400	800			150	1675		400	1620	350	5245	1:139	2645	151.9	1.43:1
	3rd 24 h	400	800		20		1350		200	2570		5340	1:123	2130	88.7	2.55:1

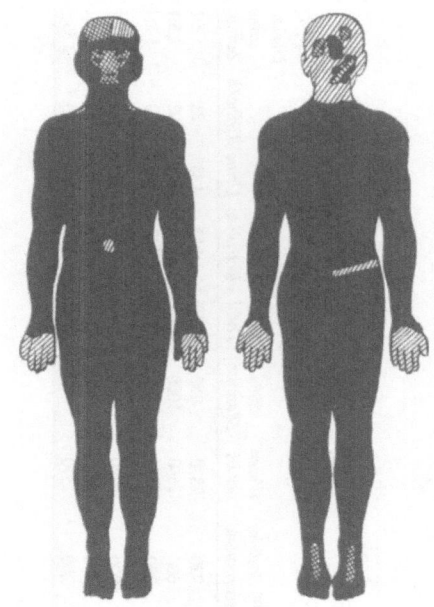

Figure 30.3   Diagram of BSA burned in Case 2

Case 2

A male, 18 years old, weighing 56 kg, sustained an extensive burn of 100% of the TBSA including 94.5% third degree (Figure 30.3). There was moderate inhalation injury (Figure 30.4). The patient was also in a state of shock at the time of

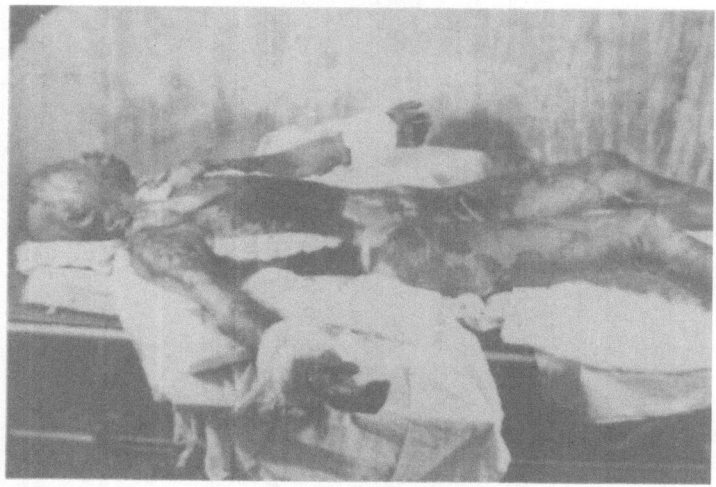

Figure 30.4   Case 2

admission with a rapid pulse of 142/min and unobtainable blood pressure. Rapid infusion of 1000 ml of balanced electrolyte solution brought back an audible normal blood pressure. His shock stage was smooth. The hemoglobinuria both enterally and parenterally gradually cleared up 7 h after the burn (Table 30.1). This patient tolerated energetic nutritional support. Parenteral fluid and antibiotic therapy were discontinued on the 21st postburn day. The wound treatment for these two cases was as follows.

Treatment of burn wounds

Burn wounds were treated by exposure in a dry warm environment. Most parts of the third degree burns (70% of the TBSA in Case 1 and 71% in Case 2) were treated with early escharectomy (Table 30.2). The surgical wound was covered with large sheets of fresh allograft or glutaraldehyde treated allograft. Small autografts, 0.3×0.3 cm in size, were inserted into holes punctured 1 cm apart in the fresh allograft 48 h later. The glutaraldehyde treated allografts were removed at a suitable moment and were replaced by autografts which achieved a 100% take in the glutaraldehyde covered area. A little more than 20% BSA of the eschar was naturally separated. The granulating wounds were grafted as the eschar was separated. Pathogenic microorganisms isolated from the wounds of both cases were quite similar – *Bacterium anitratum*, *E. coli*, and *S. albus*. No *Pseudomonas aeruginosa* or *Staphylococcus aureus* was found in a total of 126 bacterial cultures.

The devitalized cortex of the tibia was chiseled and covered with glutaraldehyde-treated allograft 90 days after the burn.

The first crop of autograft was obtained from the second degree burn wound.

Table 30.2 Escharectomy and allografting

Case	Day postburn	Escharectomy Site	Area	Skin graft types
1	5	Chest, abdomen	16	Fresh allograft
	7	Both upper extremities	20	Fresh allograft
	10	Left thigh	10	Fresh allograft
	10	Left leg	7	Glutaraldehyde treated allograft
	15	Right lower extremity	17	Fresh allograft
	Total		70	
2	4	Chest, abdomen, right upper extremity	22	Fresh allograft
	6	Back and waist	8	Fresh allograft
	9	Left upper extremity	7	Glutaraldehyde treated allograft
	12	Right lower extremity	17	Fresh allograft
	14	Left lower extremity	17	Fresh allograft
	Total		71	

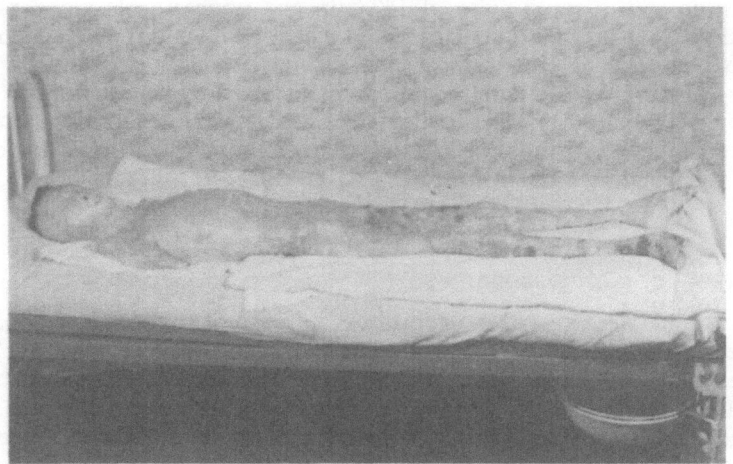

Figure 30.5   Case 1. Two months after burns

In Case 1, the waist donated its skin 7 days postburn, and the second crop was obtained from the same site 10 days later. In Case 2, the scalp was used as the donor site 7 days postburn, and the second crop was taken from the same site 10 days later. The graft take was about 85% (Figures 30.5, 30.6).

Nutritional support in the early postburn period relied mainly on the intravenous route, and was gradually replaced by nasogastric feeding of element diets. Oral intake increased to 12–21/MJ (3000–5000 kcal), with about 200 g protein, from the 15th–20th postburn days.

Although blood cultures showed negative results, six positive cultures from the intravenous catheter tips were found. The pathogenic bacteria revealed coincided well with the bacteria isolated from the wound.

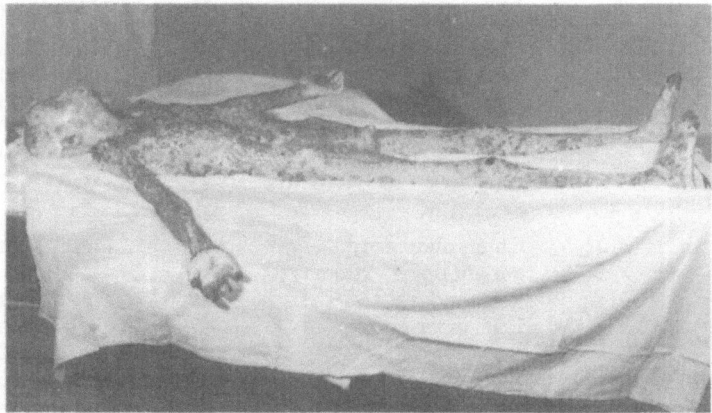

Figure 30.6   Case 2. Two months after burns

REFERENCES

1. Yang, C. C., Shi, T. S. *et al.* (1980). The intermingled transplantation of auto- and homografts in severe burns. *Burns*, **6**, 141
2. Mu Xue-xia *et al.* (1980). Successful management of a patient with 96% TBSA burned (90% BSA of third degree). *Acta Acad. Med. 2nd Mil. Med. Coll. Shanghai*, **1**(3); 70
3. Shih, T. S., Yang, C. C. *et al.* (1979). Guerison de quatre brûlures du 3e degré à plus de 90% de surface corporelle. *J. Chir. (Paris)*, **105**, 738–41
4. Wang Chang-yeh *et al.* (1979). Surgical excision in the treatment of extensive burns. *Symposium on Burns. The Third Military Med College of the PLA, Chongqing.* p. 462. (In Chinese)
5. Burn Unit, Shandong People's Hospital (1978). Successful treatment for a patient who sustained an extensive burn of 95% TBSA with 90% BSA of third degree. *Proceedings of the 9th National Surgical Congress.* p. 56. (Abstract) (In Chinese)

31 Massive Excision and Intermingled Transplantation in the Treatment of Extensive Third Degree Burns

SHIH TSISIANG, YANG CHIHCHUN, HSU WEISHI, WU SHIXIANG, XU WEIZHEN, LIU YUELIANG, XU DACHONG, LIAO ZHENGJIANG, LI BINGGUO, GU XIMING and CAO QI-DONG

Burn Unit, Rui Jin Hospital, Shanghai Second Medical College, Shanghai

INTRODUCTION

With the improvement of modern fluid resuscitation and initial care techniques, most severely burned patients will be able to survive the early phase uneventfully. Nevertheless, after successful resuscitation they may inevitably succumb to heavy protracted wound sepsis and extreme malnutrition sooner or later[1].

In the past two decades with the introduction of mafenide (Sulfamylon), silver sulfadiazine and other topical agents for the local treatment of burns, it became evident that effective topical agents, properly used, have significantly reduced morbidity and mortality[2]. However, burn wound sepsis is still a major problem in the patients with full-thickness burns of more than 50% of body surface area. In our study, mortality from burn injury, although related to the extent of burn area, was much more correlated with the amount of the body surface area affected by third degree burns. In patients with extensive full-thickness burns, the incidence of infection is not decreasing, and wound sepsis remains the major cause of morbidity and death in these patients. The reason is that the massive nonviable tissue not only serves as a favorite culture medium for microorganisms to proliferate, but also results in severe metabolic disturbances and marked depletion of host resistance[3-6].

Excision of the nonviable tissue followed by immediate closure of the wound with autografts and/or xenografts used as temporary wound dressings appears to be the only rational approach to the problem of this type of burn. There is little doubt that this method of treatment has made substantial contributions to the care of severely burned patients[7-8]. The main obstacle to this approach is that in large full-thickness burns, after removal of the eschar and allografting, definitive permanent and ultimate restoration of the integument must be accomplished by the patient's own skin, but the paucity of donor sites on a patient with extensive full-thickness burns limits its use[9].

In the early 1960s, inspired by the work of Mowlem and Jackson[10-12], we began to use a bricklaying pattern of autografts and allografts to cover the large excised wound. Later, in order to further economize the patient's own scarce skin, we began to use large sheets of allografts with punch holes in which small autografts were inlaid as a lifesaving measure. The results were encouraging. From May 1966 to 1978 the LA_{50} of third degree burns rose from 31.28% to 49.28%, which indicated an improvement achieved in the care of patients with extensive third degree burns[13]. This method, termed intermingled transplantation of auto- and allo- or xenografts, together with escharectomy, has been adopted as a routine treatment of extensive deep burns in China with satisfactory results. Although patients with third degree burns of 50% BSA might have a consistent survival rate of about 50%, those with third degree burns over 70% would have a much higher mortality[14]. The present study is devoted to evaluating this method of treatment applied to the patient group comprising those with a full-thickness burn exceeding 70% of the BSA.

CLINICAL MATERIAL AND METHODS

From January 1966 through December 1983, 96 patients with third degree burns of more than 70% of the BSA were admitted and treated at the Burn Unit, Rui Jin Hospital, Shanghai. The case records of these patients were reviewed. All patients reaching the Burn Unit alive were included. There were 76 males and 20 females, their ages ranging from 5 years to over 60 years. The mean TBSA was $93.8 \pm 5.79\%$ (range 72–100%); the mean full-thickness burn was $84.31 \pm 8.57\%$ (range 70–100%).

A protocol was proposed that early massive excision and intermingled grafting, as a method of choice, were used whenever possible for the management of these patients in order to lessen the mortality. Among the 96 patients, there were 12 children and a man over 60 years old; and they all died, including four children in whom excision operations had been carried out. Eighty-three adult patients were divided into two groups (Table 31.1). The first group comprised 28 nonoperated patients, 24 males and four females, the mean TBSA was $94.29 \pm 5.52\%$ and the mean third degree burns was $84.70 \pm 9.15\%$.

Table 31.1 Average BSA burned and extent of third degree burns in adult patients with and without excisional operation

	Cases (n)	Average BSA burned (%)	Average BSA with III° burns (%)
Patients without excision	28	94.29 ± 5.25	84.70 ± 9.15
Patients with excision	55	93.97 ± 5.58	83.64 ± 8.35

The second group comprised 55 patients, in whom the excision and inter-mingled grafting were carried out. There were 43 males and 12 females, the mean TBSA was $93.97 \pm 5.58\%$, and the mean third degree burns was $83.64 \pm 8.35\%$.

TECHNIQUES

The treatment of eschar consisted of staged excision and large sheets of allo- and/or xenografting followed by inlaying of small patches of autograft into the premade holes in the allo- and/or xenografts. Excision was done down to the fascia in all patients. In the majority of cases, the time of the first excision was within 10 days postburn, ranging from the fourth to the 23rd day after injury.

The area excised was 3–45% of the BSA per operation. The largest area excised in one patient was 65% of the BSA. The interval between two operations was usually about 3 days. As a rule, eschar excision was not performed at the end of the third week postburn, because at that time the natural separation of the eschar would have begun. After the spontaneous separation of eschar, a patchwork-grafting of small autografts and larger allografts or xenografts on the granulating wounds was needed in all cases.

Allografting and xenografting

Fresh allografts were preferred when available. Frozen allografts and fresh porcine skin were the second choice.

Autografting

In all patients the scalp was used as the donor site. The sole and even the palm were used when no other donor site was available in very severe cases. Four to six recroppings of the same donor area were often necessary.

RESULTS

Of the 96 patients, 79 died, an overall mortality of 82.3%. All the patients under the age of 14 and over the age of 60 in this series died, including four children in whom excisional operations had been carried out. Most of the children died within the first week after the burn. Shock, acute renal failure and acute fulminating septicemia were the common causes of death. Four children who died of wound sepsis on the 23rd, 26th, 26th and 28th day respectively after injury had undergone excisional operation. A man aged over 60 who died of shock had concomitant respiratory damage. In the group of adults, all the 28 patients in the first group (nonoperated) died – mortality was 100%. Twenty-seven patients in this group died of shock within 5 days after injury. The patient who died of acute fulminating septicemia also had a stormy shock phase.

Table 31.2 Comparison of results in two groups of patients, group I non-operated, group II treated with excisional operations

	Cases (n)	Survivors (n)	Deaths (n)
Group I (non-operated)	28	0	28
Group II (excisional operations)	55	17	38

In the 55 patients of the second group who had their eschars excised, 17 survived (30.9%) and 38 died – mortality was 69% (Table 31.2). Infection was the most common cause of death, since 33 patients died of wound sepsis, and another five died of pneumonia, gastrointestinal bleeding, disseminated fungal infection and postoperative shock respectively (Table 31.3).

Table 31.3 Primary cause of death (in 28 operated patients)

Causes	Deaths (n)
Shock	1
Wound sepsis	19
Septicemia	4
Pneumonia	1
Acute GI bleeding	1
Fungal infection	2

CASE REPORTS

From August to December 1983, three patients with burns of more than 90% of the BSA, including third degree burns of more than 80%, were admitted to our Burn Unit. The details and results of treatment are presented below.

Case 1

A male, aged 17, suffered from a flame injury with burns of 96% TBSA including 92% third degree burned on August 16 1983. He was admitted within 2 hours postburn, and fluid replacement therapy with catheterization of the right cephalic vein and tracheotomy were undertaken immediately. The patient was laid on a foam mattress and the wound was managed by exposure method. To hasten crust formation, an electric warm air blower was placed under the turning frame and a warm air blower was put underneath. On the second day postburn, decompression incisions were made on both sides of the chest to release the respiratory distress caused by constrictive trunk eschar. In the meantime, owing to a low P_aO_2 of 59.7 mmHg, the respiration was intermittently aided by using a high frequency jet ventilator (HFJV) and thus the P_aO_2 of the patient rose to normal. The HFJV was used for 9 days and the tracheotomy cannula was taken off on the 16th postburn day.

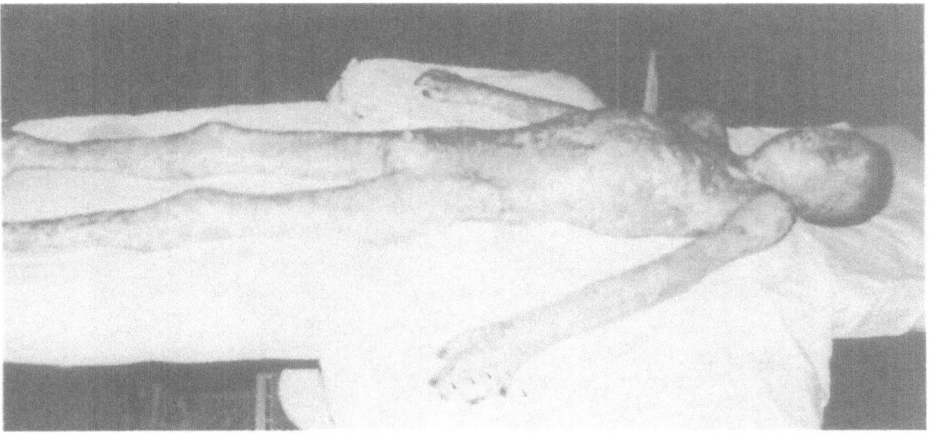

Figure 31.1 Case 1. Seventeen-year-old male with flame burns of 96% of BSA, including third degree burn of 92%. Four months after injury. All the wounds have healed. (Front view)

The third degree eschar was excised by stages; the first excision was done on the eighth postburn day, and three subsequent excisions of eschar were repeated at 2–4 day intervals, which removed the third degree area of 62% of the BSA. The wounds were covered immediately either with fresh porcine skin or freezing allograft skin, and small pieces of autograft taken from the patient's scalp and soles were inserted into the holes made on the allo- or xenograft. Ten autograftings were performed and the wound surface was completely covered with intermingled autografts, allografts and xenografts.

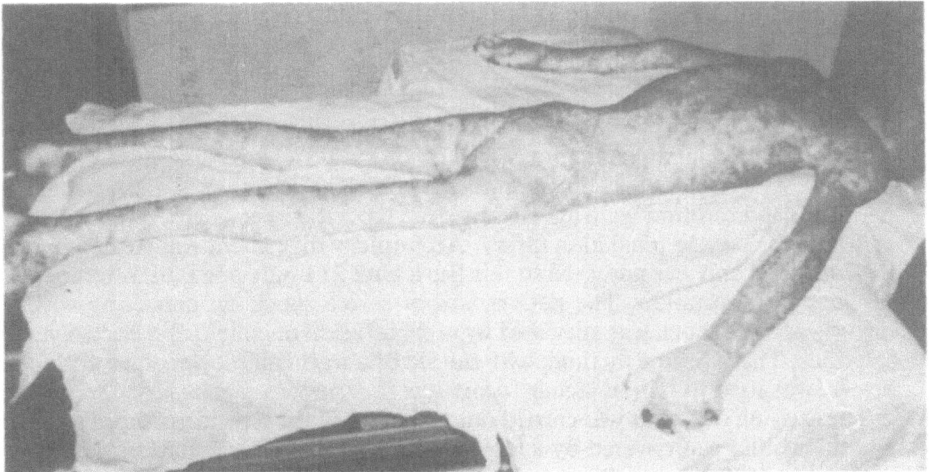

Figure 31.2 Case 1. Prone view of patient

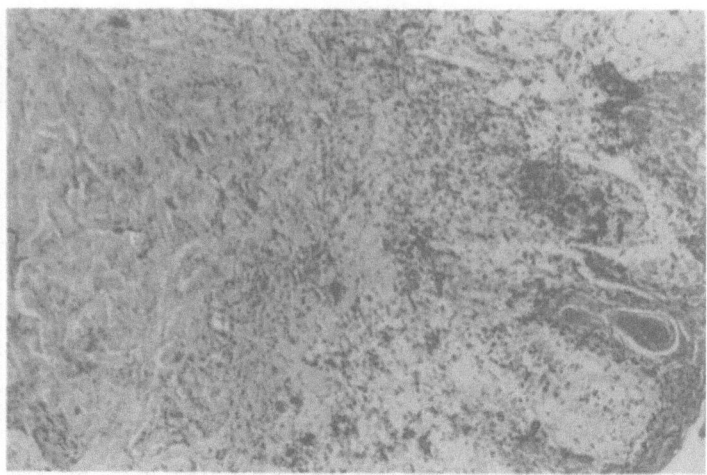

Figure 31.3 Case 1. Eighty-three days after intermingled transplantation. Remnants of the porcine collagen seen on upper left with heavy lymphocyte infiltration between xenograft and allograft

During the seventh postburn week, the patient complained of dyspnea and stridor aggravated while eating, and intercostal retractions were observed. Chest X-ray revealed nothing abnormal on the eighth postburn week, fiberoptic bronchoscopy was done, and there was a granuloma $0.7 \times 0.5 \times 0.3 \, \text{mm}^3$ in size on the anterior tracheal wall 2 cm from the carina. Pathologic evidence suggested that it might be the result of erosion of tracheal mucosa due to abutment of the tracheostomy tube tip. The granuloma was excised under general anesthesia. After excision, the symptom of dyspnea was relieved. The patient was discharged on the 182nd day after injury (Figures 31.1–31.3).

Case 2

A male, aged 34, had flame burns of 100% of the BSA, including third degree burns of 90% of the BSA, on December 2 1983. The scalp, soles, face, palms, perineum and scrotum were affected by deep second degree burns, and he also suffered from severe inhalation injury. After injury the patient was treated in a local hospital and was admitted to this Burn Unit 21 hours postburn after long distance transportation. The patient was in severe shock on admission with oliguria and the shock was alleviated by rapid infusion of colloid and electrolyte solutions. The exposure method, with the aid of a warm air blower and infrared heater, was used to hasten eschar formation.

The excision of eschar was carried out at the end of the second postburn week and the wound was covered by a large sheet of allograft. Split thickness auto-grafting and inlaying small autografts into the premade holes in the large sheet of allograft were not performed until the beginning of the fourth week postburn

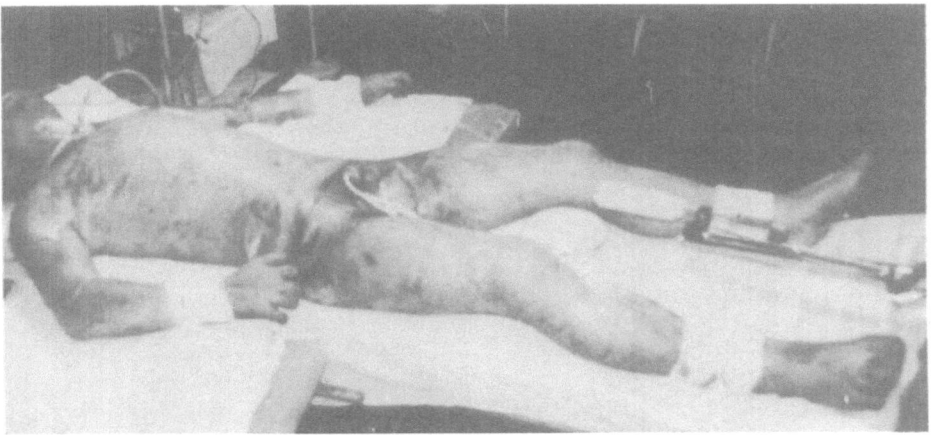

Figure 31.4   Case 2. A 34-year-old male with flame burns of 100% of BSA, including third degree burns of 90%, transferred to the Burn Unit 21 h after injury. He was complicated by severe respiratory damage. The deep second degree burns of 10% of BSA were scattered on the scalp, toes, buttocks, soles, face, waist and scrotum

when the patient's second degree burns of 2.5% of the BSA, scattered on the scalp and the soles, had healed. The autograftings were performed at an interval of 4–5 days. At the end of the fourth postburn week the eschars on the chest, back, abdomen and buttocks were cut off carefully with scissors during changes of dressing, the wounds were immediately covered with postage stamp size allograft or xenograft, and small pieces of autograft were inserted between the gaps. During the second month postburn, 12 skin graftings were carried out, and

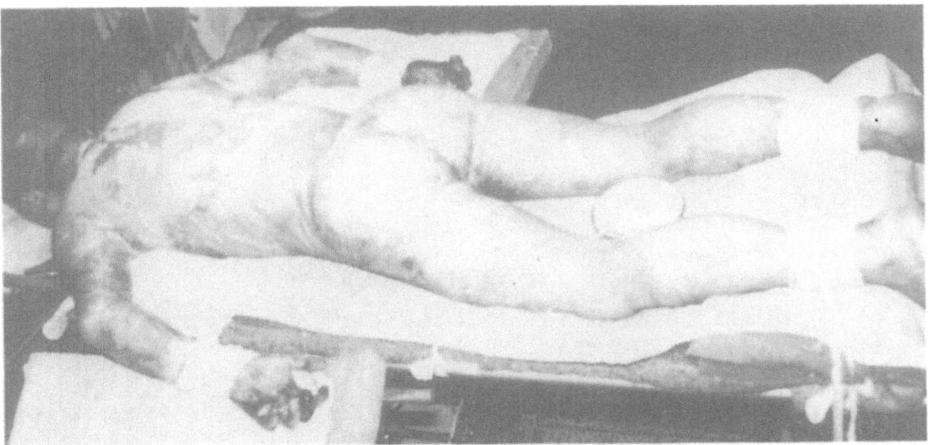

Figure 31.5   Case 1, 3 days postburn. The prone view of the patient during the early shock stage

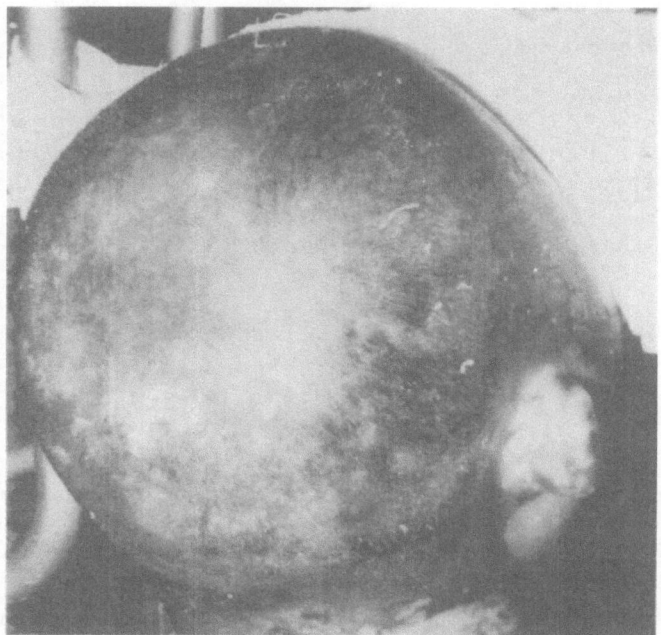

Figure 31.6 Case 1, 3 days after injury. Illustration shows third degree burn on the top of patient's scalp; the remainder of the scalp was area of deep second degree burn, which was used as a donor site after healing

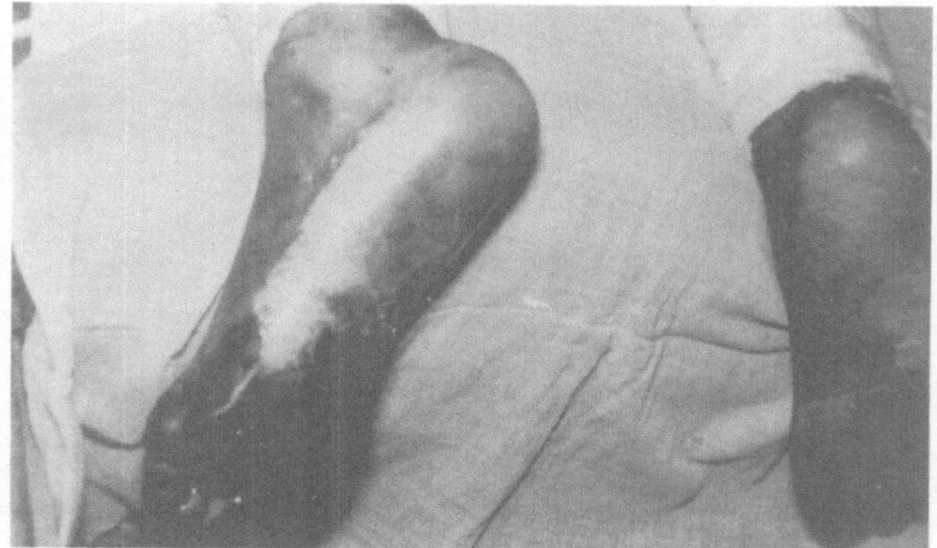

Figure 31.7 Deep second degree burns of both soles, 3 days postburn

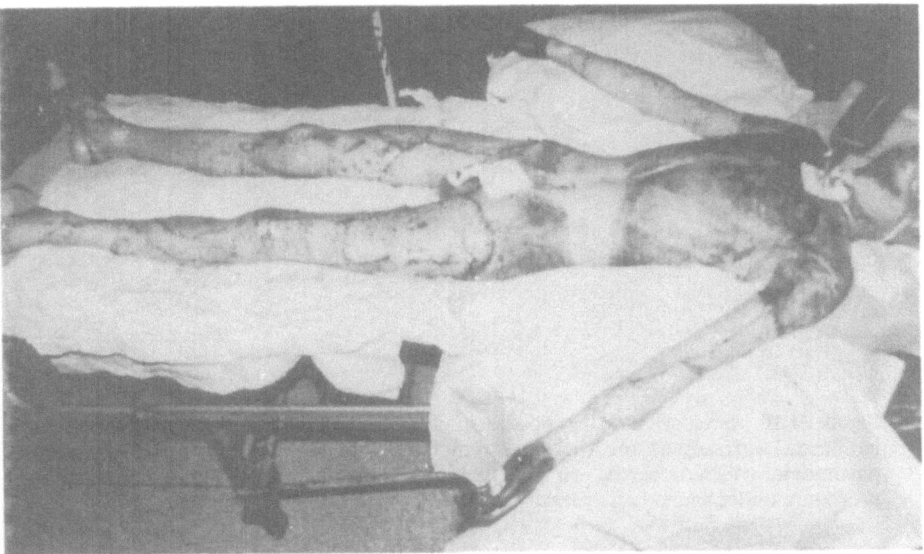

Figure 31.8 Photograph taken on ninth day postburn. Eschar excision 48% of BSA, involving four extremities, performed on sixth day after injury. The wounds were covered with large sheets of fresh allograft

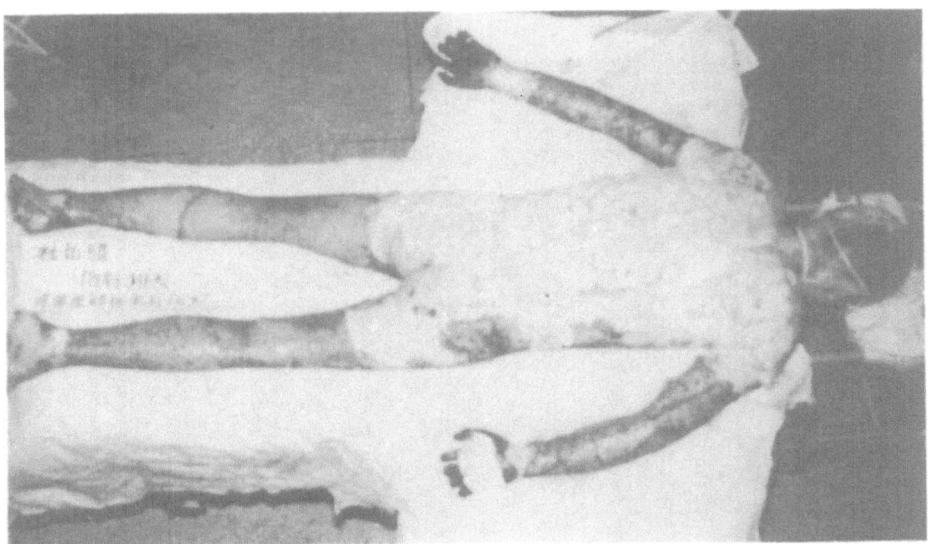

Figure 31.9 Thirty days after injury, intermingled transplantation of two upper extremities and right leg was already done. Illustration shows the granulating wound of the back covered with stamp-size patches of autografts

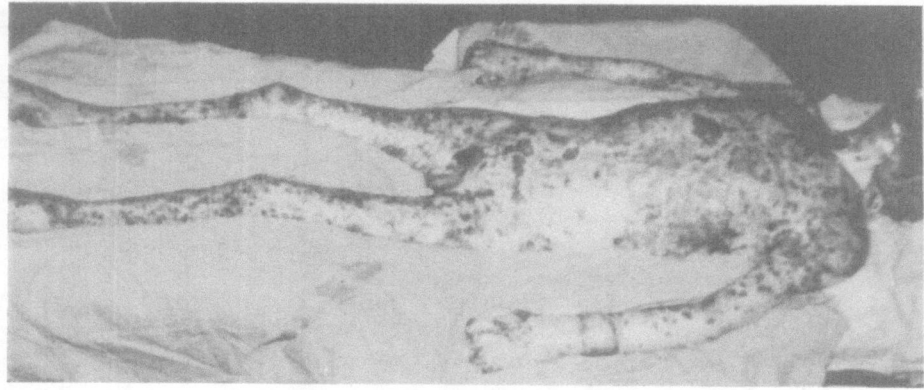

Figure 31.10 Seventy-four days postburn, only 5% eschar remaining over the right and left lateral surfaces of the thorax. At that time patient was suffering from severe pneumonia which occurred on the 68th day postburn following an autografting procedure under general anesthesia

autografts were harvested from 2.5% of the BSA to cover the third degree burn of 87% of the BSA.

The patient had a severe inhalation injury on admission. His P_aO_2 was 61.3 mmHg. A HFJV (high frequency jet ventilator) was employed until the P_aO_2 returned to normal on the tenth postburn day. Fiberbronchoscopy showed that the tracheal and bronchial mucosa were edematous, congested and

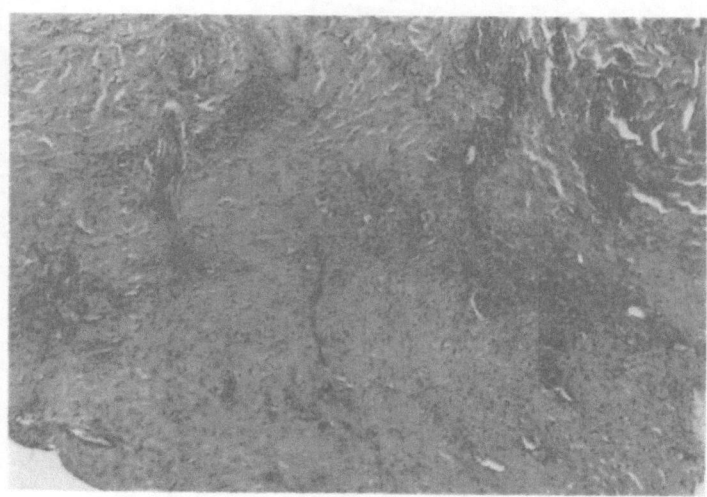

Figure 31.11 Case 2, 15th day postoperative, specimen taken from the junction of allograft and autograft, hyalinization of the collagen fibers arranged in random direction, with lymphocytes infiltration around the vessels

bleeding, the cartilage rings had disappeared and the openings of the general bronchus, lobi superior, Riedel's lobe and lobi inferior were also congested, edematous and bleeding, with necrotic mucosa. On the fifth day postburn, the necrotic tracheal and bronchial mucosa began to slough off and the 'chicken foot' bronchiolar casts of necrotic mucosa were sucked out on the seventh day postburn and the patient developed pneumonia. On the 68th postburn day, after the 11th operation under general anesthesia, his pneumonia became worse. There were moist rales disseminating in the two lungs on auscultation. Chest X-ray showed interstitial pneumonia of both lungs, the P_aO_2 was 40.5 mmHg. The patient died of respiratory failure on the 87th postburn day, despite having all the wounds successfully covered with autografts (Figures 31.4–31.11).

Case 3

A male, aged 21, had flame burns of 90% TBSA, with 81% third degree burns of the BSA. On December 6 1983, he was admitted to our Burn Unit 13 hours after injury. On admission the patient was in shock, tracheotomy was performed immediately, and a large amount of colloids and electrolyte solutions was infused. The wound was exposed to warm dry air, provided by a warm air blower and infrared heater. Fiberbronchoscopy showed lesions visualized in the trachea and both bronchi with edema and congestion of the mucosa due to inhalation injury.

The first excision was carried out on the sixth day postburn and eschars of the four extremities were excised by four surgical teams at the same time. On the 20th day, escharectomy of both sides of the chest was done, and the wounds were covered with large sheets of allograft. The area excised in two operations was 55% of the BSA. From the second to the 11th week postburn, repeated croppings from the patient's donor sites and inlaid autografting were performed, ten times in all, using the scalp, soles, waist and abdomen as the donor sites to cover the third degree burns of 81% of the BSA. Three months

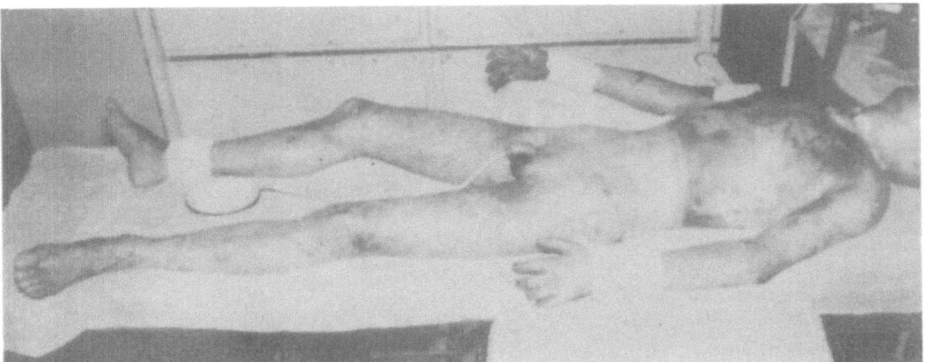

Figure 31.12 Case 3. Twenty-one-year-old male with flame burns of 90% of BSA, including third degree burns of 81%

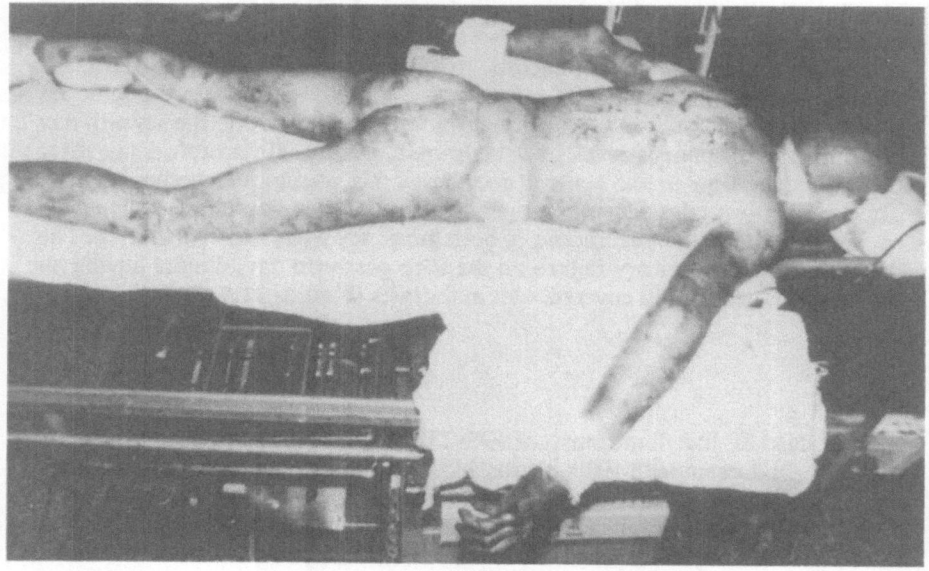

Figure 31.13 Case 3. Three days postburn (prone view)

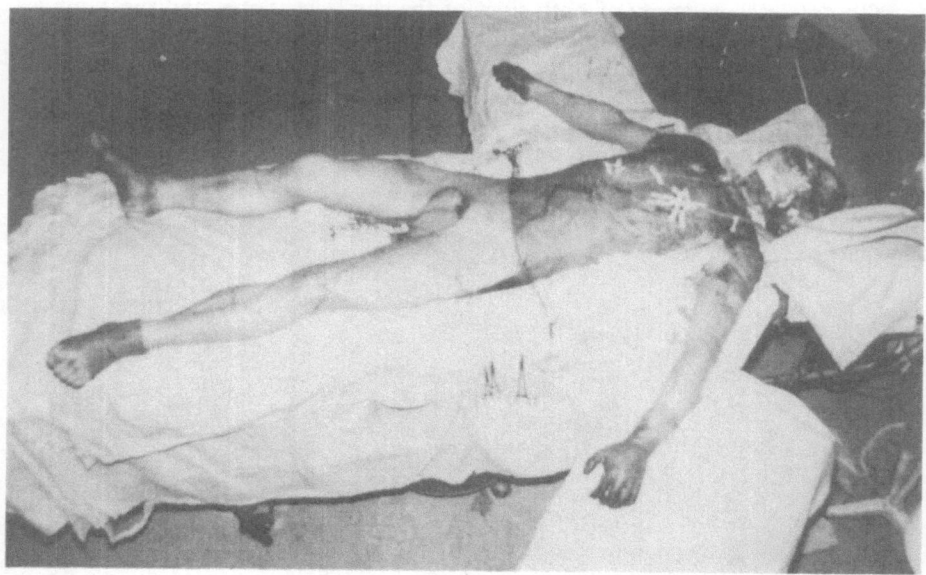

Figure 31.14 Six days after injury, the first operation involving eschar excising and transplantation of large sheet of allograft of the four extremities and lower abdomen

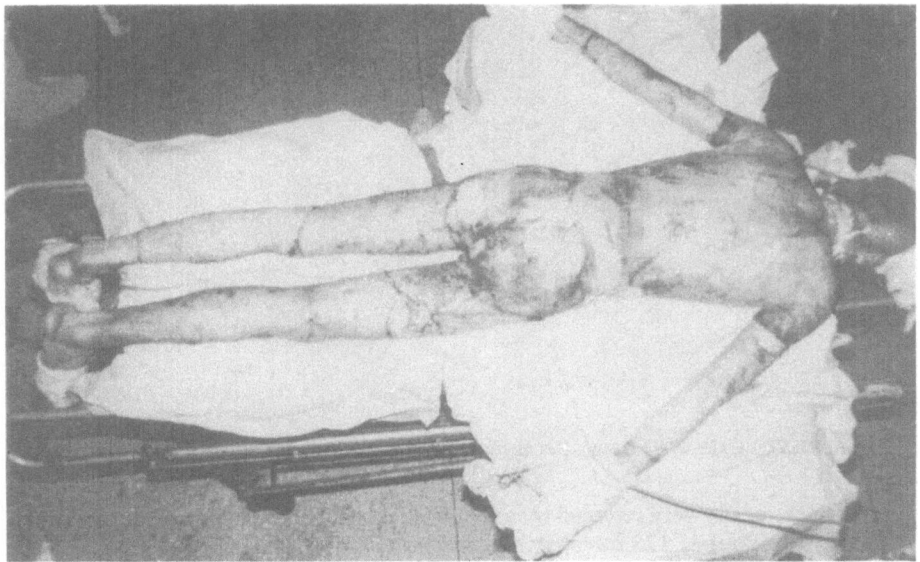

Figure 31.15   Case 3. Prone view of patient

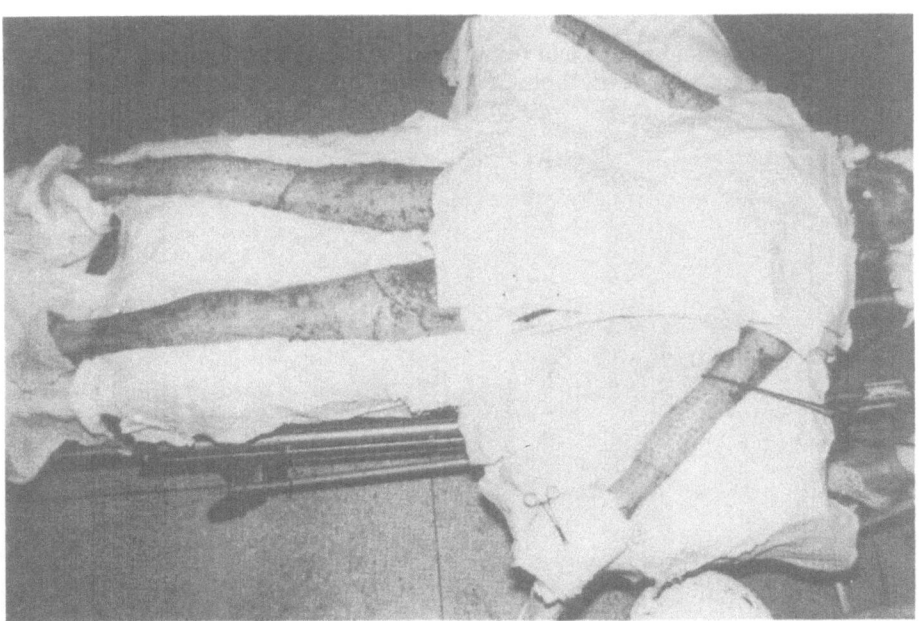

Figure 31.16   Case 3, 9 days postburn, after the first operation of eschar excision and allografting of the four extremities

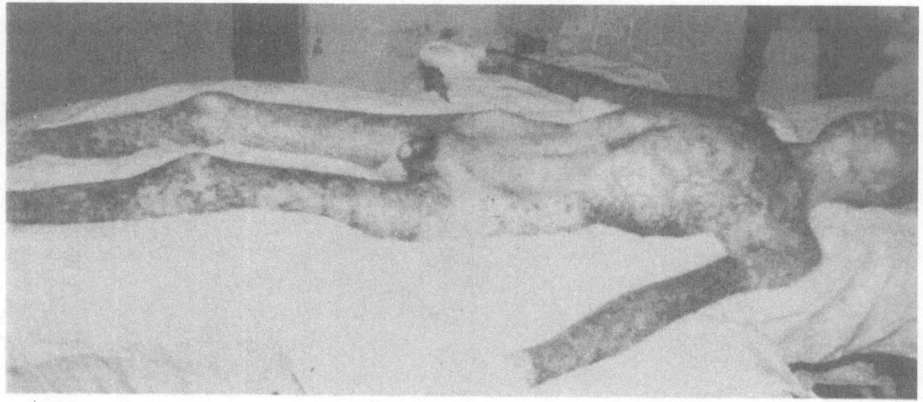

Figure 31.17   Case 3, 87 days after injury. All the wounds are covered with autografts

after the wounds were covered by autografts permanently, the patient survived and was discharged 125 days after his injury (Figures 31.12–31.18).

THERAPEUTIC MEASURES

Shock stage

The amount of fluid intake and urinary output of the three patients during the shock stage are shown in Table 31.4. During the first 24 h the total colloid

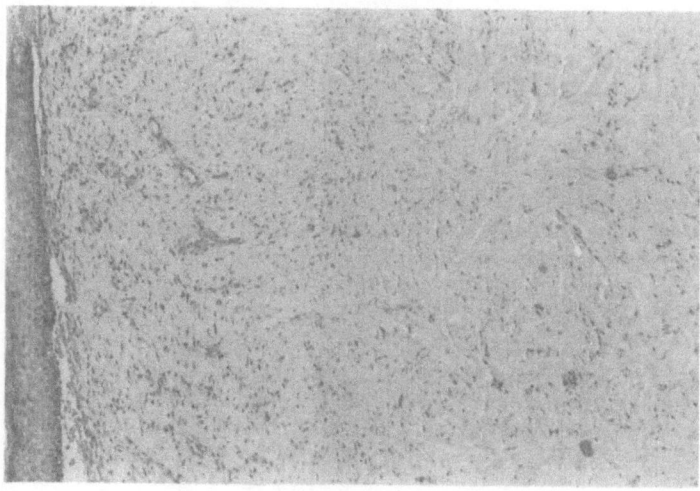

Figure 31.18   Case 3. Fifty-second day postoperative, complete epidermal healing with patient's autogenous skin

Table 31.4 Amount of fluids intake and urine of three patients within 72 h postburn

	Postburn (h)	Colloids (ml)	Crystalloids (ml)					Water (ml) Glucose sol.	Average urine volume (ml/h)
			R–L	K*–Sol	5% GNS	5% SB	Total		
Case 1	0–24	3200	3500			250	3750	5000	53
	25–48	2000	1500			125	1625	8000	98
	49–72	1000						8000	
Case 2	0–24	2300		500	3550	500	4550	4000	19
	25–48	2400		2000			2000	8000	60
	49–72	1000						8000	67
Case 3	0–24	2000		2500	4500	200	7200	3100	46
	25–48	2400		1500		125	1625	7500	41
	49–72	1000						9712	87

*1/3 1.25% sodium bicarbonate + 2/3 N.S.

solutions given in the form of whole blood and plasma amounted to 3000 ml, 2400 ml and 2000 ml respectively. Amounts of electrolyte solutions given in the first 24 h postburn were 3750 ml, 4550 ml and 7200 ml respectively. In addition, to compensate for salt-free water lost, water was given according to the daily requirement: the amounts of water given varied from 3000 to 5000 ml for the three patients during the first 24 h. During the second and third 24 h, water administered increased to as much as 8000 ml because of extra loss of water due to the dry warm air therapy. Artificial hibernation drugs, including acetylpromazine maleate, dolantin and promethazine hydrochloride, as well as diuretics (20% mannitol) were used in all cases. The average urinary output per hour was more than 40 ml in Case 1 and Case 3 during the first 24 h and in Case 2 urinary output was about 20 ml despite the diuretics used.

Table 31.5 Sodium load within 72 h postburn

	Postburn (h)	Na (mmol) total	Na mmol/ kg per 1 % BSA	Na in urine mmol/l	Total
Case 1	0–24	1086.1	0.23	—	—
	25–48	555.1	0.12	36	46
	49–72	133.8	0.02	125	291
	0–72	1775.0	0.37	—	337
Case 2	0–24	1182.3	0.18	—	—
	25–48	605.2	0.09	40	43
	49–72	167.0	0.03	47	81
	0–72	1954.5	0.30		124
Case 3	0–24	1411.3	0.26	28	30
	25–48	526.1	0.10	80	78
	49–72	133.8	0.02	114	239
	0–72	2071.2	0.38		347

The sodium load in the shock stage is shown in Table 31.5. In all cases, amounts of sodium ion infused per kilogram body weight for each 1% of the burns surface area were 0.37, 0.30 and 0.42 mmol/kg per 1% respectively within 72 h postburn. The urinary output of sodium increased every day but the total inputs of sodium during the shock stage were not completely excreted from the urine until the sixth to seventh day postburn.

The arterial blood gas studies in the shock stage are shown in Table 31.6. After high frequency positive pressure ventilation was employed, lowered P_aO_2 rose to normal levels.

In Case 1 the fluid resuscitation was administered at the second hour postburn, so the patient passed the shock stage smoothly. In Cases 2 and 3, the patients were in shock when they were transferred to our hospital, and the amounts of colloid and electrolyte solution needed were more than the calculated figure. Fortunately, as the infusion rate of fluids increased, the shock was gradually rectified.

Table 31.6 Arterial blood gases during shock stage

	Case 1			Case 2			Case 3		
	First	Second	Third	First	Second	Third	First	Second	Third
pH	7.32	7.40	7.41	7.37	7.36	7.35	7.3	7.47	
P_aCO_2 (mmHg)	44.7	36.0	32.0	36.9	52	44	31.7	36.7	
P_aO_2 (mmHg)	59.7	237.4*	72.8	61.3	80.1*	92.8	99.6	69.3	
O_2 sat. (%)	88.4	99	94.8	90.7	95.2	96.9	96.7	95	
BEB (mmol/l)	−2.6	−1.1	−2.8	−3.5	2.4	2.1	−9.5	4.7	

*Using high frequency jet ventilator

Table 31.7 Data concerning excisional operations on three patients

| | Second week postburn | | Third week postburn | | |
	Sites of excision area	%	Sites of excision area	%	Total
Case 1	Chest, abdomen, back	16	left upper extremity both groins	10	
	Right upper extremity	6	both lower extremities	30	62
Case 2	Four extremities, lower abdomen, both groins	44			44
Case 3	Four extremities, both lateral sides of the thorax	48			
		7			55

Management of the burn wound

Staged excision of eschar and intermingled transplantation of auto- and allo-grafts were performed in all cases. Details concerning excisions and auto-graftings are shown in Table 31.7 and Figure 31.19. The first excision was done on the fifth day postburn in Case 1 and on the sixth day after injury in Case 3. In Case 2, the excision was purposely delayed until the 13th day postburn and the operative autograftings procedures were done on the 25th day postburn because it was necessary to wait for the healing of the second degree wounds serving as the donor sites. Excision was done in four operations; the area excised was 62%

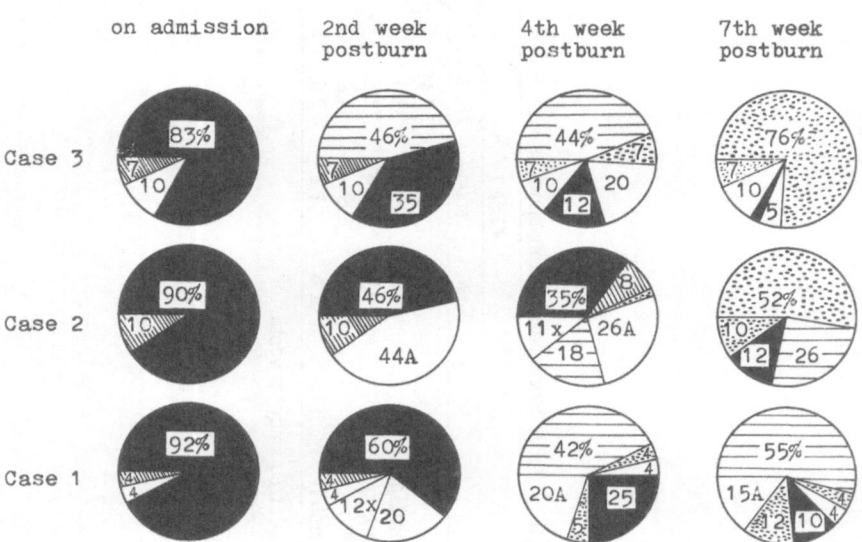

Figure 31.19 Change in the average BSA (%) of third degree burn eschar (excised and retained), intermingled grafting area and epidermal healing in three cases

of the BSA in Case 1. In Case 2, the four extremities were excised in a single operation; the area excised was 44% of the BSA. We excised the third degree eschar covering 55% of the BSA during the two operations in Case 3. In all cases the exposed wounds were covered immediately with large sheets of allo- or xeno-grafts.

As a rule, the sequence of autograftings was repeated at 3–4-day intervals. The autografts were cut into small pieces ranging from 0.3×0.3 cm to 0.6×0.6 cm and each graft was transplanted into a slit. The scalp and soles served as the principal donor sites. In each of the three patients, as many as eight to ten harvestings from the same site on the scalp and three harvestings on the sole were made. Healing of the donor sites was uneventful.

The remaining third degree eschars were scissored off immediately after their separation from the new growth of granulation tissue. Allo- and autografts were cut into small pieces and transplanted alternately in a bricklaying pattern on the granulation surface.

The evolution of the wound healing process in the three patients is shown in Figure 31.19. The major part of the eschar was excised on the fourth postburn week. The patients had ultimate wound closure with autografts at the end of the seventh, ninth and tenth postburn weeks respectively.

Bacterial monitoring of wound and rational use of antibiotics

Continuous bacterial monitoring of the wounds was carried out in every case and sensitive antibiotics, on the basis of the results of wound surface cultures and subeschar bacterial count and of their sensitivity tests, were selected and employed whenever they were necessary.

Cultures and/or biopsy quantitative cultures of subeschar were made from different sites twice or three times a week, especially after the eschar excision in the three patients. The subeschar bacterial count was negative in Cases 2 and 3. In Case 1, biopsy quantitative culture revealed a subeschar bacterial count of 10^5 per gram of tissue in 11 specimens, the maximum being 10^{11} per gram of tissue. But clinical symptoms and signs of sepsis were not noted.

Of the 66 strains of bacteria isolated from 38 burn wounds in the three patients, *Pseudomonas aeruginosa* accounted for 47% (31 strains) and *Staphyloccus aureus* 26% (17 strains). Eight strains were *Streptococcus faecalis* and ten strains were *Proteus* spp. All these strains were resistant to multiple antibiotics. *S. aureus* and *P. aeruginosa* were the bacteria found most frequently on the burn wounds.

According to the sensitive tests, the susceptibility of *Pseudomonas* to polymyxin B was high. Some Gram-negative bacilli were also sensitive to polymyxin B, amikacin and tobramycin. Some strains were sensitive to the third generation cephalosporins such as cefotaxime sodium and cefoperzone sodium. In *S. aureus* infection, vancomycin and cephalothin were the drugs of choice, while vancomycin and piperacillinum natricum were effective against *S. faecalis* infection in these cases.

In Cases 1 and 3, combinations of two or three effective antibiotics were employed as a protective measure during and after operations for 40 and 25 days

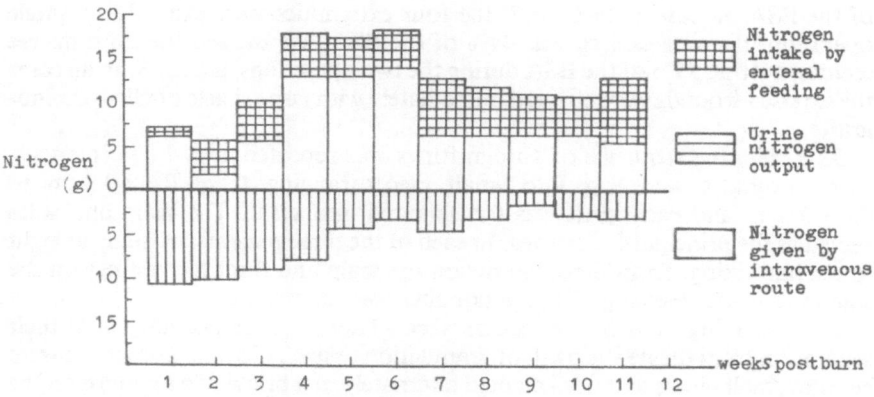

Figure 31.20   Nitrogen intake and urine nitrogen output in Case 1.

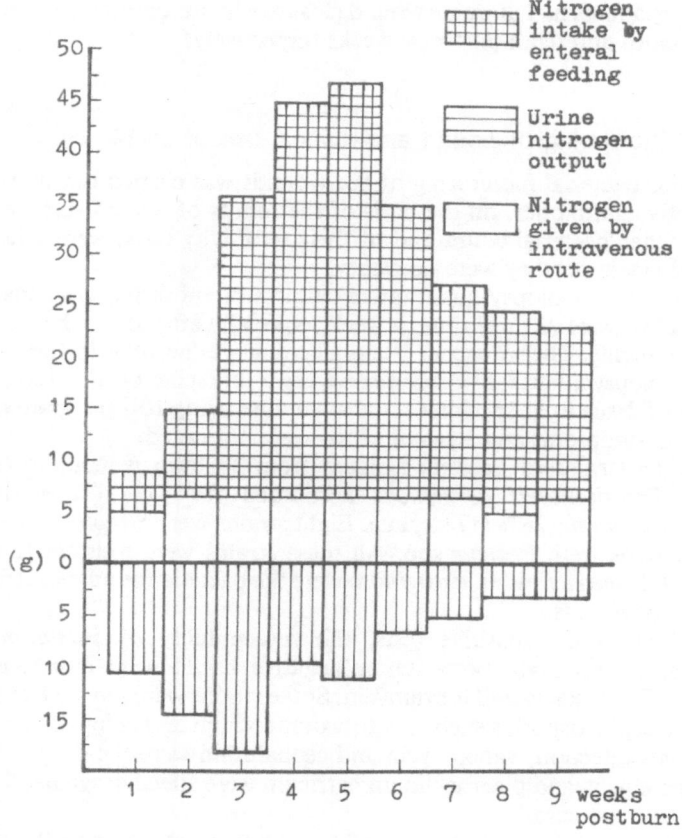

Figure 31.21   Nitrogen intake and urine nitrogen output in Case 2

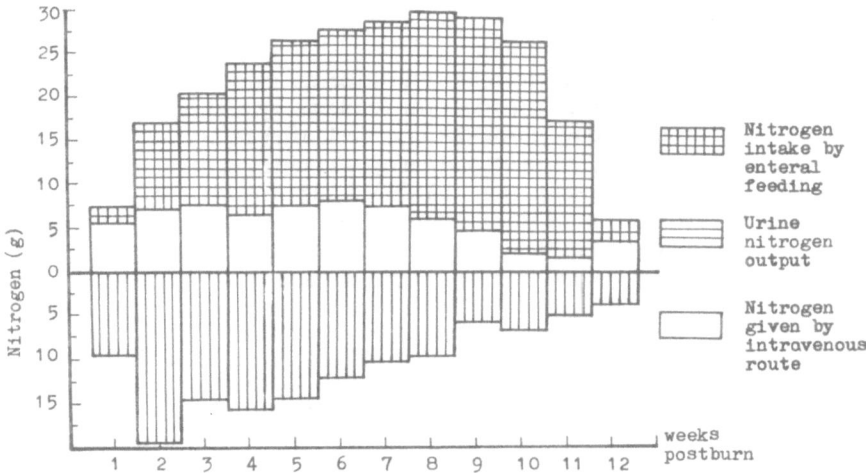

Figure 31.22   Nitrogen intake and urine nitrogen output in Case 3

respectively. Systemic antibiotics were continuously employed until death in Case 2 owing to the presence of severe inhalation injury and pneumonia.

In these patients, combined enteral–parenteral feedings (nasal tube and intravenous nutritional feeding) were usually given every day, including eggs and casein by mouth, milk, soybean milk, and element diet by a peristaltic pump and 25% glucose, human albumin and 5% crystalline amino acid solution by intravenous administration. Ten percent intralipid was used in Case 1. With the wound covered, oral and peristaltic pump nasal feeding was gradually substituted for the parenteral nutrition.

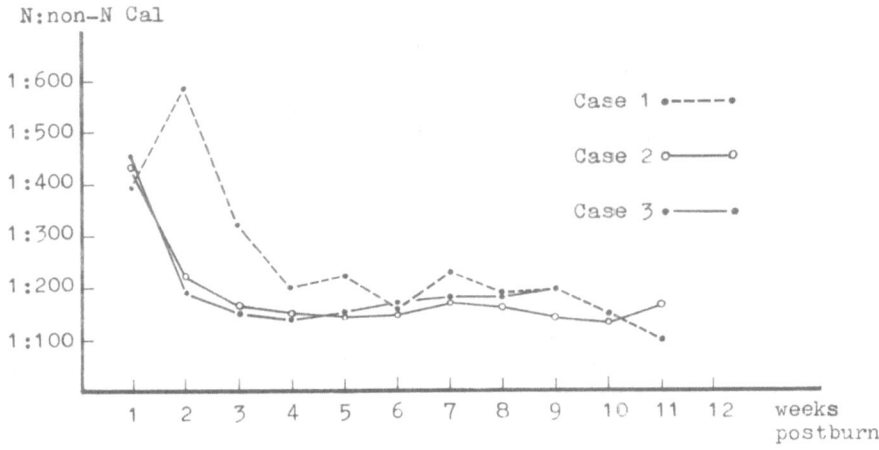

Figure 31.23   Caloric intake and calorie : nitrogen ratio in three illustrated cases

In our experience, it is better, if possible, to use peripheral venous puncture for the parenteral administration.

The total energy, nitrogen input and urine nitrogen output are shown in Figures 31.20–31.22. In each patient the total energy and nitrogen input were 12–13 MJ and 7 g per day during the first week after injury. At the second to seventh week postburn, the daily total energy and nitrogen input were 24–29 MJ, 16–47 g, 16–20 MJ, 17–28 g, and 14–29 MJ, 16–47 g in the three patients respectively. After eight weeks postburn, nutrition and nitrogen requirements decreased gradually. Positive nitrogen balance was obtained. Our dietary programs gave a kilocalorie : nitrogen ratio of about 1 : 150–200 in all patients (Figure 31.23)

FACTORS INFLUENCING THE PATIENT'S SURVIVAL

Mortality

There was only one patient over the age of 60 who died in this series, but the past results in the aged patients with less severe burns have not been encouraging. Severe burn in the aged differs in many respects from that in younger adults, and it is in these, aged, patients that at present the chance of recovery from a third degree burn over 70% of the BSA is very small. The mortality rate in the children with or without excision was also discouraging. However, in this age group, the LA_{50} of the third degree was about 40–50%[13]. The best result of the treatment in massive third degree burns in children has been reported by Burke and colleagues in 1975[14,15], but the number of patients is too small to allow a definite conclusion.

In the group of 55 patients who underwent operation, 38 died, and the overall mortality of the excisional operation was high (69%). Nevertheless, compared to the mortality of 100% for patients not operated on, we believe that the operation is still justifiable. Moreover, among the survivors, five patients with third degree burns over 90% of the BSA who would have died are alive and leading normal lives[16]. These patients' early excision followed by intermingled grafting does give a better chance of survival. Furthermore, none of the patients who died after excisional operation would have survived even if the operation had not been done. At the present time, it appears that only children and adult patients with such massive third degree burns might be benefited by eschar excision and intermingled transplantation.

Shock treatment

Some workers believe that burn shock is no longer a clinical problem and the composition and volume of fluids which should be infused make little difference for the majority of burn patients. In this series the results of shock treatment are far from satisfactory; nearly all deaths in the nonoperated group are attributable to burn shock during the shock phase. We frequently receive patients with extensive third degree burns who are transferred from other hospitals far away from Shanghai. Our experience indicates that if the patient is in shock on admission, the infusion of crystalloid solution alone is not as effective as when the colloid solution is added, especially in patients who have not received fluid therapy within 12 h after injury prior to admission. In these patients much greater amounts of both colloid and crystalloid solution are needed to ensure maintenance of the circulatory volume. However, in patients with full-thickness burns over 70% of the BSA, the shock period is still difficult to manage. Fluid resuscitation peculiar to this patient group remains to be studied. We feel that an early adequate fluid resuscitation and uneventful shock course are essential to a successful treatment.

Operation

The time of excision

Ideally, excision should be carried out during the first week after injury as soon as the patient is stable, but burn shock would often render the operation impossible. It was for this reason that 38 patients were not operated upon. Appropriate fluid resuscitation during the shock stage is essential for a successful treatment.

The depth of burns is easy to determine in a patient with third degree burns over 70% of the BSA, the full-thickness eschar is usually carbonized, and tangential excision is not practicable. In such circumstances, excision should be carried down to the fascia every time.

Selection of locality for eschar excision

As to the site of excision, we usually prefer to choose the extremities as the priority sites, provided that the trunk eschar is not infected and does not become a focus of infection.

During the excision, careful monitoring of the patient is important. But the monitoring of the arterial and central venous pressure is not always practicable. We have measured the urine output by an indwelling catheter every half-hour and a light general anesthesia is usually applied, using 'combined intravenous anesthesia' with lytic cocktail. The operation is simple; the only difficulty is massive blood loss during the excision of eschar, and it is time consuming during the insertion of small autografts. The operation can only be undertaken by a devoted team.

Wound closure

The importance of early excision and immediate wound closure has long been recognized. However, the main problem in the case of extensive deep burns is how to cover the exposed wound with graft of the patient's own skin after massive excision, since the donor site is limited.

It has been shown that one of the effective means is the use of intermingled transplantation which allows permanent sealing of the wounds with minimum autogenous skin.

Both fresh allografts and xenografts have been used as wound coverings, fresh allografts being the most effective for this approach. Unfortunately allografts are not always available when one needs them. Fresh xenografts are preferred if allografts are not available.

From 1972 to 1980, using the intermingled transplantation of porcine and human skin, we have treated 100 burn cases with promising result[17]. Fresh porcine xenograft is always available in Shanghai provided there is a butcher ready to cooperate.

The porcine skin is viable after intermingled transplantation. Its nutritional support comes from the interstitial fluid of the recipient bed within 2 weeks after grafting. The porcine epidermis can fuse with the expanded autograft epidermis to form a confluent layer of epidermal cells[17]. Later when the rejection of porcine epidermal elements takes place, the patient's epidermis can expand and creep, using the porcine collagen as a trellis frame, and the wound can avoid reexposure.

One of the disadvantages of porcine skin grafting is that the rejection usually comes earlier than that of allograft. In order to avoid wound reexposure, the slits or holes made on the large sheet of porcine xenograft should not be more than 1 cm apart, and the autograft patches should be a little larger than usual. When full-thickness burns exceed 60% of the BSA, wound closure with porcine skin is not so efficient, and significant open wounds may persist after autolysis of the grafted porcine skin.

A tourniquet is always used when excision is performed on the extremities. Eschar of the four limbs can be excised at the same time by four surgical teams, the advantage of this being that we can excise a larger surface area of eschar within a relatively shorter time. Eschar over as much as 40–45% of the BSA has been removed at one time.

The subsequent operation may be carried out 3 days after the first operation, and the chest and the abdomen are usually chosen as the sites for excision. An average amount of 2500–3000 ml blood transfusion is needed for eschar excision of the four limbs, and 2000–2500 ml blood should be transfused for the operation on the chest and abdomen. The back of the body and the buttocks are usually spared, because the skin of these localities is much thicker, some dermal remnants may remain in the subcutaneous tissues. With the help of intermingled patchwork grafting of auto- and allografts, skin regeneration may be possible despite the carbonized appearance of the eschar or an obvious granulation wound, which might easily make one believe that no regeneration would be possible in such a wound. Usually, two subsequent operations take the 70–80% third degree burns of the BSA down to about 30–40% of the BSA. In such circumstances, the wound infection is more easy to control by using topical agents. It is interesting to note that after excision had been applied to the 17 survivors, the average BSA of the remaining third degree burn eschar not excised was $35.03 \pm 11.42\%$, while in the 38 patients who died the average BSA of the remaining eschar area was $52.49 \pm 16.26\%$ (Table 31.8).

The more eschar excised, the less the bacterial colonization of the wounds and

Table 31.8 Comparison of average BSA of third degree burn eschar (excised and retained) between survivors and deaths in excision group

Excision group	Cases (n)	Average BSA with III ° burns (%)	Average BSA of III ° burns excised (%)	Average BSA of III ° burn eschar retained
Survivors	17	80.84 ± 7.82	45.8 ± 13.96	35.03 ± 11.42
Deaths	38	84.94 ± 8.11	31.92 ± 15.08	52.49 ± 16.26
			$p < 0.001$	$p < 0.001$

the greater the chance of patient survival. We all realize that not every survival represents a therapeutic triumph. There are many factors which influence the patient's survival. Patients who died had less eschar excised because they usually had a stormy shock phase or suffered from early sepsis which would make massive excision hazardous.

Despite the improved method of intermingled transplantation, mortality in patients with extensive full-thickness burns over 70% of the BSA was still extremely high. The fact that several patients died in spite of having all the wounds successfully covered with autografts suggests that in the treatment of massive third degree burns many problems such as shock, infection, nutrition and hypercatabolism remain to be solved.

REFERENCES

1. Baxter, C. (1974). The current status of burn research. *J. Trauma*, **14**, 1
2. Monafo, W. W. and Ayvazian, V. H. (1978). Topical therapy. *Surg. Clin. N. Am.*, **58**, 1157–71
3. Howard, R. J. and Simmons, R. L. (1974). Acquired immunologic deficiencies after trauma and surgical procedures. *Surg. Gynecol. Obstet.*, **139**, 771
4. Miller, C. L. and Baker C. C. Changes in lymphocyte activity after thermal injury. *J. Clin. Invest.*, **63**, 202–10
5. Li, B. G., Feng, S. J., Sun, Y. M., Shih, T. S., Yang, C. C. and Hsu, W. S. (1983). Change in T lymphocytes and its subpopulations after extensive thermal burns. In Yang, C. C., Sheng, Z. Y. and Shih, T.S. (eds.) *The Treatment and Research in Burns*. pp. 323–31. (Beijing: Science Press; and New York, Chichester, Brisbane, Toronto, Singapore: Wiley Medical)
6. Xu, D. Z., Xu, Y. P., Shih, T.S., Yang C. C. and Hsu, W. S. (1983). PMN chemotaxis and burn infection. In Yang, C. C., Sheng, Z. Y. and Shih, T. S. (Eds.) *The Treatment and Research in Burns*. pp. 332–9. (Beijing: Science Press; and New York, Chichester, Brisbane, Toronto, Singapore: Wiley Medical)
7. Burke, J. F., Bondoc, C. C. and Quinby, W. C. Jr. (1974). Primary burn excision and immediate grafting: A method shortening illness. *J. Trauma*, **14**, 389
8. Chang, T. S. and Shih, C. H. (Shih, T. S.) (1963). Study of debridement in cases of extensive burns. *Chinese J. Surg.*, **11**, 117–19
9. Tong, F. C., Shih, C. H. (Shih, T. S.), Chu, T. A. and Chang, T. S. (1963). Successful management of 11 cases of extensive burns involving more than 80 percent of the body surface. *Chinese Med. J.*, **82**, 104–16
10. Jackson, D. (1954). A clinical study of the use of skin homografts for burn. *Br. J. Plast. Surg.*, **7**, 26–43

11. Colson, P. and Prunieras, M. (1960). Traitement de grands brûlés. *Lyon Chir.*, **56**, 182-9
12. Colson, P., Leclercq, P., Merigot, P., Gangolphe, M., Houot, R. and Prunieras, M. (1962). Du rôle de l'homogreffe dans le procédé de Mowlem-Jackson. *Acta Chir. Belg.*, **54**, 751
13. Shih, T. S., Yang, C. C. and Xu, W. S. (1983). The treatment of burns (summing up experience of 22 years). In Yang, C. C., Sheng Z. Y. and Shih, T. S. (Eds.) *The Treatment and Research in Burns.* pp. 3-100 (Beijing: Science Press; New York, Chichester, Brisbane, Toronto, Singapore: Wiley Medical)
14. Burke, J. F., Quinby, W. C., Bondoc, C. C., Cosimi, A. B., Rusell, P. S. and Szyfelbein, S. K. (1975). Immunosuppression and temporary skin transplantation in the treatment of massive third degree burns. *Ann. Surg.*, **182**, 183
15. Cosimi, A. B. and Burke, J. F. (1982). Skin transplantation. In Morris, P. J. (ed.) *Clinical Surgery International.* Vol. 3, *Tissue Transplantation.* pp. 161-175 (Edinburgh, London: Churchill Livingstone)
16. Shih, T. S. *et al.* (1979). Guérison de quatre brûlures du 3ᵉ degré à plus de 90% de la surface corporelle. *J. Chir.* (*Paris*), **105**, 738-41
17. Yang, C. C., Xu, W. S., Yang, B. Z. and Dong, H. L. (1982). Intermingle transplantation of porcine and human skin in extensive burns. *Chinese Med. J.* **95**, 261-6

32 Mechanism and Management of Repeated Recurrence of Residual Wounds in Severely Burned Patients – Role of Sweat Glands

WANG LIANGNENG, ZHONG DECAI, HONG ZHOUYUAN and LIU JIEWU

Department of Plastic Surgery and Burns, Fourth Military Medical College of the PLA, Xian

On the basis of the treatment of 12 cases of severely burned patients with complicated residual wounds and 20 successive biopsies of the wounds at different stages in two cases, we have observed the recurrences and the healing process of the wounds, their histologic changes, and an appropriate treatment has been suggested in treating these recurrences of wounds.

CLINICAL FINDINGS

All cases were adults. Three patients had burns of 40–50% of the BSA with 50% third degree burn, one had burns above 30% BSA and five had burns of less than 29% BSA. The remaining three patients had deep second degree burns only. Nine cases had 2–7% BSA of residual wounds and the other three were admitted for more extensive residual wounds of 20%, 20% and 16% BSA respectively. All patients suffered also from emaciation, stiffness of joints and contractures. Most of the residual wounds were distributed on the lower extremities (nine instances) and the trunk (11 instances), but a few were on the upper extremities (three instances) and the scalp (two instances). The repeated recurrences of residual wounds appeared most frequently in the healed area of deep dermal burns.

The most frequent causal microorganism of the wounds was identified as *Staphylococus aureus*, while *Staphylococus albus* and *Pseudomonas aeruginosa* were sometimes the causal bacteria. Wound recurrence started from pyogenic foci seated under the scabs of the healed epithelium. Sometimes the infection began at the margin of the previous graft. The infective foci broke down and the wound became a small ulcer by destroying the nearby epithelium within 3–5 days. This phenomenon could appear during different stages in the same patient. Sometimes the ulcer after specific therapy would heal spontaneously by epithelialization, whereas in some other areas the infective foci were just forming the ulcer.

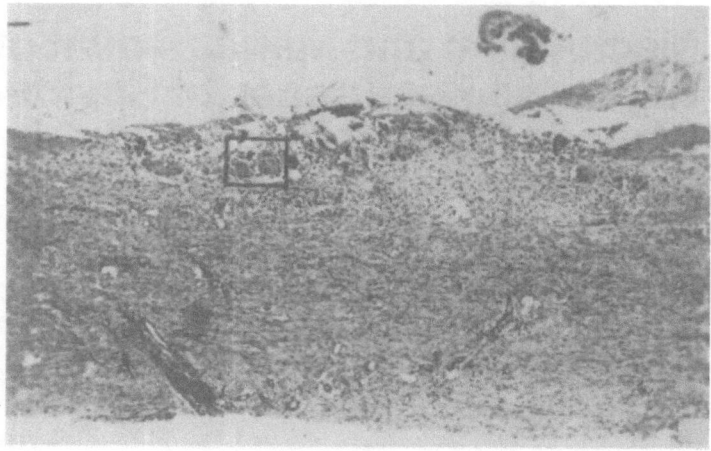

Figure 32.1 The epithelium was destroyed by pyogenic organisms under scab, the debris of the epithelial cells were phagocytized by numerous macrophagocytes with slight inflammatory reaction. No hair follicle and sweat gland were seen. HE × 32

Biopsy specimens taken from the ulcer under the broken epithelium showed a granulation tissue with cell infiltration among which there were numerous phagocytes containing the debris of broken epithelial cells, and a thin layer of epithelium at the margin of the ulcer (Figures 32.1, 32.2). In the deep layer, sweat glands and a few hair follicles were seen. Inflammatory reaction might reach the subcutaneous tissue. Vasodilatation, perivasculitis and periadenitis of

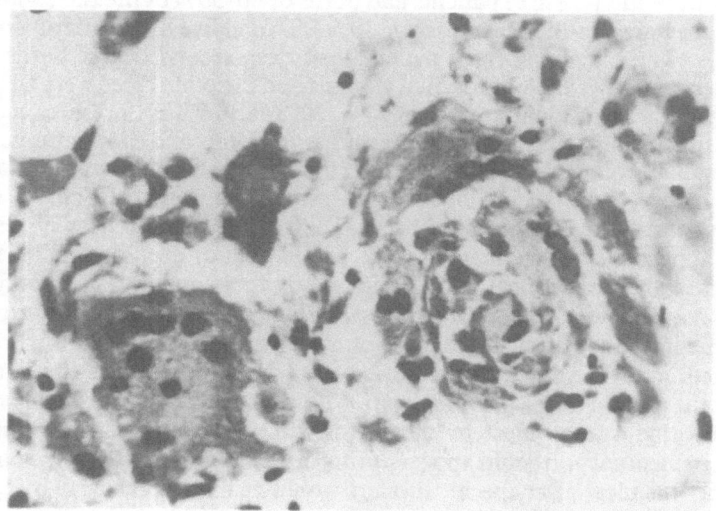

Figure 32.2 Macrophagocyte in Figure 32.1. × 215

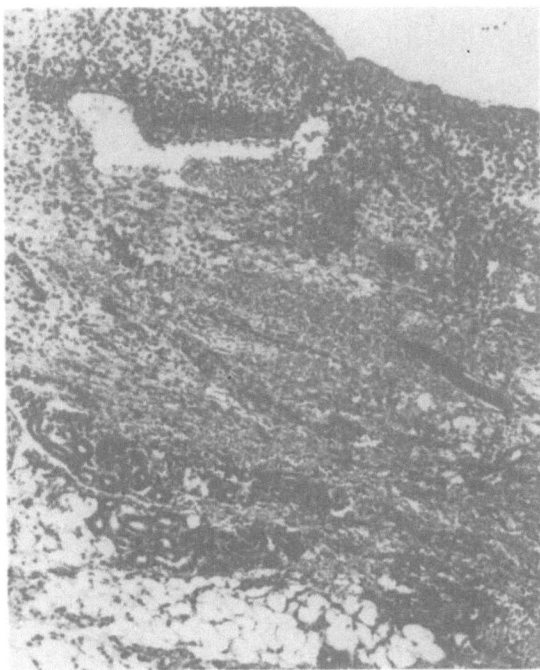

Figure 32.3 Inflammatory infiltration under granulation deepened to subcutaneous fat tissue. Many sweat glands and a few follicles were noted in the dermis with vessels dilated. HE × 68

the sweat glands were noted (Figures 32.3, 32.4). When the infection was under control, the pathologic section showed the reepithelialization from the canaliculous epithelial cells of the sweat glands (Figure 32.5). After a long period of repeated infections and ulcerations, patients would suffer complications – anemia, hypoproteinemia, and even severe emaciation. In spite of the application of topical agents, antibiotics, traditional herbal medicine or skin grafting, the wounds might recur overnight in the nearly healed area and then treatment would have to be started all over again. Having treated these cases with meticulous care, we found that it was essential to abide by the following surgical principles in the care of these wounds.

(1) It is important to improve the general condition of the patient with additional nutritional support and also give repeated small blood transfusions.

(2) Daily tub bath is mandatory, with careful washing of the crusts and scabs of the wound in order to facilitate wound drainage and reepithelialization.

(3) Large wounds may not heal spontaneously by cicatrization and epithelialization; the granulation of the wound should be scraped off down to the fibrous base, and autografting of skin may be performed right away.

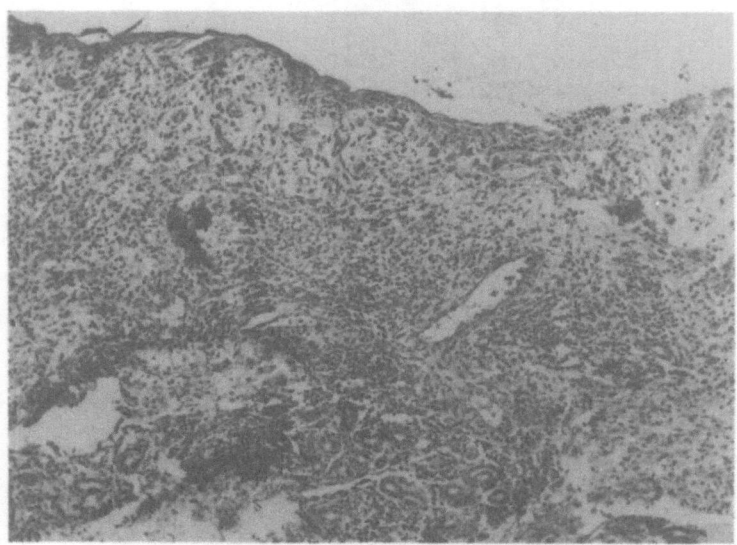

Figure 32.4 Periadenitis of sweat glands and perivasculitis at the edge of the chronic wound. HE × 68

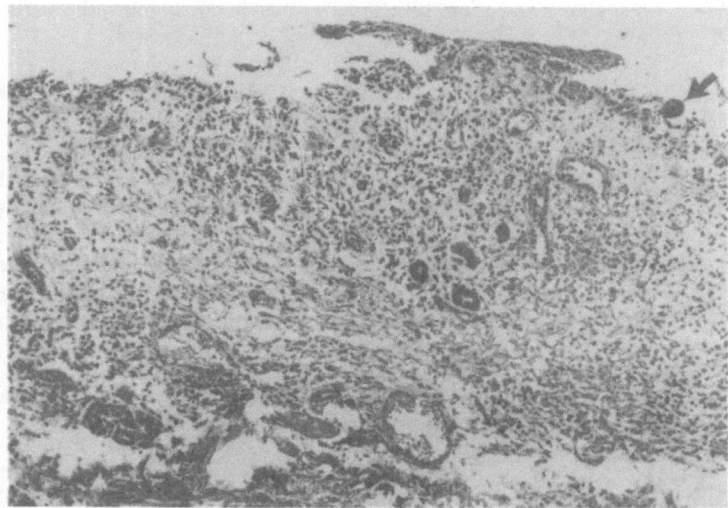

Figure 32.5 Inflammatory reactions obviously reduced, vessel dilation subsided. Some ducts of sweat glands regenerated and reached the wound surface. No hair follicle was noted. HE × 68

(4) Suitable antimicrobial agents may be used topically, and antibiotics may be administered systemically if indicated.

In two cases, the remnant wounds healed completely within 16 and 38 days by skin grafting. In the other ten cases (12 recurrent instances), healing took 2–4 months (an average of 3.2 months).

Two to ten years after injury all but two patients were in good condition and returned to their former work. The healed scars were thin, soft, whitish and short of elasticity.

DISCUSSION

Wound healing, infection and reepithelialization of deep partial thickness burns

In deep partial thickness burns, the hair follicles and sebaceous glands are usually destroyed (burn to half or two thirds thickness of skin). The wound is usually healed by epithelialization from the hair follicles and sweat glands within 3 weeks. If the burn is deeper than two thirds thickness of skin, the only viable epithelial element left is in the sweat gland, and healing usually takes the longer time of 4–5 weeks. If a tiny scab is formed on the wound and the remaining glands might be infected by the pathogenic microorganisms harbored in the coiled canaliculi, the infection would flare up, once the general resistance of the patient decreases. A pinpoint pyogenic focus at the very beginning may enlarge and form a large ulceration. Treatment by cleansing the wound and drainage decreases the number of bacteria and the administration of antibiotics might enable the wound to heal up again.

Crust and scabs

Crust and scabs may cause aggravation of the infection. Often a vicious circle is formed with this kind of wound. Crust and scabs – infection – pyogenic foci – ulceration – reepithelialization – reinfection – and so on. Daily gentle washing of the wound and careful peeling of the crusts and scales would break the circle, and the wound would heal eventually. Using this program, seven cases of chronic wounds healed completely within 3 weeks.

Sweat glands

Sweat glands in humans develop well, with an average of 143–339 per cm^2 of skin sited in the deeper part of the dermis. In the deep partial thickness burn, the remaining viable epithelial elements in the sweat glands may provide the epithelium for healing a fairly large wound. Whether the infection of the remaining sweat glands is conducive to the formation of trophic or hypertrophic scars needs further study.

33 Refrigerated Human Amnion as a Burn Dressing: Clinical Application and Histologic Observations

LI JIEYING, TANG QINGLAN and WU JIAYUN
Department of Surgery, Zhong Shan Hospital, Shanghai First Medical College, Shanghai

Human amniotic membrane has been shown to be an effective biologic dressing both clinically and experimentally. This biodressing may (1) alleviate pain, (2) minimize evaporative and exudative losses and (3) prevent further contamination of the wound, with resultant accelerated healing[1-4]. In animal experiments[5], bacterial counts decreased in virtually all infected burn wounds treated either with allogenic skin or human amniotic membrane. However, the degree of decreased bacterial counts was a thousandfold greater with amniotic membrane.

The purpose of this study is to observe the efficiency of refrigerated human amniotic membrane in the local management of burns, especially deep burn and, at the same time, to evaluate the bacteriologic cultures taken at regular intervals and the histologic studies on the refrigerated amniotic membrane.

MATERIALS AND METHODS

Preparation of the amniotic membrane

All membranes are obtained from normal, healthy pregnant women with no history of infectious diseases. The amniotic fluid must not be contaminated. The fresh placenta is immediately put in a sterile container and refrigerated. The amniotic membrane is stripped off the placenta within 12 h employing aseptic technique and flushed with sterile normal saline. It is then rinsed with 0.25% sodium hypochlorite and washed again five times with normal saline. The membrane is finally transferred to a sterile jar containing 0.5% chloramphenicol (Chloromycetin) in normal saline. The membrane may be kept in a refrigerator for as long as 8 weeks. During this period, a weekly check for sterility is done by culture for aerobic and anaerobic organisms. Both light and electron microscopy studies are conducted before and 4 and 8 weeks after refrigeration.

Application of the amniotic membrane

The wounds are washed with 1:1000 benzalkonium and debrided. The amniotic membrane is then applied. Trapped fluid or air must be expelled to afford intimate contact of the wound with amniotic membrane. The membrane edge should overlap the normal skin to leave no wound exposed. When the membrane is applied to the face fenestrations should be made to accommodate the nostrils, the mouth and the eyes. Another piece of amnion is applied to the ears. Adjacent amnion should overlap. As secretions tend to be present within the first week postburn, a dry sterile cotton pledget is put at the corners of the eyes and the mouth and changed when needed to take up such secretions. When amnion is applied to the hand, the fingers should be wrapped separately. After application, the wound may be left exposed and kept dry by an infrared lamp. Sometimes fine mesh gauze and bandage are used for wounds on extremities. Swab cultures are made before application of the amnion and thereafter when necessary.

A single application is often adequate. Local drainage and reapplication are needed whenever fluid or pus has collected beneath the membrane.

Clinical material

From January 1981 to September 1982, 22 cases with 32 burn wounds were treated by application of refrigerated amniotic membrane. Fluid resuscitation and other therapeutic measures were applied as needed. Ages of these 22 cases ranged from 13 to 73 years, with TBSA burned 8–60%, averaging 29%, and burnt surface covered with the membrane ranged from 3–40% of the BSA. Distribution of the burn sites was: face and neck, ten; upper extremities, nine; lower extremities, six; trunk, seven. Depth of burn injury was: superficial burns, 5 areas; deep second degree burns, 10 areas; deep dermal with scattered small third degree burns, 17 areas. The initiation of amnion application in most cases was 6 h to 4 days postburn. Only two had the amnion applied on the eighth and 12th postburn days respectively. Swab cultures before application showed bacterial growth in ten cases. The organisms found were *Staphylococcus epidermidis*, *Staphylococcus aureus*, *Enterobacter aerogenes*, *Pseudomonas aeruginosa* and *Escherichia coli*.

RESULTS

Clinical

As soon as the membrane was applied, pain was promptly relieved. The patients felt well and had a good appetite. Body temperature elevated to 38–39 °C and gradually returned to normal after 4–7 days. The wound exudation decreased soon after the application of the membrane. The pale color of the deep burns turned reddish after 12–24 h. In 2–3 days, an eschar was formed and edema subsided. No inflammatory reaction was seen. The eschar spontaneously sloughed off when the wound reepithelialized. A smooth scar was formed with

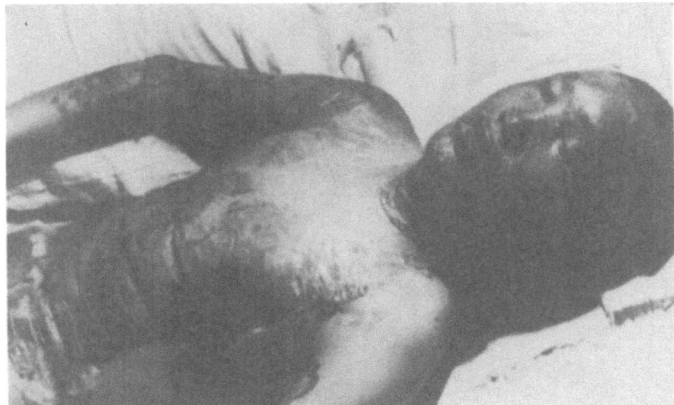

Figure 33.1 Thirty-one-year-old male suffered from hot steam burns with 30% deep dermal and full thickness burns of BSA. Most of the burns were covered with amniotic membrane on the second postburn day. The photograph was taken on the 14th day postburn

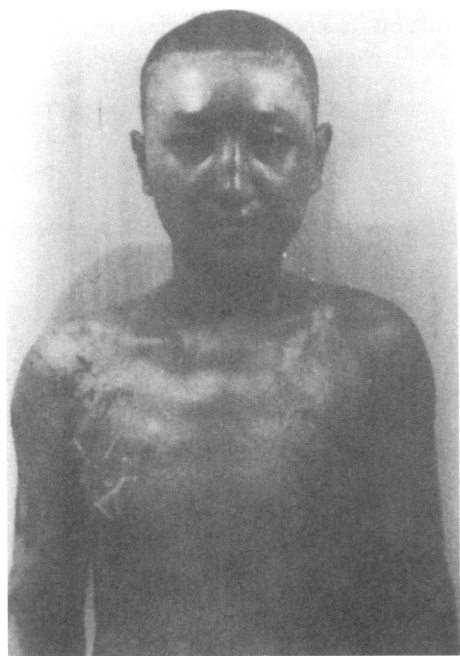

Figure 33.2 Same patient as in Figure 33.1. Four weeks postburn, most of the burned wounds were healed. Scattered granulating wounds were spontaneously healed after further changes of the dressing

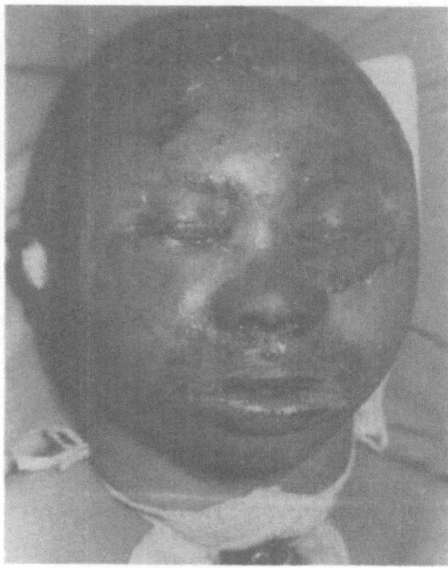

Figure 33.3   Twenty-eight-year-old male, with flame burns to 37% of BSA. The deep dermal burns of face with full thickness burns on the forehead, nasolabial portion, cheeks and ears were covered with amniotic membrane

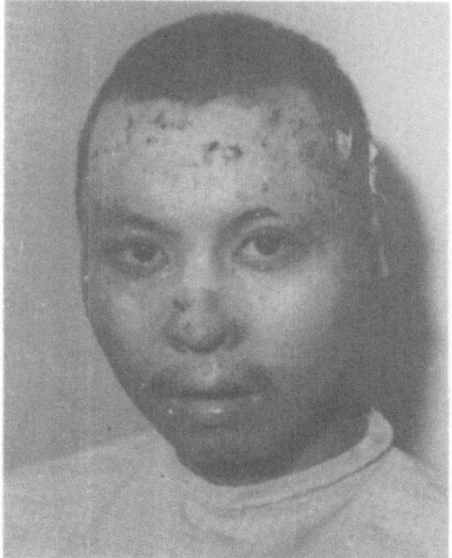

Figure 33.4   Same patient as in Figure 33.3. Four weeks postburn, most of the burned wounds were healed. Scattered granulating wounds were spontaneously healed after further changes of the dressing

some pigmentation. The superficial burns healed spontaneously under the eschar in 5–7 days. Among the ten deep dermal burns, five healed and four still had small wounds with islands of epidermis when the eschar separated. The small wounds healed in 10–14 days after two or three further dressings. A 67-year-old man with circumferential burns on both legs was severely infected before application of the membrane. The amnion autolyzed 24 h after the application and the method was abandoned. In 17 deep dermal burns, four healed after a single application in 14–21 days; 12 still had small, granulating wounds after the spontaneous separation of the eschar (Figures 33.1, 33.2); four were autografted because the wounds were either on the face (Figures 33.3, 33.4) or on the dorsum of the fingers and hands; and the other eight healed within 1 week with conventional treatment. One case of this group of 17 was a man sustaining 53% of the TBSA burned. The amnion was applied to an extent of 40% of the BSA. On the fifth postburn day, the amnion dressing on the posterior surface of the lower extremities autolyzed. Wound sepsis set in and infection soon spread to the anterior surface aspect of the lower extremities. Subsequently, the amniotic membrane treatment was given up for this case.

The incidence of wound infection decreased in comparison with the control areas; the wound healing was shortened by 2–5 days. Scattered areas of full-thickness burns may heal spontaneously under the amniotic membrane.

Ten of the 22 cases have been followed up for 6 months to 1 year. Superficial

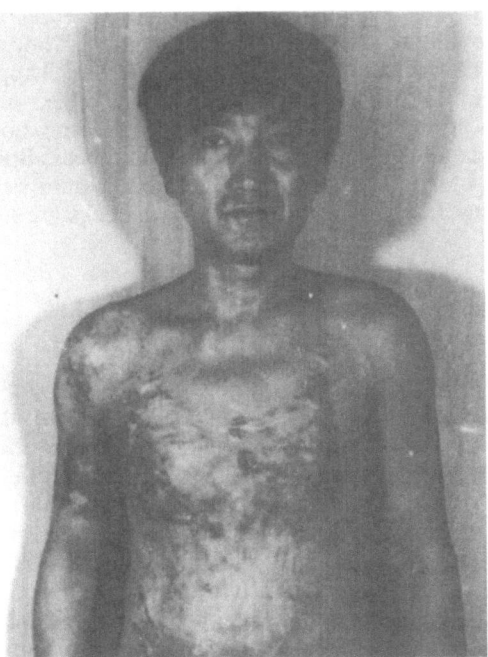

Figure 33.5 Same patient as Figures 33.1, 33.2. One year postburn, scattered hypertrophic scars are seen on the arm, chest and abdomen.

burns left no trace whatsoever. Deep dermal burns had scar formation with, however, only mild hypertrophy. The scars of deep dermal with scattered full-thickness burns were uneven, with scattered hypertrophic areas 0.5 cm above the rest of the skin surface (Figure 33.5). However, hypertrophy was mild in comparison with those patients in whom other nonsurgical methods were used.

Bacteriology

Aerobic and anaerobic bacterial cultures of the preserved amnion showed no growth up to 7 weeks after refrigeration. By the eighth week, candida were isolated in two of the four specimens.

Microscopy

Under light microscopy, the epithelium of the fresh amnion is a single layer of cuboid cells. The nuclei are round and clear. After 4 weeks of refrigeration, some epithelial cells become detached and the nuclei are small or crenated. By the eighth week no further change is noted.

Electron microscopy shows intact clear cell and nuclear membranes in a fresh amnion membrane. The chromosomes are uniformly distributed in the cytoplasm. Part of the heterochromatins gather together under the nuclear membrane. Microvilli are seen clearly on the surface. They are long and thin. The desmosomes between the cells are clear. As for the cell apparatus, numerous microfilaments and fat droplets can be seen. After 4 weeks under refrigeration, only mild changes are observed, i.e. the microvilli become shorter and flattened, and the chromosomes are blurred, with mild autolysis. Structure of the cell apparatus is also blurred, fat droplets decreased in number and vacuoles are present. The changes in amnion preserved for 8 weeks are similar to those for 4 weeks.

DISCUSSION

The clinical effects of refrigerated amniotic membrane in the treatment of burn wounds are immediate relief of pain, decrease in exudation, lessening of systemic reactions and shortening of healing time. Among the 22 cases studied, most wounds were deep dermal burns, some with scattered full-thickness burns. Moreover, in ten of the 22 cases, swab cultures of the burnt surface revealed bacterial growth before application of the amnion dressing. Most of these wounds healed after a single amnion dressing. It is presumed that the application of the amnion membrane facilitates both the control of infection and the protection of the residual epithelial cells. The burnt surface, while looking pale on admission, becomes reddish 12–24 h after application of amnion. This may be an indication that effective circulation in the burn wound has been restored. The control of infection and restoration of effective circulation will provide an optimal environment for healing.

Follow-up results on the 15 wounds of ten cases showed that there was less hypertrophic scar present on the deep dermal burns even with scattered third degree burns.

Most of the membranes used were refrigerated. The duration of refrigeration ranged from 2 days to 8 weeks. No difference was noted with regard to their therapeutic effects.

Bacteriologic examination revealed that our method of preparation and preservation proved to be sterile for 8 weeks. As for the fungal colonization found by the eighth week, it could be due to contamination from the frequent samplings. Nevertheless, to play safe, it may be wise to use only the amnion refrigerated for less than 6 weeks.

The mechanisms for the control of infection and promotion of epithelialization by amnion membrane are still uncertain. Some investigations have been made. Pigeon[2] mentioned that the amniotic membrane was formed by the ectoderm of the fetus. Electron microscopy[6] demonstrated that in early pregnancy, the amnion and fetal skin have many similarities. So it was suggested that amnion possesses functional properties similar to those of skin. Robson et al.[5] postulated that the antibacterial effect of amniotic dressing was due to the effective sealing of the wound which allowed the host immunologic activity to work at its peak efficiency. Dino et al.[1] found that biopsies of the burnt skin revealed massive infiltration of phagocytes under the membrane. Furthermore, Galask and Snyder[7] demonstrated that a number of antimicrobial factors were present in the amniotic fluid. Bose[8] indicated that amnion as a biologic dressing decreased evaporative losses. Thereby desiccation was avoided and conversion of a 'zone of stasis' to a 'zone of necrosis of full-thickness burns' was prevented.

In this study we have found that the clinical effects of the fresh and refrigerated amnions are alike. Histologic examinations demonstrate that after refrigeration the cell membrane and nuclear membrane of the amnion are intact but varying degrees of degeneration of the nucleus, cytoplasm and cell apparatus are observed. It seems that the therapeutic properties of the membrane are not related to its cell structures.

SUMMARY

Refrigerated human amnion has been used as a biologic dressing in the treatment of fresh burn wounds. Its clinical effects are immediate relief of pain, decreased exudation, fewer and milder systemic reactions and shortened healing time. Among the 22 cases (32 wounds) most wounds are deep second degree or deep second degree with scattered full-thickness burns. Most of these wounds healed in 10–21 days after a single dressing with the membrane. Ten of the 22 cases have been followed-up for 6–12 months. The deep burns had scar formation but the degree of hypertrophy was much less than that when other nonsurgical methods were applied.

A weekly check for sterility of the preserved fluid of the amnion by culture of aerobic and anaerobic organisms revealed no bacterial growth up to 7 weeks of refrigeration. Histologic examination of both fresh and refrigerated amnions demonstrated that after refrigeration both cell and nuclear membranes of the amnion were intact but varying degrees of degeneration of the nucleus, cytoplasm and cell apparatus did occur. It seemed that the therapeutic properties of the membrane were not related to its cell structures.

REFERENCES

1. Dino, B. R. *et al.* (1965). The use of fetal membrane homografts in the local management of burns. *J. Phili. Med. Assoc.*, **41**, 890–8
2. Pigeon, J. (1960). Treatment of 2nd degree burns with amniotic membranes. *Can. Med. Assoc. J.*, **83**, 844
3. Robson, M. C. *et al.* (1973). Amniotic membrane as a temporary wound dressing. *Surg. Gynecol. Obstet.*, **136**, 904
4. Joseph, S. G. *et al.* (1978). Human amniotic membrane. A versatile wound dressing. *Can. Med. Assoc. J.*, **188**, 1237
5. Robson, M. C. (1972). Quantitative comparison of biologic dressings. *Surg. Forum*, **23**, 503
6. Ursula, M. L. (1968). Ultrastructure of the human amnion, chorion and fetal skin. *J. Obstet. Gynecol. Br. Commonw.*, **75**, 327
7. Galask, R. P. and Snyder, I. S. (1970). Antimicrobial factors in amniotic fluid. *Am. J. Obstet. Gynecol.*, **106**, 59
8. Bose, B. (1979). Burn wound dressings with human amniotic membrane. *Ann. R. Coll. Surg. Eng.*, **61**, 444

34 Evaluation of Various Topical Chemical Antimicrobials in Burns: An Experimental Study

GE SHENGDE, FANG ZHIYANG, CHEN YULIN and XIANG XIUE

Burn Unit, Changhai Hospital, The Second Military Medical College, Shanghai

TU SHIZHONG, HAN GONGYU and XIU BINRONG

Pharmaceutical Department, The Second Military College, Shanghai

Burn wound infection is the main cause of sepsis and septicemia which threaten the lives of burn patients. Teplitz emphasized that management of the burn wound should be improved to meet the need to minimize the inherent bacterial strains[1]. New approaches were made[2] following the successful clinical use of mafenide (Sulfamylon)[3], silver nitrate[4] and silver sulfadiazine[5]. Drug sensitivity testing of some silver, zinc and cerium salts of the sulfa drugs and polyanamine and its derivatives against pyogenic bacteria commonly seen in burn infection was carried out in our Burn Unit in 1979[6]. The most sensitive drugs, silver sulfadiazine, silver sulfamerazine, and silver sulfamethazine, were picked out for further experimental study in *Pseudomonas* would sepsis in burned rats[7]. The present study was designed to make *in vitro* tests of the sensitivity of 17 chemical agents, most of them silver salts[8]. The sensitive drugs so selected, together with silver 2-sulfahydryl-4-nitropyridine-*N*-oxide, silver pipemidate and pipemidic acid, were tested on burned mice which were seeded with *Pseudomonas aeruginosa*.

MATERIAL AND METHODS

Drug sensitivity test

Source of bacterial strain

A strain of *P. aeruginosa* was obtained from the infected wound of a burn patient.

Culture medium

Common nutrient broth was used.

Topical antimicrobial agents

Sixteen silver salts were used. They were silver salts of *p*-methoxybenzoate, *p*-aminobenzoate, *p*-hydroxybenzoate, benzoate, fumarate, succinate, citrate, aspartate, sulfadimozine, sulfamethoxypyrazine, sulfamethoxydiazine, nicotinate, salicylate, pipemidate, sulfadiazine, and 2-sulfahydryl-4-nitropyridine-*N*-oxide. The only non-silver agent used was the pipemidic acid (which was prepared by the Pharmaceutical Department of the Second Military Medical College).

Method of determination

Tube dilution method was employed, and the working stock was prepared by adding 10 mg of each testing agent to 5 ml of distilled water to make a concentration of 2 mg/ml. The tubes were sealed, autoclaved and preserved in a refrigerator. Upon testing, the stock agents were further diluted by sterilized broth to 200 μg/ml, 100 μg/ml, 50 μg/ml, 25 μg/ml and 0.78 μg/ml in nine serial dilution tubes. The tenth tube was a blank which served as the control.

With highly potent antimicrobial agents, a hundred times dilution 20 μg/ml of the stock was first made, and then followed by a serial dilution as described above.

Bacterial inoculation was prepared by inoculating the strain of *P. aeruginosa* into a broth culture medium, and incubating for 6 h.

An 0.05 ml quantity of the bacterial inoculum was added to each testing tube and incubated under 37 °C for 24 h.

Topical treatment of the infected burn wound

Preparation of topical antimicrobial cream

Constituents of the cream base were: stearic acid, 11.25 g; glycerine monostearate, 7 g; glycerine 8.50 g; Vaseline, 8.50 g; sodium lauryl sulfate, 1 g; nipagine A, 0.10 g; dimethylsulfoxide, 2 ml; and distilled water, 61 ml.

Each 100 g of antimicrobial cream base contained 6 mmol of different silver salts, or 6 mmol pipemidic acid.

Preparation of broth culture

The same strain of *P. aeruginosa* as in the sensitivity test was employed. The bacteria were transferred into a broth medium the day prior to the experiment and were diluted to 10^9 microorganisms per milliliter on the day of experiment.

Topical treatment experiment

Preparation of animal model

Mice, irrespective of sex, weighing 14–22 g, were anesthetized with intraperitoneal sodium pentobarbital, 7 μg/g body weight. A deep second degree burn was inflicted by immersing the mouse's tail into a 70 °C water bath for 8 s. One hour after scalding, the burned tail was dipped into the *Pseudomonas* broth culture for 1 min. The seeded burned tail was then put into a plastic tube, 10–12 cm long and 0.6–0.8 cm in diameter, fixed by interrupted sutures to the surrounding skin.

Topical antimicrobial therapy

One hundred forty mice were divided into seven groups. Topical therapy was started 5 h after seeding. The cream base and the cream of antimicrobial agents were given to the animals of corresponding groups except the control group. An adequate amount of cream was injected with a syringe into the plastic tube, until the burned tail was in full contact with the cream. A silk ligature was made at the distal end of the plastic tube to prevent the cream from leaking out. The animals were then caged in groups, with food and water taken *ad libitum*. The observation lasted 2 weeks. Some animals died within the observation period and date of death was recorded. Heart blood was drawn and cultured after death.

RESULT

The sensitivity of the antimicrobial agents determined by the tube dilution method showed that the minimal inhibitory concentration (MIC) of silver aspartate and silver nicotinate appeared to be the lowest. They were the highly sensitive agents against the strain of *P. aeruginosa*. The silver salts of succinate,

Table 34.1 MIC of topical antimicrobial agents

Topical antimicrobial	MIC (μg/ml)
Silver p-methoxybenzoate	3.125
Silver p-aminobenzoate	3.125
Silver p-hydroxybenzoate	3.125
Silver benzoate	3.125
Silver fumarate	1.563
Silver succinate	1.563
Silver citrate	1.563
Silver aspartate	0.781
Silver sulfadimozine	3.125
Silver sulfamethoxypyrazine	3.125
Silver sulfamethoxydiazine	6.250
Silver nicotinate	0.781
Silver salicylate	1.562
Silver 2-sulfahydryl-4-nitropyridine-*N*-oxide	3.125
Silver sulfadiazine	3.125
Silver pipemidate	1.563
Pipemidic acid	6.250

fumarate, citrate, and salicylate ranked second (Table 34.1). The MIC of 2-sulfahydryl-4-nitropyridine-N-oxide in the present study was similar to that determined in our laboratory in 1980, it being the most sensitive agent among polyanamine and its derivatives. Pipemidic acid and silver pipemidate were the effective topical antimicrobial agents with less toxicity[8] which were recently prepared by the Pharmaceutical Department of our college.

The concentrations of the selected topical antimicrobial agents and their therapeutic results in mice are listed in Table 34.2.

Each group comprised 20 animals. In both the control and the cream base groups 19 out of 20 animals died. All positive blood cultures of P. aeruginosa were obtained from the dead animals. The number of animals in the silver pipemidate, silver nicotinate, pipemidic acid, silver 2-sulfahydryl-4-nitropyridine-N-oxide and silver aspartate groups was one, two, four, four and five respectively. Growths of P. aeruginosa in blood cultures proved to exist in all but three pipemidic acid groups.

DISCUSSION

The problem of drug resistance of silver sulfadiazine has been reported in the literature[9,10]. Yet it remains the most effective antimicrobial agent among the metallic salts of sulfa drugs[6,11–13]. The result of in vitro screening of 17 chemical antimicrobial agents (16 being silver salts) showed that the sensitivity of some of the non-sulfa silver salts against P. aeruginosa far exceeded that of silver sulfadiazine. Among these 17 agents, five were selected for the therapeutic study on P. aeruginosa infection of burned mouse tails.

Experimental results showed that there were 19 deaths in both the control and cream base groups. The number of deaths was obviously minimized in all the therapeutic groups, which indicated the efficacy of the treatment. Among the antimicrobial agents, silver pipemidate and silver nicotinate were the most effective. Dead animals in the pipemidic acid, silver 2-sulfahydryl-4-nitropyridine-N-oxide and silver aspartate groups numbered four, four and five respectively. Growth of P. aeruginosa was demonstrated in all groups except the silver pipemidate group, in which three out of four were negative.

The present study offers effective topical antimicrobial agents which were proved by therapeutic experiment to be more effective than silver sulfadiazine. These agents may be considered for clinical trial.

CONCLUSION

The study reported in this chapter was designed to determine the drug sensitivity of 17 topical antimicrobial agents against P. aeruginosa in order to select effective agents for the prevention of P. aeruginosa burn wound sepsis. The results demonstrated that all the agents were sensitive; silver aspartate and silver nicotinate showed the lowest MIC. The latter two drugs, together with the recently formulated pipemidic acid, silver pipemidate, and the silver 2-sulfahydryl-4-nitropyridine-N-oxide, were selected for therapeutic study on

Table 34.2 Therapeutic results of topical antimicrobial cream

Group	Cream conc. (%)	Animals	Deaths (n) 1st wk	2nd wk	Total	Positive blood cultures of P. aeruginosa
Control	—	20	17	2	19	19
Cream base	—	20	19	—	19	19
Silver nicotinate	0.7	20	2	—	2	2
Silver aspartate	0.5	20	5	—	5	5
Pipemidic acid	0.9	20	4	—	1	1
Silver pipemidate	1.2	20	1	—	1	1
Silver 2-sulfahydryl-4-nitropyridine-N-oxide	0.8	20	4	—	4	4

burned mouse tails infected with *P. aeruginosa*. The antimicrobial agents were applied in the form of cream with the model group, with the cream base group as the control. Significant therapeutic efficacy was shown in silver pipemidate and silver nicotinate. The present study offers effective topical antimicrobial agents for the prevention and treatment of *Pseudomonas* burn wound sepsis and probably septicemia.

REFERENCES

1. Teplitz, C. *et al.* (1964). Pseudomonas burn wound sepsis. I. Pathogenesis of experimental Pseudomonas burn wound sepsis. *J. Surg. Res.*, **4**, 200
2. Modak, S. M. *et al.* (1981). Sulfadiazine silver-resistant Pseudomonas in burns. New topical agents. *Arch. Surg.*, **116**, 854
3. Lindberg, R. B. *et al.* (1965). The successful control of burn wound sepsis. *J. Trauma*, **5**, 601
4. Moyer, C. A. *et al.* (1965). Treatment of large human burns with 0.5% silver nitrate solution. *Arch. Surg.*, **90**, 812
5. Fox, C. L. Jr. (1967). Silver sulfadiazine. Addendum to local therapy of burns. *Mod. Treat.* **4**, 1259
6. Ge, S. D. *et al.* (1980). Drug sensitivity test of N^1-metal sulfa drugs and zincpolyanemine and its derivatives against commonly seen pathogenic bacteria in burns. *Acad. J. 2nd Mil. Med. Coll. PLA*, **1**, 35
7. Ge, S. D. *et al.* (1980). Study of antibacterial therapy of burn wound sepsis. *Acad. J. 2nd Mil. Med. Coll. PLA*, **1**, 38
8. Tu, S. Z. *et al.* (1982). The preparation of 22 kinds of silver, zinc organic salts and their antibacterial actions. *Acad. J. 2nd Mil. Med. Coll. PLA*, **3** (*Suppl.*). **58**
9. Veisfw, K. *et al.* (1977). Drug resistance in relation to the use of silver sulphadiazine cream in a burn unit. *J. Clin. Pathol.*, **30**, 160
10. Heggers, J. P. *et al.* (1978). The emergence of silver sulphadiazine resistant Pseudomonas aeruginosa. *Burns*, **5**, 184
11. Fox, C. L. Jr. *et al.* (1979). Metal sulfonamides as antibacterial agents in topical therapy. *Scand. J. Plast. Reconstr. Surg.*, **13**, 89
12. Pegg, S. P. *et al.* (1979). Clinical comparison of maphenide and silver sulphadiazine. *Scand. J. Plast. Reconstr. Surg.*, **13**, 95
13. Salisbury, R. E. *et al.* (1980). Burn wound sepsis: Effect of delayed treatment with topical chemotherapy on survival. *J. Trauma*, **20**, 120

35 Early Diagnosis of Burn Wound Infection with *Aspergillus* by the Use of Tissue Sliver Culture

XIAO GUANGXIA, WANG DEWANG, ZHANG YAPING, LIU MINGZHEN and QIN XIAOJIAN
Burn Center, Southwestern Hospital, The Third Military Medical College, Chongqing

Since topical antibacterial agents have become widely used in treatment of burn wounds, the incidence of fungal infections caused by *Aspergillus* and *Mucor* have become an increasing problem for burn patients in recent years. The clinical manifestations of these fungal infections are quite different from those caused by *Candida*. Invasion into the burn wound appears to be common and rapid, often followed by a poor therapeutic result. Therefore, a means of early diagnosis is urgently needed. In our clinical practice, it has been shown that organisms recovered from either swabs or biopsy specimens taken from burn wounds were often a mix of bacteria and fungi. However, since the common cultural media (blood, agar etc) are more favorable for the rapid growth of common bacteria, the existence of fungi was often overlooked. From February 1981, a modified cultural procedure – tissue sliver culture – has been used for 100 biopsy specimens, 38 culture results of which were compared with those of common cultures and histologic findings of the tissue biopsy. It has been found that the tissue sliver culture method appears to be the best for the recovery of *Aspergillus* from the wound.

METHODS

Under aseptic conditions, a tissue sliver (nearly 0.5 g in weight) is taken from the wound and placed on the slope of Sabouraud culture medium. Along the slope of the medium 1–2 ml amikacin solution (1000 μg/ml) is added. It is incubated under 37 °C and examined daily. Positive growth is identified by the appearance of fungal hyphae, and the isolated fungal species should be further identified.

RESULTS

From February to July 1982, a total of 100 biopsy specimens suspected of fungal infections was taken for tissue sliver cultures, 47 of which revealed the emergence of fungi. The pathogenic organisms were *Aspergillus*, totalling 37, and *Candida, Mucor* and *Penicillium*, comprising the other ten.

Thirty-eight biopsy specimens were simultaneously studied by using three different procedures, i.e. silver swabs, surface technique tissue biopsies and tissue sliver cultures. The recovery rates were quite different (Table 35.1).

Table 35.1 Recovery rate of *Aspergillus* from 38 biopsy specimens using three different methods

Method	Specimens (n)	Positive growth (n)	%
Swabs and surface cultures	38	3	8
Tissue biopsy	38	10	26
Tissue sliver cultures	38	23	61

Ten specimens proved to be fungal invasions by the histologic examination of tissue biopsy. Similar specimens were taken for common and tissue sliver cultures, the results of which are shown in Table 35.2.

DISCUSSION

Fungal infections of the burn wound are tending to increase, but diagnosis of such infection has often been overlooked or delayed. This is probably related to the lack of an accurate diagnostic method. In clinical practice, the identification of pathogenic organisms and the decision on therapeutic measures are usually based on the results of common cultures, which are unsuitable for satisfactory growth of fungi, especially in the case of concurrent bacterial infection. The rapid growth of bacteria in common culture interferes with the growth of fungi. As shown in Table 35.2, 38 biopsy specimens suspected of fungal infection were simultaneously studied by three methods, the positive rates of which were 61% in tissue sliver cultures, 26% in tissue biopsies and only 8% in common cultures. Ten biopsy specimens which had been histologically proved to be invasive fungal infections were subjected to tissue sliver cultures, all of which revealed fungal growth, while in the common cultures, eight revealed only heavy growth of *Pseudomonas aeruginosa, Staphylococcus pyogenes,* and *Serratia*. Fungal growth was demonstrated in two specimens, but they accounted only for 1–3% of the colonies found. It should be pointed out that, in most of these biopsy sections, a large number of spores or hyphae have been demonstrated under microscopic examinations, and in some of them evidence of vascular invasion has been found. This denotes that the common cultural method could not meet the need for the monitoring of fungal infection. Pruitt suggested the timely histologic examination of the biopsy of burn wounds, which attracted our attention, and since 1981, we have used both HE stain and PAS stain for histologic preparations. While the histologic examinations yield better results than the common cultures, however, once the fungal invasion was identified by histologic section, not infrequently it would be seen that diagnosis was already

Table 35.2 *Aspergillus* detection by common cultures and tissue sliver cultures from ten biopsy specimens with histologic evidence of *Aspergillus* invasion

No.	Sample	Histologic exam. (HE + PAS stain)	Common culture		Tissue thread culture	
			Aspergillus Bacteria		Aspergillus	Culture day
1	Leg muscle	Aspergillus invasion	−	S. pyogenes	+	3
2	Leg muscle	Aspergillus invasion	1%	S. pyogenes 98%	+	2
3	Thigh muscle	Aspergillus invasion	−	Pseudomonas 1% Pseudomonas S. pyogenes	+	3
4	Thigh subeschar	Aspergillus invasion	−	Pseudomonas	+	4
5	Forearm subeschar	Aspergillus invasion	−	Pseudomonas	+	2
6	Leg subeschar	Aspergillus heavy growth	3%	S. pyogenes 97%	+	1
7	M. pectoralis major	Aspergillus heavy growth	−	Serratia	+	2
8	Upper limb muscle	Aspergillus vascular invasion	−	Serratia	+	3
9	Thigh muscle	Aspergillus vascular invasion	−	Serratia	+	3
10	Forearm muscle	Aspergillus vascular invasion	−	Serratia	+	1

too late, and extensive debridement, even amputation of the infected limb, would not be able to save the patient's life. Fungal infections have their own pattern of onset and development. Clinical manifestations often give us an impression that fungal infection in burn wounds appears insidiously severely and late. The reason probably lies in the fact that an accurate and quicker method for the identification of fungi isolates is still lacking. We found the use of tissue sliver cultures for fungal growth seems to improve the method for monitoring fungal infection of burn wounds.

The higher yield of tissue sliver culture may contribute to the fact that the tissue itself may serve as an ideal medium for the growth of fungi and, in addition, the utilization of Sabouraud culture medium and addition of amikacin solution to inhibit the concomitant common bacteria might further provide a favorable environment for the rapid growth of fungi.

36 The Toxin of Decomposed Burn Tissues

ZHANG MINGLIANG, XIAO YONGAN, LI HESHENG, SUN YONGHUA and CHANG ZHIDE

Burn Unit, Ji Shui Tan Hospital, Beijing

Every burn surgeon must face the challenge of a still puzzling syndrome, burn toxemia. The role played by bacteria and their toxins in so-called 'burn toxemia' has been made clear during recent years. Burn infection has its own special character since it is related, without a single exception, to the existence of burn eschar. In view of these characteristics, it seems imperative to search into the interactions between the bacteria, eschars and the host as a whole in order to verify the nature of 'burn toxemia'. The experiment reported in this chapter was thus inspired and designed.

MATERIALS AND METHODS

Mice weighing 20–25 g were used in this experiment. The bacteria employed were *Staphylococcus albus*, *Staphylococcus aureus*, *Bacillus subtilis* and *Pseudomonas aeruginosa*.

The mice were divided into four groups.

(1) Eschar bacteria group. The mice were depilated and immersed in a 80 °C bath for 30 s to produce a third degree burn covering 80% of the BSA. The eschars were excised immediately and put in Petri dishes. The broth of the bacteria which had been cultured at 37 °C for 16–20 h was added to the dishes. These dishes were placed in a 37 °C incubator for 6 d. The contents of the dishes were homogenized and then extracted with normal saline at 40 °C overnight and centrifuged. The supernatant was collected and sterilized in a boiling water bath for 30 min. The samples were centrifuged and the supernatants were stored for use.

The burn area of a mouse was 80% of the body surface; the eschars produced from this were about 2.5 g in weight; the amount of the extract prepared from 1 g of eschar was 1 ml.

(2) Bacteria control group. The bacteria were cultured in the broth at 37 °C for 6 days, heated in a boiling water bath for 30 min, and stored.

Table 36.1 Toxicity of eschar bacteria

Extracts	Animals (n)	Amount of extract (ml)	Dead (n)	Time of death
Eschar + *S. aureus*	10	1	10	
Eschar + *S. albus*	9	1	7	within 12 h
Eschar + *S. albus* + *B. subtilis*	14	1	14	
Eschar + *P. aeruginosa*	10	1	10	

(3) Eschar control group. The eschars were put in Petri dishes. A similar amount of broth without bacteria was added with penicillin and streptomycin. The extracts were prepared as in group 1.

(4) Normal skin bacteria control group. The mice were depilated. Normal skin of 80% of the BSA was excised and cultured with *S. albus*. The extracts were prepared in the same way.

All procedures were performed under strict aseptic conditions. The extracts were repeatedly cultured to show that the bacteria were original. The extracts of eschar (group 3) were proved sterile before use. One milliliter of various extracts prepared was used to attack the mice by intraperitoneal injection. The mice which received intraperitoneal injections were caged and observed for 7 d.

RESULTS

Eschar bacteria

Five minutes after injection, the mice looked ill (weakness, dyspnea, twitch etc). Most of them died in 30 min, some in 12 h (Table 36.1).

Table 36.1 shows that the eschar bacteria can make most of the mice die, even when the eschar is incubated with nonpathogenic organisms such as *B. subtilis*. Death was caused neither by the living bacteria nor by the thermolabile exotoxin which was readily destroyed at 80 °C for 30 min.

Bacteria control

The mice were attacked with heated bacteria broth. The results are shown in Table 36.2.

Table 36.2 Toxicity of heated bacteria broth

Bacteria	Animals (n)	Attacking dose (ml)	Dead (n)	Time of death
S. aureus	10	1.0	0	
	4	2.0	0	
S. albus	9	1.0	0	
	4	2.0	0	
B. subtilis	4	1.5	0	
	4	2.0	0	
P. aeruginosa	11	1.0	11	12–36 h

It can be seen from Table 36.2 that none of the heated cultures of *S. aureus*, *S. albus* and *B. subtilis* could cause death in any of the animals. However, heated culture of *P. aeruginosa* killed all animals; obviously it was caused by endotoxin which was thermostable and was not destroyed by boiling. But the animals killed by heated *P. aeruginosa* died in 12–36 h, whereas the animals in the eschar bacteria group of *P. aeruginosa* died in 30 min to 12 h. The lethal effects were quite different.

Simple eschars

Both the eschar extracts and the extracts of eschars which were pretreated with pancreatin were used to attack the mice. The results are illustrated in Table 36.3.

This part of the experiment demonstrates that the simple eschar extracts have no toxicity.

Table 36.3 Toxicity of simple eschar extracts

Extracts	Animals (n)	Dose for attack (ml)	Dead (n)
Eschar	15	1.5	0
Eschar + pancreatin	10	1.0	0

Normal skin bacteria controls

The extracts of *in vitro* incubation of normal skin with *S. albus* were used to attack mice; the doses used were 1.5 ml per animal. Two mice died and eight survived. This shows the toxicity is less than that of eschar bacteria extracts.

Table 36.4 shows us the conclusion that the mortality with extracts of eschar Gram-positive bacteria in the mice is 94%. Only a few animals in group 4 are killed. There are statistical significances between group 1 and the other control groups ($p < 0.005$). It is considered that the high death rate of the animals resulted from decomposed elements of 'eschar bacteria'.

Table 36.4 Comparison of toxicity among various extracts

Group	Extract	Animals (n)	Dead (n)	Mortality	χ^2	p
1	Eschar + Gram-positive bacteria	33	31	94%		
2	Heated Gram-positive bacteria	35	0	0	60.4	< 0.005
3	Simple eschar	25	0	0	50.4	< 0.005
4	Normal skin + Gram-positive bacteria	10	2	20%	16.2	< 0.005

Estimation of lethal doses of eschar bacteria extracts

B. subtilis and *S. albus* were selected to make eschar bacteria extracts (Table 36.5).

The lethal dose of 0.05 ml/g body weight is equivalent to about 34% BSA of the infected eschars and the lethal dose of 0.04 ml/g body weight is equivalent to about 28% BSA of the infected eschars.

Table 36.5 Lethal doses of extracts

| | Eschar – S. albus extract | | | | Eschar – S. albus – B. subtilis extract | | |
Animals (n)	Amounts of extracts (ml/g body weight)		Results	Animals (n)	Amounts of extracts (ml/g body weight)		Results
7	0.054	0.053	All died	12	0.050	0.048	All died
	0.053	0.052			0.047		
	0.052				0.045	0.045	
	0.051				0.043		
	0.050				0.041	0.041	
					0.040	0.040	
					0.040	0.040	
2	0.048	0.048	All died	5	0.036	0.036	All died
					0.034	0.034	
					0.032		
5	0.047	0.043	All survived	5	0.036	0.036	All survived
	0.043	0.042			0.034	0.031	
	0.039				0.022		

Table 36.6 Composition of extracts

Composition	Eschar + Gram-positive bacteria	Normal skin + Gram-positive bacteria	Simple eschar	Culture of S. albus	Culture of S. aureus
Indole	+	+	–	–	–
Hydrogen sulfide	+	+	–	–	–
Phenol	–	–	–	–	–
Sulfate	+	+++	+	+++	+++
Phosphate	+++	+	+	+++	+++
Chloride	+	+	+	+	+
Ammonia (mg%)	25	12.4	5	7.43	6.08
Amines (mg%)	769	89.3	5	42.3	42.3

+ + + large amounts; + + moderate amounts; + small amounts; – negative

Composition of the toxin and pathology

The compositions of the various extracts were analyzed and are listed in Table 36.6.

Except for ammonia and amines, the quantities of the remaining constituents of various extracts are nearly the same. The ammonia in the eschar bacteria extracts is one to three times the amount of other extracts. The amounts of amines in the eschar bacteria extract equal about 150 times that of the simple eschar extract, about 18 times that of the bacteria cultures, and about eight times that of the normal skin bacteria extract. Amines are strongly toxic to organisms. A large quantity of these substances is produced after the eschar has decomposed by bacterial action. Suppose amines are the major toxic substances lethal to the animals. The normal skin produces a small quantity of amines of low toxicity, after the skin has incubated bacteria. Simple eschar extract of bacteria cultures also contains a small amount of amines, which are not enough to cause the death of animals.

Autopsies were performed immediately after death of the animals. Specific pathologic changes were not found, except for edema and leukocyte infiltration of the heart, liver, spleen, lungs, kidneys, and intestines.

DISCUSSION

Rosental[1] and Fedorov et al.[2] first presented the theory of 'burn toxin'. They described the burnt skin as a toxin which could cause the poisoning of the body. Recently, investigators have refined the 'burn toxin' theory[3,4] but some authors consider that the metabolites of certain bacteria may be the cause of death[5] of those patients who died of 'burn toxemia'.

From the present experiment we found that the eschars decomposed by bacteria might produce a group of toxic substances, which we named 'the toxin of decomposed burn tissues'. The major component of these toxic substances is amines. If severe infection is developed on a wound covering more than 30% of the BSA, the toxic substances formed might be lethal to the body. It should be noted that the extracts were roughly prepared. Otherwise we might expect to have extracted substances of stronger toxicity. Since the mechanism of burn toxemia is complex, in addition to the effect of bacteria and their toxins the role played by 'the toxin of decomposed burn tissues' must be considered.

REFERENCES

1. Rosental, S.R. (1959). Substances released from skin following thermal injury, 'burn toxin'. *Surgery*, **46**, 932
2. Fedorov, N.A. *et al.* (1959) Experimental investigationon burn autoantigens. *Pathophysiol. Exp. Ther.*, **6**, 53
3. Schoeuenber, G.A. *et al.* (1975). Experimental evidence for a significant impairment of host defence for Gram-negative organisms by a specific cutaneous toxin produced by severe burn injuries. *Surg. Gynecol. Obstet.* **4**, 555

4. Aoyama, H. *et al.* (1980). Toxic effects of extracts from burned skin, serum and blister fluid of burned patients on mitochondrial function. *Burns*, **47**, 33

5. Artz, C.P. *et al.* (1979) Review of mechanisms for toxemia associated with bacteremia. In Artz, C.P. *et al.* (eds.) *Burns, A Team Approach*. p. 70. (Philadelphia, London, Toronto: Saunders)

37 The Common Organisms of Invasive Infection in Burns and the Choice of Antibiotics

XIAO GUANGXIA, WANG DEWANG, ZHANG YAPING, LIU MINGZHENG and QIN XIAO JIAN

Burn Center, Southwestern Hospital, The Third Military Medical College, Chongqing

Colonization of burn wounds soon after injury seems inevitable. However, as a matter of fact, most of them are superficial or noninvasive. Whenever the organisms were found to be from the adjacent unburnt tissue, the nature of the infection would turn out to be invasive, and a different clinical significance would emerge. In our unit, during the period from April 1980 to April 1982, a total of 226 strains of organisms isolated from cultures of the subeschar unburnt tissue were collected. These data may reflect some clinical aspects of the common invasive organisms of burns in the early 1980s. Meanwhile, thorough investigations of drug sensitivity to 17 antibiotics were carried out. A reference scheme of antibiotic choice can thus be presented.

RESULTS

Organisms discovered from cultures of subeschar unburnt tissue

As shown in Table 37.1, 226 strains including 21 species were identified.
The following conclusions are reached from the data in Table 37.1.

(1) The number of Gram-negative rods exceeded that of the strains isolated. Gram-negative rods accounted for 117 strains and Gram-positive cocci 92 strains. The ratio between them was 1.27:1.

(2) From the 117 strains of Gram-negative rods, 13 bacterial species were differentiated, of which *Pseudomonas, Serratia, Klebsiella* and *Escherichia coli* accounted for 92 strains and were responsible for 83.8% of the Gram-negative rods infections. Therefore, due attention should be paid to these four rods so far as prevention and treatment of Gram-negative rods infection are concerned.

(3) In preventing and treating Gram-positive coccal infections, attention should be paid to *Staphylococcus pyogenes, Staphylococcus albus,*

Table 37.1 Organisms isolated from cultures of subeschar unburnt tissue*

Organisms	Positive No.	Positive rate %
Gram − rods:		
Pseudomonas	57	25.2
Serratia	17	7.5
Klebsiella	14	6.2
E. coli	10	4.5
Proteus	4	1.8
Citrobacter	4	1.8
B. anitratus	3	1.3
E. cloaca	2	0.9
M. polymorpha	2	0.9
B. alcaligenes	1	0.4
Flavobacterium	1	0.4
Aeromonas liquefaciens	1	0.4
Aerogenes	1	0.4
Subtotal	117	51.7
Gram + cocci:		
S. pyogenes	50	22.1
S. albus	20	8.9
S. faecalis	14	6.2
Streptococci	6	2.7
Tetragena	2	0.9
Subtotal	92	40.8
Others:		
Fungi	11	4.9
Diphtheroid	3	1.3
B. subtilis	3	1.3
Total	226	100%

*226 strains, April 1980–April 1982

Streptococcus faecalis and Streptococci, because these four species accounted for 90 of a total of 92 strains, and were responsible for 97.9% of the Gram-positive coccus infections.

Drug sensitivity of the common invasive organisms in burn wound infection

As stated above, the predominant invasive pathogens of burn wounds were four in Gram-negative rods and four in Gram-positive cocci. Therefore, analyses of drug sensitivity deal chiefly with these eight pathogens to 17 antibiotics being used now in our unit. These 17 antibiotics are penicillin, erythromycin, oxacillin, tetracycline, kitasamycin (leucomycin), lincomycin, chloramphenicol, metronidazole, ampicillin, kanamycin, amikacin, gentamicin, tobramycin, polymyxin B, carbenicillin, sulbenicillin and cephradine. For the sake of

Table 37.2   The common invasive organisms of burns and drug sensitivity*

Organisms	Antibiotics (sensitivity rate %)†
Pseudomonas	Amika. (100), poly. B (93), tobra. (42.3)
Serratia	Amika. (96.2), poly. B (96.2), tobra (61.5)
Klebsiella	Amika. (100), poly. B (93.8), tobra. (81.3), cephra. (50)
E. coli	Amika. (100), poly. B (90), tobra. (80), genta. (70), cephra. (60), kana. (50)
S. pyogenes	Amika. (96.2), kita. (leuco.) (88.8), linco. (87.5), cephra. (83.8), oxacil. (77.5), tobra. (70), sulbeni. (57.5), genta. (53.8)
S. albus	Kita. (leuco.) (100), carbeni. (100), cephra. (94.1), linco (88.2), amika. (88.2), genta. (70.6), oxacil. (70.6), erythro. (70.6), ampicil. (52.9), tetra. (52.9)
S. faecalis	Amika. (88.5), cephra. (69.2), kita. (leuco.) (50)
Streptococci	Oxacil. (100), ampicil. (100), carbeni. (100), penici. (90.9), kita. (leuco.) (90.9), tobra. (90.9), sulbeni. (90.9), linco. (80.2), chlora. (80.2), genta. (80.2), erythro. (80.2), kana. (80.2), amika. (72.7)

*Only drugs with a sensitivity rate > 50% are listed
†For full drug names, see text

convenience in consultation, only those drugs with a sensitivity rate exceeding 50% are listed, in Table 37.2.

Brief comments on kanamycin, gentamicin, polymyxin B and amikacin

Since 1960, the antibiotics recommended by our unit for the prevention and treatment of Gram-negative rods infections were kanamycin, gentamicin and polymyxin B. However, with the exception of polymyxin B, their sensitivity rates have been declining sharply. For example, in the early 1960s, kanamycin was the first choice in treating Gram-negative rods infections, except *Pseudomonas*, as it maintained a sensitivity rate exceeding 80%, but by now its sensitivity rate to *Serratia*, *Klebsiella* and *E. coli* has decreased to only 26.9%, 18.8%, and 50% respectively, and we plan to abandon it. Gentamicin, once extensively used in this unit, is also going to be dropped, because its sensitivity to strains of *Pseudomonas* (28.2%), *Serratia* (34.6%) and *Klebsiella* (31.3%) has fallen dramatically. There is an interesting finding that, although polymyxin B has been used for more than 20 years in this unit, its sensitivity rate to strains of *Pseudomonas*, *Serratia*, *Klebsiella* and *E. coli* is still high, up to 93.6%, 96.1%, 93.8% and 90% respectively. At present, the sensitivity rate of amikacin to eight of the above organisms is markedly high, i.e. to *Pseudomonas* 100%, *Serratia* 96.2%, *Klebsiella* 100%, *E. coli* 100%, *S. pyogenes* 96.2%, *S. albus* 88.2%, *S. faecalis* 88.5%, and Streptococci 80.2%. It is, by far, the only drug found effective against a majority of both Gram-negative rods and Gram-positive cocci. It is proposed that rational use of this drug should be figured out in order to keep up its potency longer.

Table 37.3 Reference scheme for choice of antibiotics in invasive infection of burn wounds

Organisms	Ordinary infection	Serious infection
Gram − rods:		
Pseudomonas	Polymyxin B	Amikacin
Serratia	Tobramycin	Amikacin, polymyxin B
Klebsiella	Tobramycin, cephradine	Amikacin, polymyxin B
E. coli	Tobramycin, gentamicin, cephradine	Amikacin, polymyxin B
Gram + cocci:		
S. pyogenes	Oxacillin	Kitasamycin (leucomycin), lincomycin, cephradine
S. albus	Oxacillin	Kitasamycin (leucomycin), lincomycin, cephradine
S. faecalis	Cephradine, kitasamycin (leucomycin)	Amikacin
Streptococci	Penicillin, oxacillin	Cephradine

Choice of antibiotic in treating invasive infection of burns

For convenience in choosing drugs, we have worked out a reference scheme (Table 37.3) based on the following two points.

(1) Drugs selected should be those of higher sensitivity rate.

(2) Because of the frequent existence of mixed infection of burn wounds, the drugs with a comparatively broader antimicrobial spectrum were given preference.

In addition, considering the cost and supply of the drugs, we divided the infections into two groups: in cases of minor and moderate burns without critical clinical pictures, drugs in the 'ordinary infection' category should be chosen, while in extensive full-thickness burns or cases with critical clinical pictures, drugs in the category of 'serious infection' should be chosen.

38 Early Surgical Treatment of Severely Burned Hands

ZHONG DECAI

Department of Plastic Surgery and Burns, The First Hospital, The Fourth Military Medical College, Xian

Early escharectomy (or tangential excision) followed by immediate grafting is a preferred treatment in the management of deep burns of the hand. This kind of treatment gives not only a better functional result, but may also reduce the amputation rate. However, exposed burned phalangeal bones and joints might often lead to a partial or complete amputation subsequently. The object of our present work is to establish the appropriate measures to preserve the digital length. This chapter presents a report of our recent clinical experiences in the early surgical treatment of severely burned hands. There were nine cases with 14 hands and 66 digits, and fine results were achieved in all.

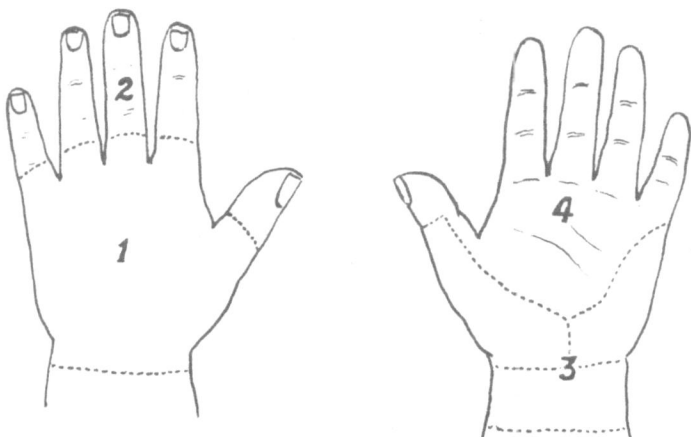

Figure 38.1 Regional areas of burned hands. 1, Dorsum of hand; 2, dorsum of digit; 3, thenar–wrist area; 4, volar–digit area

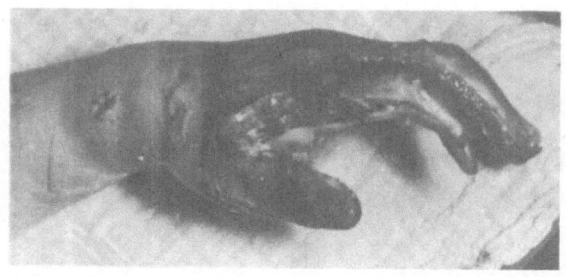

a

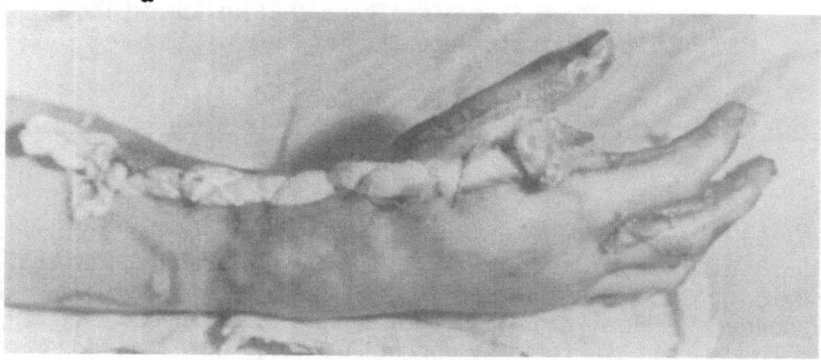

b

Figure 38.2   a, Escharotomy of digits. **b**, Escharotomy of third degree burned hand

THERAPEUTIC MEASURES

Anatomic characteristics and management

Based on its anatomic characteristics, the hand may be divided into four areas (Figure 38.1).

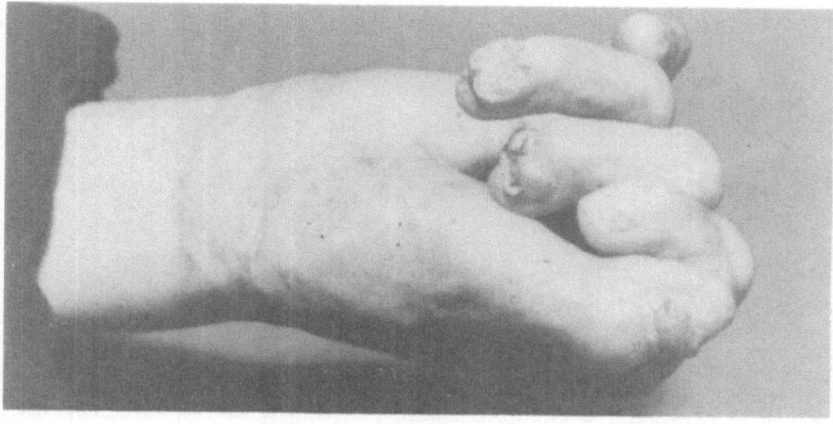

a

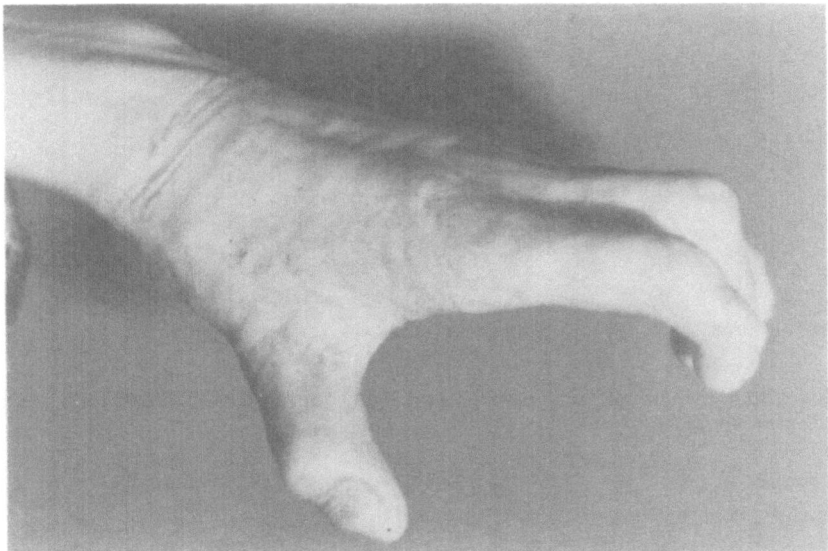

b

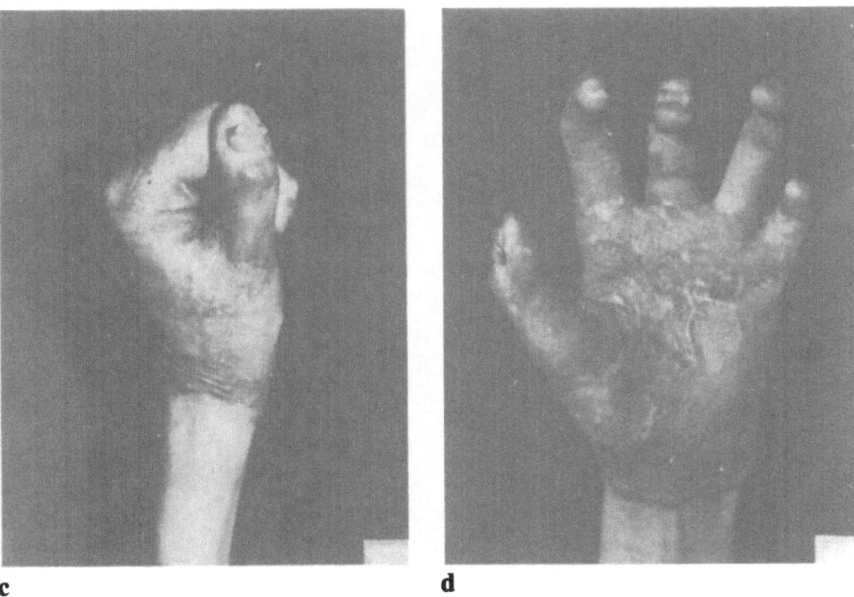

c   d

Figure 38.3 a,b, Results of escharectomy and immediate skin graft of a whole hand suffering from third degree burns; followed up for 1½ years. **c,d,** Primary excision and prompt graft of a total hand, postoperation for 1 year

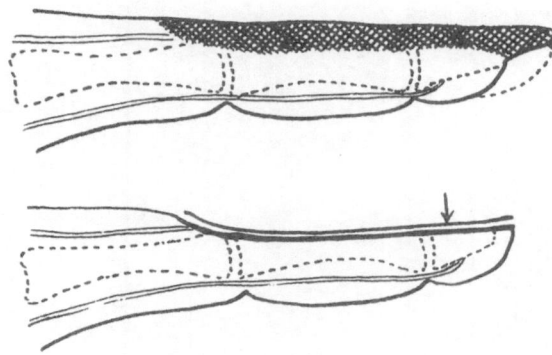

Figure 38.4 Management of exposed bones and joints with fingertip repair. Arrow indicates skin graft

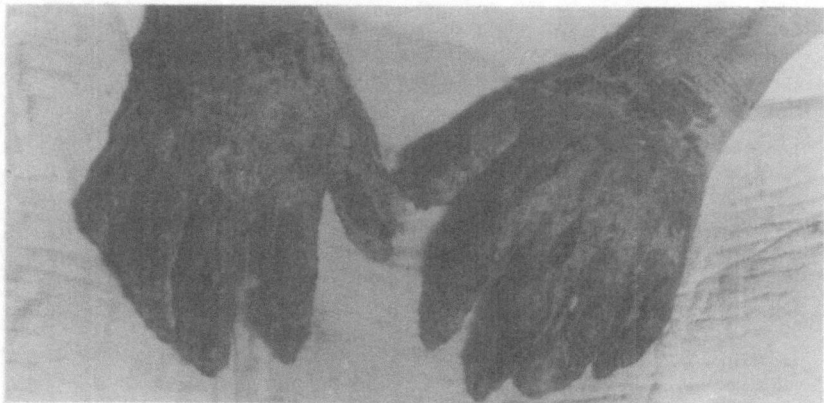

a

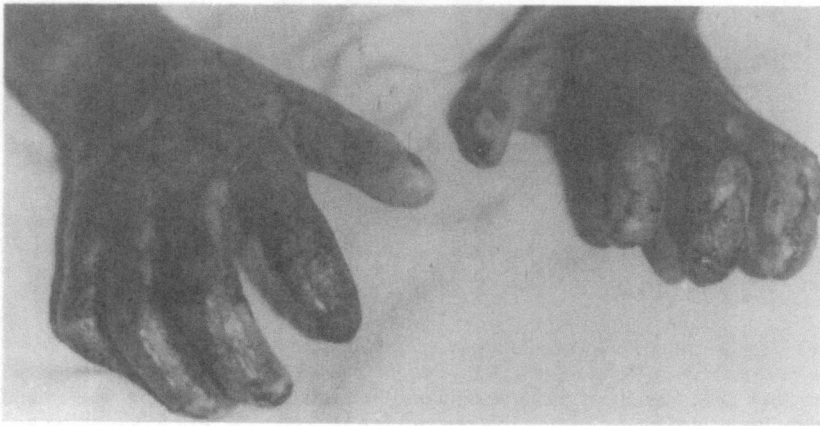

b

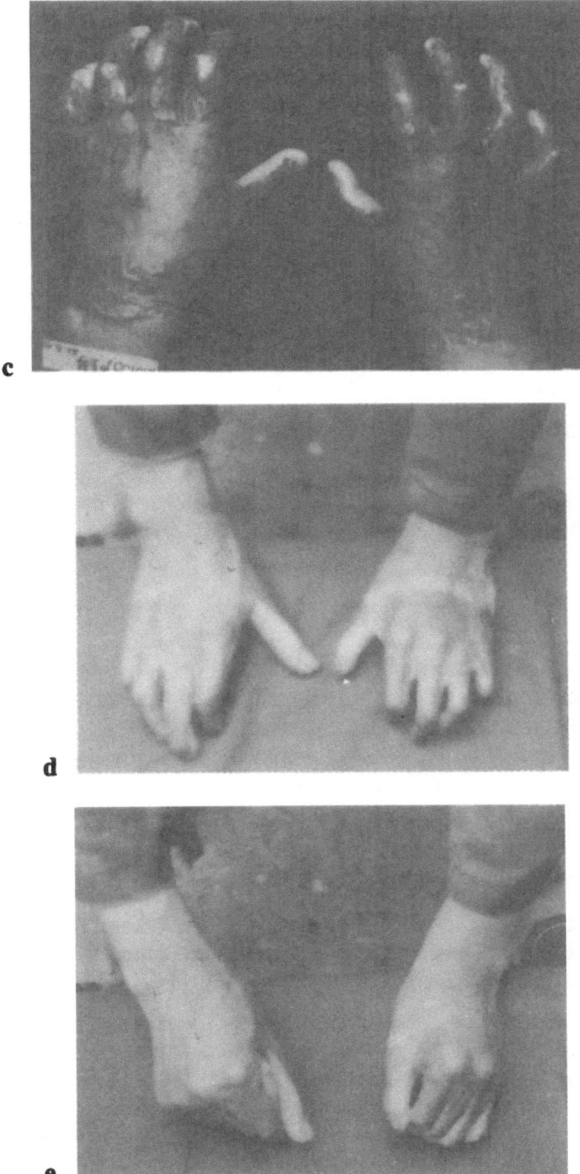

Figure 38.5 Severely burned hands with infection for 9 days. **a,** On first operation, necrotic tissue and granulation were excised. Dorsum of digit burns deepened to bones and joints. Fingertips necrosed and shrank. **b,** Wound healed completely after 10 days of bone marrow surface graftings. **c,** Followed up for 6 months postoperation with excellent functional and cosmetic result; grasp power was 8–9 kg initially. **d,e,** Good function after 1 year follow-up

(1) Dorsum of hand including proximal three fourths of the first phalanx. This
     site is the most easily burned in burn hand patients. Skin grafting and web
     repair are the objects of management.

(2) Dorsum of digits involving extensor tendons, bones and joints. Deep burn
     of this part presents particular problems. It may directly affect the digital
     length and function.

(3) Thenar–wrist area. Sometimes thenar muscles may be partially damaged.

(4) Volar–digit area. Third degree burn of this area is rare. If it does occur, the
     skin and superficial part of the soft tissue are often involved.

Early treatments

Immediate measures

In deeply circumferential burns, escharotomy of hand and fingers should be
performed on admission. Unilateral or bilateral incisions up to the fingertip will
promptly release the digital circulation (Figure 38.2).

Escharectomy and skin grafting

In deep second degree burns, tangential excision is performed down to the
subdermal layer. In third degree burns, excision of the eschar should be carried
out down to the fascia routinely. In our series, there was a patient with third
degree burn of both hands, and we were able to restore good function with
improved cosmetic results (Figure 38.3).

Reconstruction of web spaces

After escharectomy of the whole hand, skin grafts on the dorsum and palmar
surface of the hand are sutured together in the web spaces, but the first web is
covered by grafting with Z-plasty.

Management of exposed bones and joints

If the volar skin is intact and soft tissue is present, decortication and arthrodesis
should be carried out, using a rongeur for decortication followed by arthrodesis
and immobilization of digits in full extension. A thin split skin graft may be
grafted immediately on the fresh bone marrow surface (Figures 38.4, 38.5).

Incomplete amputation of the digits

In severely burned cases, the dorsum of the finger was entirely destroyed including the nail and fingertip. Under such conditions, the terminal phalangeal bone should be partly excised leaving the very end for attachment of the flexor tendon, and the volar flap is turned over the dorsum part to form a new fingertip (Figure 38.6). If a larger area of bone and joints is exposed, decortication with immediate grafting and fingertip repair should be carried out rather than shortening of the digit with volar flap coverage. In this way, the digit would preserve its maximal length (Figure 38.6).

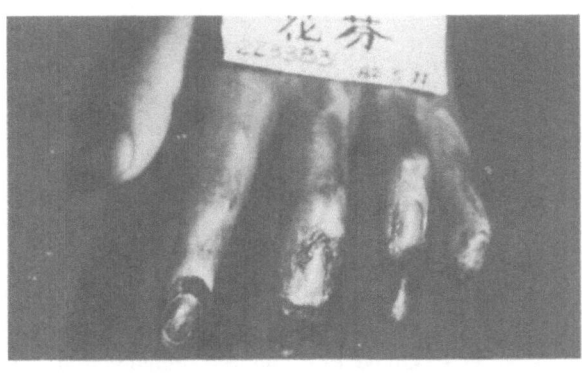

a

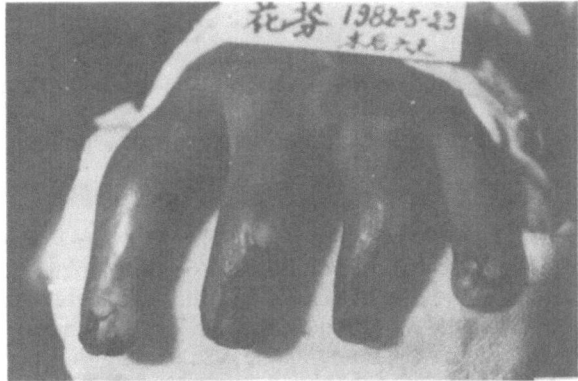

b

Figure 38.6 **a**, Hot press burn of the left hand for 4 months. Distal portion of 2–5 fingers necrosed with exposed bones and joints. **b**, incomplete amputations. Index and small fingertips were repaired

Postoperative care

It is important to immobilize the hand in a functional position, MP joint at 60° flexion, and PIP and DIP joints at full extension. This immobilization is accomplished by an aseptic volar splint put in the inner layer dressing. The hand is elevated in order to reduce edema of the finger. Physiotherapy and exercise should be continued after the healing of the wound for 8 weeks or longer to restore the function of the MP joints.

RESULTS

Correct assessment of results

Incomplete amputations of burned digits were classified in six grades (Figure 38.7).

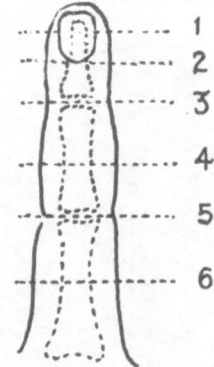

Figure 38.7   Grades of incomplete amputation of finger

Grade 1:   loss of distal phalangeal bone within 0.5 cm
Grade 2:   all the nail bed destroyed, but the end of the tendon remained
Grade 3:   amputation at DIP joint
Grade 4:   amputation at the midpoint of second phalanx
Grade 5:   amputation at PIP joint
Grade 6:   amputation at the midpoint of first phalanx

There were nine cases with 14 hands and 66 fingers treated with the described procedure, including 100 exposed bones and 68 open joints (Table 38.1), of which 11 hands had successful closure of grafting on the bone marrow surface. Only three hands required second grafting. No suppurative arthritis or osteomyelitis had been noted in any of the cases during the course of therapy.

Table 38.1   Results of treatment of burned digits deepening to bones and joints

Type of burn injury	Digits (n)	Digits preserved (n)	Incomplete amputations					
			1	2	3	4	5	6
Dorsum of digits and fingertips	50	7	12	11	14	6*	—	—
Dorsum of digit	6	6	—	—	—	—	—	—
Fingertip	10	1	7	2	—	—	—	—

*Distal phalanxes of small digits were almost destroyed

Follow-up

Eight cases with 12 hands were followed up for more than 6 months, involving 78 phalanges and 42 interphalangeal joints with bone marrow surfaces grafting. These thin grafts have held up well, and none of the patients complained of undue sensibility of the graft in daily work. The fingertips were oval in shape, without discomfort. The interphalangeal joints were stiff at the functional position.

39 8-Year Experience on the Use of Skin Stored in Liquid Nitrogen

ZHU ZHAOMING and SHENG ZHYONG

Department of Burn, Trauma Center, Postgraduate Medical College and 304 Hospital of the PLA

Since 1973, we have successfully used homologous skin stored in liquid nitrogen for the treatment of patients with extensive full-thickness burns. The method of storage was reported elsewhere in 1979[1].

Some 405 000 cm² of skin from adult cadavers and 25 000 cm² of skin from stillborn cadavers have been harvested and stored in a period of 8 years. The stored skin has been used in 158 burn patients in our hospital. The extent of burns was over 50% TBSA in 75 patients and over 90% TBSA in 30 patients. Large sheets of stored skin were most frequently used after excision of eschars, and the allograft used at one time was about 10–30% TBSA. Altogether 313 allograftings of preserved skin have been done, and 90% take was recorded in 80% of cases, 80–90% take in 10%, 50–80% take in 4% and a take of 50% or less in 6%.

After escharectomy, a large sheet of stored skin with multiple evenly placed small holes was applied to the wound, and small pieces of autografts were subsequently inserted into the holes; or the wound was covered by stamp grafts of mixed allo- and autografts. The autografts enlarged gradually and coalesced in due time, so that the wound did not reopen. However, the wound might reopen, if the distance between two of the autografts was too great, and the rejection phenomenon of stored skin occurred about 4–5 weeks postoperatively.

The cases of two patients with major burns illustrate the outcome of the use of the frozen skin.

Case 1 is that of a 23-year-old female admitted in August 1975, who sustained a flame burn of 95% TBSA (third degree 75% TBSA and deep second degree 20%). Escharectomy was done on the right upper and left lower limb on the fifth postburn day and about 2160 cm² of frozen skin stored for 19 days was applied to the wounds. The eschars on the anterior thorax and abdomen were excised on the seventh postburn day and the wounds were covered with 1860 cm² of frozen skin stored for 21 days. The eschars on the left upper and right lower limb were excised on the ninth postburn day and 4000 cm² of frozen skin stored for 23 days was applied to the wounds. All the frozen skin took well. Small pieces of autografts were inserted into the small holes of the frozen allografts 48 h after allo-grafting. These wounds healed in $1\frac{1}{2}$ months postburn. The patient survived.

Case 2 is a 28-year-old female admitted in October 1980, who sustained a flame burn of 95% TBSA (third degree 90% and deep second degree 5%). Escharectomy was performed in stages on the fourth, ninth and sixteenth post-burn days on the right upper and left lower limb, left upper limb and anterior thorax, right lower limb and abdomen; frozen skin stored for 1 year was applied to the wounds. The percentage of graft taken was over 95%. The wounds healed in 2 months, and the patient survived.

From our results it appeared that there were no significant differences between the use of frozen and fresh skin for covering the excised burn wounds, except the following: (1) pinkish recolorization was obviously delayed in frozen skin, (2) occasionally the epidermis of the frozen skin peeled off in time and (3) frozen skin did not take well on heavily colonized wounds or granulation. Among the many causes which contributed to failure of grafting, the technique of grafting and the quality of frozen skin were the most important ones.

Grafting of frozen skin required much more meticulous care; all necrotic tissues including deep fascia with questionable blood supply should be excised thoroughly, and hemostasis should be perfect. Pressure dressing should be used in order to put the graft in good contact with the underlying wound surface, especially at the edge of the wound. The stored allograft, after thawing, should be kept in normal saline solution at 4 °C, and be used as soon as possible, and contact with germicidal agents or hot liquid should be prevented.

The determination of succinic dehydrogenase (by modified Hershey's method) and the trypan blue dye exclusion test (modified Praw's method) showed that the viability of the preserved skin was only 50% of the prestorage value. The results coincide with the reports of Lawrence[2]. The results illustrate that the viability of skin is significantly decreased after being frozen, hence the current techniques used for storage need further improvement.

To attain the best effect, the following points should be observed.

(1) Cadaveric skin exceeding 6 h at room temperature, or 24 h under refrigeration after death, or of doubtful quality, should not be accepted for storage.

(2) Every step in the process of storing should be strictly controlled.

(3) We recommend that 10% DMSO and 1:5000 nitrofurazone (Furacin) in Krebs–Ringer phosphate buffer solution be used as the cryoprotective solution, its pH being 7.2.

     Since 1979, the new cryoprotective solution has been used in place of the previous one. The results have apparently been improved.

(4) Cooling must be controlled at the rate of 1–3 °C/min. The skin is folded into two layers and put into a plastic bag, then transferred into the container of solid CO_2. Our experimental results indicate that the ultra-structure of frozen skin of guinea pig is better preserved by slow cooling at the rate of 1 °C/min than by a process of rapid freezing[3]. A purpose built unit in which the cooling rate can be controlled to 1–3 °C/min is used.

(5) The faster the thawing time, the better the results will be, because the damage due to recrystallization of ice will be minimized.

Bondoc[4] recommended 37 °C as the thawing temperature, but we recommend thawing in a 40 °C water bath and the frozen skin will become soft within 1–3 min.

SUMMARY

We have successfully used allologous skin stored in liquid nitrogen in the treatment of major burns for 8 years. The effect of frozen skin is similar to that of fresh skin. However, the viability of the frozen skin is only 40–50% of that of unfrozen skin. This shows that the method of storage needs further improvement.

REFERENCES

1. Sheng Zhiyong *et al*. Preservation of skin in liquid nitrogen. *Chinese J. Surg.*, **217**, 53
2. Lawrence, J. C. (1972). Storage and skin metabolism. *Br. J. Plast. Surg.*, **25**, 440
3. Zhu Zhaoming *et al*. Cooling rate and the ultrastructure of skin of guinea pig. *Chinese J. Surg.*, **20**, 275
4. Bondoc, C. C. *et al*. (1971). Clinical experience with viable frozen human skin and a frozen skin bank. *Ann. Surg.*, **173**, 371

40 The Experimental Study on Acute Respiratory Failure Caused by Burn Associated with Inhalation Injury

YANG ZONGCHEN, LI AO, JIANG KUNYUAN, CHEN FAMING, WANG TIANYI, LIAN WEIKUN, WU ZHENZHONG, YOU ZHONGYI, LI JINNIAN, XIAO LIMIN and QIN XIAOJIAN

Burn Center, Southwest Hospital, The Third Military Medical College

Burn associated with inhalation injury usually ends in acute respiratory failure which involves a very high postburn mortality. Retrospective and uncontrolled clinical studies seem unable to offer clear-cut insights into this confusing problem. The experiment reported in this chapter was designed to evaluate and analyze the clinical, pathophysiologic and pathologic changes with well-controlled dogs which sustained extensive burns associated with inhalation injury.

MATERIAL AND METHODS

The experiment was conducted under intravenous sodium pentobarbital anesthesia. Fourteen male mongrel dogs, weighing 9.8–15.2 kg, were arbitrarily divided into two groups. Group I received 5% glucose solution 40 ml/kg within 24 h after the burn, while group II were resuscitated with Ringer's lactate solution 4 ml/kg per 1% of body surface area burned (Parkland formulae).

Respiratory steam burns were inflicted on dogs of both groups by the method of our laboratory[1]. Third degree burns were produced on their backs by burning with 3% napalm for 20 s.

The items shown in Table 40.1 were monitored in both groups of animals before the burn and 2, 8 and 24 h after the burn.

RESULTS

The changes of various parameters listed in Tables 40.2 and 40.3 were similar in both groups of animals.

Table 40.1   Items studied

Items	Remarks
HB	
HT	
pH	
BE	
P_aO_2	
P_aCO_2	
P_vO_2	
CVP	Right heart catheterization through jugular vein
PAP	Ditto
PAWP	Ditto
PV (plasma volume)	Dye (T-1842) dilution method
CI (cardiac index)	Impedance wave method
SVR (systemic vascular resistance)	
PVR (pulmonary vascular resistance)	
Oxygen availability	
Pathologic examination of lungs*	Both LM and EM
Chest X-ray film	A-P and right oblique view
Lung water content†	By weighing
Bacteriologic study of lung tissue*	Both qualitative and quantitative

* Including animals which died 24 h and were sacrificed at the end of 24 h
† Right lung

Hemodynamic characteristics of hypovolemic shock were observed. The average FAP, CI and PV markedly decreased and remained at a low level throughout the experiment. Changes in CVP, PAP and PAWP were not significant. They fluctuated within their normal ranges. No apparent pulmonary hypertension or fluid overloading was observed in either group of animals. (Tables 40.2, 40.3).

Progressive impairment of pulmonary function was noticed. Tachypnea and hyperventilation occurred right after the burn. The P_aCO_2, P_aO_2 and BE values decreased and A-aDO$_2$ and pH values increased within 2 h and 8 h postburn. By the end of the 24th postburn hour, P_aO_2 decreased to 55.7 mmHg and A-aDO$_2$ increased to 56 mmHg (animals breathing on room air) in group I; and P_aO_2 and P_aCO_2 decreased to 61.98 mmHg and 36.28 mmHg respectively in group II. A low P_aCO_2 and high pH persisted; although the latter showed a tendency to decline, it was still higher than its preburn value at the end of the experiment.

At the end of the experiment, the water contents of the lungs in these two groups of dogs rose respectively to $81.2 \pm 1.21\%$ and $81.5 \pm 1.36\%$ which were significantly higher than normal ($78.53 \pm 1.06\%$, $p < 0.001$).

No changes in either plasma protein or its albumin fraction were observed. They leveled with their preburn values.

Bacteriologic studies on the lung tissue were performed immediately after the death of five dogs in group I and six dogs in group II. Pathogenic bacteria were isolated in all the specimens submitted to culture. The bacterial count exceeded 10^5 per gram of lung tissue in four dogs.

As shown in Table 40.4, in both groups of dogs, 2 h postburn, the lung fields

Table 40.2 Hemodynamic and pulmonary changes in Group I dogs

	Preburn	Postburn (h)		
		2	8	24
FAP (mmHg)	129.43±6.86	102.86±8.65	112.62±10.41	87.8±9.97
CVP (cmH$_2$O)	2.20±0.62	2.27±0.61	1.14±0.36	0.9±0.75
PAP (mmHg)	16.29±1.42	17.24±2.37	18.93±2.72	16.30±1.99
PAWP (mmHg)	3.21±0.54	4.54±0.63	6.93±1.57	7.00±1.55
CI (l/min per kg)	2.03±0.18	1.62±0.09	1.67±0.29	1.54±0.26
PV (ml/kg)	53.14±3.88	42.34±5.14	38.16±3.82	36.78±3.87
P_aO_2 (mmHg)	87.48±11.06	68.49±20.81	74.66±16.85	55.74±21.68
A-aDO$_2$ (mmHg)	15.62±12.25	35.4±22.73	38.94±16.15	50.56±23.6
P_aCO_2 (mmHg)	41.72±4.90	31.49±5.89	31.70±4.53	31.94±7.86
Respiration rate	17.0±7.0	44±16	45±17	46±17
BE$_b$	-6.4±3.2	-6.9±3.5	-6.7±3.4	-9.7±4.8
pH	7.274±0.059	7.37±0.086	7.328±0.052	7.309±0.027

Table 40.3 Hemodynamic and pulmonary changes in Group II dogs

	Preburn	Postburn (h)		
		2	8	24
FAP (mmHg)	130.57±5.13	116.43±7.24	113.57±9.21	109.50±8.06
CVP (cmH$_2$O)	1.30±0.32	1.80±0.41	1.99±0.41	3.65±0.78
PAP (mmHg)	19.87±1.55	22.57±2.35	21.36±1.93	22.93±3.87
PAWP (mmHg)	3.71±0.46	4.47±0.59	7.31±1.10	5.68±1.68
CI (l/min per m^2)	2.80±0.4	1.75±0.28	1.83±0.17	2.37±0.32
PV (ml/kg)	53.18±3.88	45.78±6.80	44.23±5.95	46.82±4.41
P_aO_2 (mmHg)	83.94±10.68	71.07±17.46	73.0±17.46	61.93±26.96
A-aDO$_2$ (mmHg)	15.68±12.25	33.17±13.59	38.06±23.1	36.28±25.4
Respiration rate	19±4	37±19	43±17	37±22
BE$_b$	-4.9±2.6	-6.5±4.5	-8.6±5.2	-8.6±3.4
pH	7.295±0.049	7.354±0.043	7.315±0.072	7.325±0.063
P_aCO_2 (mmHg)	43.59±7.67	33.86±7.15	32.11±4.51	31.97±8.20

Table 40.4   Findings of chest films

Postburn hour	Group	Animals (n)	Main findings		
			Pulm. edema	Atelectasis	Pulm. infection
8	I	6	3	2	1
	II	6	4	4	1
24	I	5	3	2	2
	II	6	5	4	3

were clear. Some dogs showed evidence of pulmonary edema and/or atelectasis 8 h postburn. There were signs of pulmonary edema and atelectasis in the majority of dogs 24 h postburn; shadow-characterized bronchopneumonia was found in some of them.

Two dogs in group I and one in group II expired before the end of the experiment (Table 40.4); the remaining 11 survived and were exsanguinated to death. The pathologic findings were similar in these 11 dogs. They were congestion, edema, hemorrhage of tracheobronchial mucosa with scattering ulcerations or necrotic sloughings. Congestion and edema of peribronchial and interstitial tissues, alveolar edema and collapse of the lung were observed. Hyaline membranes were formed in the alveoli of several dogs. The ultrastructural changes consisted of interstitial edema, swelling of type I pneumocytes, increase in number and vacuolation of type II pneumocytes. The alveolar spaces were filled with edematous fluid, fibrins, white blood cells and sloughed type II pneumocytes.

DISCUSSION

Pulmonary insufficiency induced by 30% BSA burn accompanying severe respiratory burns was characterized by gradual progression of hypoxia. The clinical pictures were as follows.

(1) Respiration increased immediately after the burn. Two hours postburn, P_aCO_2 dropped markedly with an increase in pH value. The P_aO_2 and BE values decreased slightly. No abnormal breathing sound was detected. Chest films were clear.

(2) Eight hours postburn, most of the dogs experienced dyspnea. Rales were evident. Chest film revealed evidence of pulmonary edema in about half the dogs. Lesions of atelectasis were found in some of them. The P_aO_2, P_aCO_2 and BE values dropped progressively. The A-aDO$_2$ values increased. However the P_aO_2 value remained at the lower limit of the normal only in most of the animals. The pH values tended to decrease, yet exceeded their preburn values.

(3) Twenty-four hours postburn, the dogs' general state deteriorated. Most showed severe respiratory distress. Respiration became shallow and rapid. Inspiratory and expiratory rhonchi and rales were evident. There was roentgenographic evidence of pulmonary edema, bronchopneumonia and atelectasis. Hypoxia became aggravated, P_aO_2 decreased to less than

60 mmHg, and A-aDO$_2$ increased to above 50 mmHg (animal breathing on room air). In the majority of dogs, P_aCO_2 still stayed below the normal value, and BE decreased significantly. The water content of the lungs increased. Postmortem findings revealed that, in addition to tracheo-bronchial mucosal lesions, the most frequent and striking findings were interstitial and alveolar edema, not infrequently intermingled with atelectasis and bronchopneumonia. Although these features were similar to conventional acute respiratory disease syndrome (ARDS), they might be considered as a special pattern of ARDS.

The predominant pathologic finding of the present study was pulmonary edema. It is generally accepted that pulmonary edema after inhalation injury is primarily caused by increased pulmonary vascular permeability. However, a question is raised: 'Does it bear any connection with pulmonary hypertension or decreased plasma osmotic pressure?' Our results showed the PAP values of either group of dogs fluctuated within their normal ranges. It indicated that the etiologic factor of pulmonary hypertension was not involved. In the present experiment, although the oncotic pressure had not been measured, based on the fact that the total serum protein and albumin only slightly decreased, it might be proposed that the pressure did not play an important role in the development of pulmonary edema.

Additional factors other than tracheobronchial mucosal damage, such as shock and sepsis, might be superimposed on the development of respiratory distress. In this study, 11 dogs survived the experiment, six of them having the complication of severe hypoxia ($P_aO_2 < 60$ mmHg, A-aDO$_{20}$ > 50 mmHg), while the other five survivors were well oxygenated ($P_aO_2 > 70$ mmHg). Their main differences were that the former sustained an eventful shock period and early infection. For example, at the end of the experiment, the blood pressure of the former was 85.36 ± 15.37 mmHg and of the latter was 118.75 ± 17.3 mmHg. It was found that the postburn lung tissue culture of four out of the six hypoxic dogs revealed a bacterial count of more than 10^5 per gram. None of the cultures of the five well-oxygenated dogs had a bacterial count exceeding 10^5/g. Probably the respiratory distress and shock interplayed with each other to make the condition worse.

It is well known that fluid replacement is essential to burn shock resuscitation but fluid overload may initiate or be deleterious to pulmonary edema. In the present experiment, pulmonary edema developed early and gradually became severe. However, no significant differences in the severity of pulmonary edema were demonstrated between these two groups with different modes of fluid supply. This indicates that the intravenous infusions set by the conventional formulae do not show any significant effect on the development of pulmonary edema in the dog suffering from 30% BSA flame burn associated with steam inhalation injury.

REFERENCES

1. Zhu Peifang, Li Ao *et al.* (1981). A canine model of severe steam respiratory burns. In *Abstracts of International Burn Seminar (Shanghai)*, p. 95

41 Multisystem Organ Failure Complicating Major Burns

LIU SHIHENG and JIA XIAOMING
General Hospital of the PLA
SHENG ZHIYONG (SHENG CHIH-YONG)
Trauma Center, Postgraduate Medical College and 304 Hospital of the PLA

Since the 1970s, surgeons have been aware of the emergence of a syndrome which is characterized by significant dysfunction of more than two organ systems, subsequent to serious traumas, prolonged and extensive operations, major burns, or systemic infections. This syndrome has been named 'multisystem organ failure' by many investigators[1]. We have reviewed retrospectively all burn patients who manifested clinical pictures indicative of this syndrome and who were admitted to our burn service in the past 10 years, in an attempt to analyze its causative factors and to work out measures for its prevention.

CLINICAL MATERIALS

From 1970 through 1980, 108 patients with burn areas exceeding 50% TBSA and full-thickness injury over 20% TBSA were admitted. Among them, 20 patients developed failure of two or more organs during the course of the disease, comprising an incidence of 18%. Five patients survived. The mean age of the 20 patients was 30 years, mean extent of burn 78.8%, and mean area of full-thickness burns 51%. The mean quantity of fluid replacement during the first 24h was 111.8 ml/1% and that of whole blood 8.7 ml/1%; during the second 24h, fluid replacement amounted to 78.8 ml/1% and whole blood 814 ml/1%. Depending upon the general condition of the patient, the first excision of eschar, followed immediately by allografting, was performed 3–5 days postburn, and the second operation 2–3 days later. Generally, autografting was done 2 days after allografting. The patients were usually covered with appropriate antibiotics, such as gentamicin and cephalosporins, preoperatively.

The criteria for the diagnosis of organ failure are as follows.

(1) Pulmonary failure. Hyperpnea, dyspnea, presence of rales, tachycardia etc appear after the injury or an operative procedure; $P_aO_2 < 60$ mmHg, progressive anoxemia despite inhalation of high concentrations of oxygen,

and the support of ventilation with the use of a ventilator; X-ray film shows mottled infiltration in both lungs later in the course.

(2) Cardiac dysfunction. The status of the peripheral circulation remains poor in spite of energetic resuscitation after an injury or operation, central venous pressure rises to over $20\,cmH_2O$ while the arterial pressure remains low, the pulse is as rapid as 160 or more a minute, assuming a gallop rhythm; in some cases there is a slow pulse inconsistent with the general condition of the patient, together with a weak heart sound and decreasing urinary output. The electrocardiogram reveals a sinus tachycardia, arrythmia, myocardiac anoxemia, and deviation from axis etc.

(3) Acute renal failure. Urinary output decreases to less than 17 ml/h with more or less fixed specific gravity of 1020 or lower, or a normal or even high urinary output with progressively rising BUN. The ratio between UUN and BUN is less than 15:1 and that of urinary creatinine and blood creatinine less than 20:1. There is evidence of hyperkalemia, hyponatremia and acidosis.

(4) Hepatic dysfunction. SGOP rises to twice normal value, or jaundice appears with serum bilirubin $> 2\,mg/dl$. Prothrombin time is prolonged. Elevation of blood ammonia level in severe cases and even the symptoms of hepatic encephalopathy may be seen.

(5) Stress ulcer. The chief clinical manifestation is the upper gastrointestinal bleeding.

(6) Coagulopathy. Abrupt appearance of widespread bleeding with rapid fall in platelets down to less than 50000/cm, signs of hypercoagulability or hypocoagulability, lowering of prothrombin activity, positive plasma protamine paracoagulation test and fall in fibrinogen content ($< 200\,mg/dl$) are seen.

As judged by the above criteria, six patients developed significant dysfunction in two organs, eight cases in three organs, four in four organs, and two in five organs. Dysfunction was most frequently seen in the lung (16 times), kidney (15 times) and liver (nine times), and less seen in the heart (eight times), blood coagulation (seven times), stomach (six times) and brain (once). In about half the cases, renal failure was the earliest to appear, and in 20% of the cases, pulmonary failure occurred first. The time at which dysfunction appeared varied in different organs: on average, renal failure manifested 5 days, lung 8.3 days, liver 10.3 days, and bleeding stress ulcer 11.4 days after the injury.

In nine out of the 20 patients, there was either significant shock at the time of admission, stormy shock phase, or lowering of systolic blood pressure to less than 80 mmHg with pulse rate over 160.

Blood culture was positive in 15 of the 20 patients, and Gram-negative rods accounted for 18 (*Pseudomonas aeruginosa* in 13 cases). In ten, multisystem organ failure occurred before positive blood culture, while in ten it occurred after it, and in five they occurred on the same day. Burn wound sepsis occurred in two cases, and invasive *Mucor* infection in one case. Seven of the 20 patients had received respiratory burns.

DISCUSSION

Extensive deep burn is such a serious injury that it gives rise to a series of strong systemic reactions which may predispose to derangement of functions of different organs. Li Ao[2] in 1978 reported multisystem organ failure with an incidence of 16.2% in major burns of over 50% TBSA. The incidence was 18% in the present series.

Based on the clinical data of the present series, multisystem organ failure after major burns can be divided into two types, sequential and fulminating.

Sequential multiple organ failure

In this type, the kidney is usually the first organ affected, followed by the liver. Sometimes, pulmonary failure appeared first. The symptoms generally manifest themselves as early as 2–3 days after the injury. Usually, in the wake of renal and hepatic dysfunction, bleeding stress ulcer follows, and finally fatal systemic bacterial or mycotic infections set in. In this series of 20 patients, 16 belong to this type.

Case report

A male, aged 59, total burn area 70% TBSA, with 58% full-thickness injury, was admitted 4 h after burn, shock phase uneventful.

Escharectomy was performed on the left upper and lower limbs under general anesthesia 3 days postburn. Large sheets of perforated allograft were used to cover the resulting wounds. Symptoms of systemic infection appeared soon after the operation, and it was controlled after adjustment of antibiotics. The eschar on the chest was excised on the fifth postburn day. Signs of renal dysfunction were detected soon after the operation, BUN rose rapidly from 28 mg/dl to 115 mg/dl on the 30th postburn day, with the blood creatinine level as high as 6.8 mg/dl. Average daily urinary output was 1080 ml, urine specific gravity hovered around 1020, and UUN was 258 mg/dl.

The sclera and skin became icteric on the 16th postburn day, the serum bilirubin was 22 mg/dl, SGOP 650, alkaline phosphatase 50.5, and trans-peptidase 316, and both urine bilirubin and urobilinogen were positive. Jaundice subsided 2 weeks later under treatment. Twenty days after the injury, the patient developed dyspnea and sense of oppression, the respiratory rate reaching 32–38/min. X-ray film of the chest revealed scattered patchy infiltrations in both upper lungs. The blood was pH 7.46, $P_a CO_2$ 47 mmHg, HCO_3^- 25.5 mmol/l, and BE + 3.5 mmol/l. Ventilation was employed, to no avail. Abdominal distension appeared on the 28th postburn day, and the patient vomited coffee ground material and passed tarry stools, and hemoglobin content rapidly fell from 11.2 g to 6.5 g. On the 31st postburn day, temperature abruptly rose to 39.5 °C. Black necrotic patches were seen on the left upper extremity and dorsum. Culture of the wound exudate manifested the growth of *Mucor*. The left upper limb was then amputated. The general condition deteriorated rapidly postoperatively, and the patient died 24 h after the amputation.

Fulminating multisystem organ failure

Failure of the lung, heart, liver, kidney etc all develops at the same time after shock or systemic infection. The onset is early and fulminating, and it carries a high mortality rate. Four patients fall into this category.

Case report

A male aged 47, total burn area 59%, with 38% full-thickness, accompanied by respiratory burn, was admitted 1 h after the injury. Despite immediate tracheostomy and energetic resuscitation, his shock phase was stormy. His electrocardiogram revealed a reversed T wave and depressed ST segment. Dyspnea developed on the second postburn day with the symptom of oppression. His respiratory rate was 30–40/min. Rales were heard in both lungs. Chest X-ray film showed areas of opacity over both lung fields. Blood pH was 7.603, P_aO_2 39.1 mmHg, P_aCO_2 29.5 mmHg, HCO_3^- 28 mmol/l, and BE + 9 mmol/l. Respiration was assisted with a ventilator. Jaundice developed, serum bilirubin raised to 29 mg/dl with direct component of 21 mg/dl and SGOP was 260 u. Urine bilirubin was positive, BUN 50 mg/dl, and UUN 246 mg/dl. The eschar on the chest and left lower limb was excised on the third postburn day under general anesthesia, and the resulting wounds were covered with large sheets of perforated allografts. Respiratory symptoms became more marked, jaundice persisted, and urinary output decreased after the operation. Blood culture showed positive growth of *P. aeruginosa* 19 h postoperatively. The patient died 57 h after the operation.

Pathogenesis of multisystem organ failure

This has not been entirely elucidated. However, repeated clinical observations suggest that it is closely related to prolonged deficient tissue perfusion and severe systemic infection.

In our series of 20 patients, four were in profound shock on admission, and five were in an unstable hemodynamic state during the shock phase. All these nine patients also suffered from respiratory burn. Fulminating multisystem organ failure developed in all the former four patients, while sequential organ failure ensued within 10 days after the burn in the latter five, and all of them died of septicemia or burn wound sepsis 5–22 days after the injury.

Case report

A male, 20 years of age, with total burn area 86%, including 67% full-thickness injury, was referred from another city, and arrived 14 h after the injury. On admission, the patient was restless, BP unobtainable, pulse rate 140, heart sound weak, extremities cold, with an empty urinary bladder. Hemoglobin was 19 g/dl, and HCO_3^- 9 mmol/l. After massive infusion of fluids and diuretics,

BP rose to 138/100 and urinary output recovered to 30–50 ml/h. However, BUN steadily rose from 31.3 mg/dl on the first postburn day to 135 mg/dl on the seventh, with blood creatinine level of 11 mg/dl. UUN was 600 mg/dl and serum potassium 7.9 mmol/l.

The patient developed abdominal distension and hiccough on the third day, soon followed by coffee ground vomitus and tarry stools. He was delirious with cloudy sensorium on the fourth day. Body temperature became subnormal. Blood grew *Bacillus alcaligenes* on culture. He died on the ninth postburn day.

Preoperative and peroperative problems

Early excision of full-thickness wounds and good coverage afterwards have been accepted by many experienced surgeons as an effective therapeutic modality for extensive deep burns. However, negligence in reevaluating the general condition and functional status of different internal organs of the patient, resulting in inadequate preoperative preparation, or insufficient replacement of blood volume during the operation resulting in hypovolemia, might precipitate multisystem organ failure after the operation. Fry[4] pointed out that multisystem organ failure can be attributable to certain major operations or abdominal surgery with inadequate preparation. He reported that in 553 cases of major emergency operations, 38 developed such complication.

In our series, there were five patients who developed multisystem organ failure in 3 days after an extensive escharectomy, and three of them died respectively on the second, third and 18th postoperative day. The mean age of these five patients was 37 years, mean extent of burn area was 80.2%, and mean area of full-thickness burn was 55.1%. Two patients had a history of hepatitis or biliary calculi; three had hypertension, rheumatic heart disease, or chronic duodenal ulcer; and two patients were complicated with inhalation injury. In one case, we considered retrospectively that the excision was too extensive so that his heart rate rose to 190/min at one time.

Case report

A male, 49 years of age, with burn area 80% TBSA, full-thickness 50%, was admitted half an hour after the injury. It was reported that he suffered from 'rheumatic heart disease' and 'chronic duodenal ulcer' 2 years previously. After admission, a left side pneumothorax was accidentally produced during intravenous catheterization of the subclavian vein. Aspiration of 1400 ml of air from the left pleural cavity cleared up the pneumothorax. Bilateral lower extremity escharectomy was performed on the fifth postburn day. The extent of excision was 34%. Excessive blood loss during the procedure once brought up the heart rate to 190/min. Rapid transfusion of 1200 ml whole blood lowered the heart rate to 150 but dyspnea developed, and the respiratory rate was 32–40/min 24 h after the operation. Roentgenogram showed patches of haziness in both the upper and middle lung fields. SGPT level was normal before the operation, and rose to 250 u 4 days postoperatively, with an icterus index of 40 u.

On the sixth postoperative day, the SGPT level was further elevated to 305 u, icterus index 40 u. On the ninth postoperative day, although the SGPT dropped to 170 u, the serum bilirubin rose to 7.8 mg/dl. Jaundice persisted up to 30 days after the operation, and the SGPT level stood at 270 u. The preoperative electrocardiogram was normal, but after the operation it showed a depressed T wave in leads II, III, and AVF. The electrocardiography remained abnormal 6 days postoperatively, and the chest film showed enlargement of heart shadow. Thereafter, signs of pulmonary infection were revealed. *P. aeruginosa* were isolated from the sputum and the wound. Although the patient presented the symptom of systemic infection, repeated blood cultures were negative. He passed tarry stools on the 35th and 38th postoperative days with lowering of hemoglobin. He finally survived after aggressive systemic treatment and repeated graftings.

As this patient reached the age of 49, had a history of rheumatic heart disease and chronic duodenal ulcer, and an iatrogenic pneumothorax was inflicted upon him soon after admission, it was quite obvious that it was difficult to achieve a stable *milieu intérieur* by instituting the same resuscitative measures as in other burn patients. Though the time of operation was postponed to the fifth postburn day, an extensive excision was nevertheless undertaken, and the patient lapsed into shock during the operation. Soon after the operation, the patient manifested signs of dysfunction of the lung, liver, heart, and upper gastrointestinal tract, followed by bouts of systemic infection. A high price was paid to save the patient.

Serious infections

Eiseman[3] and Fry[4] asserted that serious systemic infection may predispose to multisystem organ failure. In Li Ao's[2] series of 50 cases, 24 cases occurred simultaneously with or subsequently to a positive blood culture, usually of a Gramnegative organism.

In our series of 20 cases, multisystem organ failure was closely related to septicemia in five, and in one case it occurred after the development of burn wound sepsis. Gram-negative bacilli accounted for all the organisms recovered.

Two patients in our series developed fulminating multisystem organ failure due to transfusion of contaminated bank blood. One patient, whose organ failure ameliorated when systemic infection was brought under control, survived. The other, whose infection ran rampant with organ failure worsening, finally died.

In some patients, episodes of infection occurred because of the protracted existence of burn wounds. As a consequence, dysfunction of the lung, liver and kidney would relapse again and again until septicemia or burn wound sepsis was brought under control or the burn wounds were sealed by grafting.

Principles of management

Multisystem organ failure carries a formidably high mortality of 74–91.5%[2,4]. Inasmuch as shock and infection are the major predisposing causes of multisystem organ failure, we would suggest that, in the light of the present retrospective study, the following precautions should be taken in the management of a major burn.

(1) Adequate early resuscitation is of paramount importance in the prevention of multisystem organ failure. Unfortunately, as yet we are lacking some precise yet noninvasive and simple-to-interpret bedside parameters to indicate that the replacement therapy is really reacting favorably and little damage has been done to the various vital organs. Similarly, we are rather incapable of giving a burned patient, who has lapsed into a profound shock for a certain period of time, a treatment so effective that it would help the injured organs recover to normalcy in a short period of time. Much research in these areas is necessary.

(2) It cannot be overemphasized that a comprehensive reevaluation of the patient and careful perusal of the patient's past history are necessary in order to make a proper decision on the time for excisional surgery and extent of excision, and to make a plan to prevent ventilatory and circulatory disturbances during and after the operation.

(3) Removal of eschar and covering of wounds with skin grafts as early as feasible, appropriate use of antibiotics, and effectual remedies for local and systemic infections are important measures in both prevention and treatment of multisystem organ failure.

(4) Dysfunction of the lung and kidney usually precedes that of other organs. Therefore, it seems likely that early successful management of pulmonary or renal insufficiency may abort the sequential development of functional failure of other organs.

SUMMARY

One hundred and eight cases of burn exceeding 50% TBSA (third degree in excess of 20%) were admitted from 1970 through 1980. Of these, 20 patients developed multisystem organ failure. The average area of thermal injury of these 20 patients was 78.8%, and that of full-thickness injury 51%. Five patients survived.

Failure of two organs occurred in six patients, three organs in eight, four organs in four, and five organs in two. The lung, kidney, and liver were most frequently affected. Renal failure manifested 5 days, lung failure 8.3 days, hepatic failure 10.3 days, and bleeding stress ulcer 11.4 days, on average, after the injury.

Fifty percent of the patients either experienced profound shock at the time of admission, or a stormy shock stage, or shock during excisional surgery. Five out of 20 had concurrent inhalation injury. Fifteen patients had had a positive blood culture either shortly before or simultaneously with the onset of multiple organ failure. Thus, we believe that shock and invasive infection played important roles in the development of multisystem organ failure.

In the light of the foregoing analysis, we would suggest that timely and adequate resuscitation shortly after the injury, careful planning in regard to the date of operation and extent of excision on the basis of a comprehensive reevaluation of the patient are imperative so as to avert any hemodynamic disturbance which might occur during the operative procedure. Early and adequate covering of burn wounds, prevention and treatment of invasive infection with appropriate topical and systemic antimicrobial agents, and prevention and early treatment of pulmonary insufficiency constitute the essential measures in guarding against the occurrence of multisystem organ failure after an extensive thermal injury.

REFERENCES

1. Bauer, A. (1975). Multiple, progressive or sequential systems failure. A syndrome of the 1970s. *Arch. Surg.*, **110**, 779
2. Li Ao *et al.* (1979). Multiple organ failure in severe burns. In Li Ao (ed.) *Symposium on the Treatment and Research in Burns. The 3rd Military Medical College, Chongqing.* (Medical Science Pub.)
3. Eiseman, B. (1977). Multiple organ failure. *Surg. Gynecol. Obstet.*, **144**, 323
4. Fry, D. E. (1980). Multiple system organ failure: The role of uncontrolled infection. *Arch. Surg.*, **115**, 136

42 A Report on Five Cases of Burns Associated with Mechanical Injuries

Burn Unit, 159 Army Hospital, PLA

Burns associated with mechanical injuries largely happen in industrial and traffic accidents. In modern war, these associated injuries may be more complicated and difficult to manage because of the use of various sophisticated weapons. Since 1978, five cases of burns associated with mechanical injuries have been admitted to our hospital and they all recovered (Table 42.1). The present chapter describes their hospitalized course, with some comments.

PROBLEM OF ASSOCIATED INJURIES

Attention must be paid to the existence of associated injuries when the severity of a burn does not coincide with the clinical condition, or the patient responds poorly to the therapies adopted.

Case reports

Case 1

A man of 30 was knocked down by gas waves in a furnace explosion, and his trunk and left lower extremity buried by hot bricks. He lost consciousness for about 15 min and was sent to hospital within 30 min. On admission, the patient was in a state of compensated shock. The burn covered 19% TBSA with 10% of full-thickness burn. There were nine lacerations on his scalp. Roentgenogram showed fractures of the left ribs (4–7), right clavicle, left transverse process of the vertebrae (L1–4) and hemopneumothorax. Transfusions of 1000 ml 5% glucose saline, 500 ml moderate molecular dextran, 200 ml plasma and 200 ml 5% sodium bicarbonate were immediately performed. His blood pressure rose from 80/60 mmHg to 120/90 mmHg in 1 h. Then 1000 ml of gas and a little blood-like liquid were drained out through a closed drainage of the pleural cavity. The wounds on the scalp were debrided and sutured. The chest was fixed

Table 42.1 Clinical data of five associated injuries

Case	Sex	Age	Cause of injury	Burn size (% TBSA/III° burn)	Blood pressure on admission (mmHg)	Main mechanical injuries associated with burns
1	M	30	Furnace explosion	19/10	80/60	Lacerations of scalp; II° brain injury; fracture of ribs; hemopneumothorax; rupture of jejunum
2	M	45	Traffic accident	18/5	80/70	Fracture of rib; laceration of lung; hemopneumothorax; dislocation of L4 vertebra; incomplete paraplegia
3	M	38	Gunpowder explosion	22/7	70/40	High-explosive injury; crush injury of limb; splintered fracture of femur
4	M	38	Traffic accident	8/5	120/78	Fracture of ribs; hemopneumothorax
5	F	7	Electric burn in open heart operation	25/20	90/50	Operative injury in chest and abdomen

with thorax bandaging. Six and a half hours later, the patient complained of a pain in the abdomen and vomited some coffee-ground gastric content, then blood pressure fell again to 90–78 mmHg. There were general tenderness and muscular tension on the abdominal wall; 3 ml of pus-like liquid were drawn out from the peritoneal cavity. In an ensuing laparotomy, a rupture of the jejunum was found and repaired; drainage of the peritoneal cavity was carried out. After the operation, the patient's condition was for a time better, but began deteriorating on the fourth postoperative day. He ran a high fever and the left lower extremity swelled and became inflamed. Escharectomy was carried out on the burned limb and followed by allografting. In the operation, posterior muscles of the limb were found to have been devitalized with 15 abscesses of various sizes. Blood culture made on the operating day showed *Staphylococcus aureus*. Following the operation, septicemia was controlled. After four autografts, the patient recovered.

This patient had a minor burn of 19% TBSA, but he was in a state of evident shock on admission. The combination of careful inquiry into his history and systematic examination showed multiple injury comprising fractures, hemopneumothorax, intestinal rupture etc. The patient was saved by correct diagnosis and planned treatment.

Case 2

A man of 45 was involved in a traffic accident. His tractor turned over and his trunk and both lower extremities were injured. Simultaneously the boiling water in the engine splashed on his abdomen and right upper and lower extremities. He was given first aid in a local hospital including the transfusion of 500 ml low molecular dextran and 500 ml 5% glucose solution. He was admitted to our hospital 14 h postburn, when he was in shock. The size of his scald was only 18/15 (% TBSA burn/third degree burn). Roentgenogram showed a projecting vertebra (L4). Even after transfusion of a total of 2700 ml liquid had been carried out within the first 6 h in hospital, his blood pressure progressively fell from an initial 80/70 mmHg to 0. Further radiographic examination revealed fracture of a rib (left 9) and pleurisy with effusion. Therefore, pleuracotomy was indicated and 3 liters of blood-like liquid were drained out with closed pleural drainage. These procedures combined with transfusions of 600 ml whole blood, 200 ml blood plasma and 500 ml normal saline improved the patient's condition. His blood pressure rose to 120/80 mmHg after 1 h 45 min. On the fifth postburn day he developed *S. aureus* septicemia and on the next day a suppurative pleurisy was diagnosed. His burn wound was infected. The patient was treated with antimicrobial drugs, continual drainage from the pleural cavity and staged escharectomy followed by autografting. Finally, he recovered and was discharged on the 57th postinjury day.

This patient had also a minor burn of 18% TBSA, but was in serious shock on admission. The patient showed poor response to routine treatment, which made us think of injuries other than burn insult. Further examination confirmed a hemorrhage in the pleural cavity. Pleurocentesis and other active procedures were accordingly performed and the patient was saved.

DISCUSSION

In simple burns, the patient's condition usually fits with the severity of the burns. So far as a young patient with less than 20% of TBSA burn is concerned, he rarely develops shock, or if the shock does occur, it is easily rectified with routine treatment. Both the above patients developed evident shock, which could hardly be explained by their burns. The main cause of their shock was concealed hemorrhage in the viscera, which also accounted for their poor response to routine treatment based on burn size. These cases therefore teach us to pay attention to associated injuries when the patient's condition does not coincide with his burn size, or routine treatment does not work well.

SKELETAL TRACTION

Skeletal traction should be taken as the treatment of choice when burns are associated with closed fracture of the same limb.

Case report

In Case 3 the patient, a man of 38, suffered a splintered fracture of his femur and burn on his face and limbs following the collapse of his house. Although the burn size was 27% of TBSA with 7% third degree burns, the patient was in serious shock when admitted to our hospital. After successful resuscitation, skeletal traction was performed through third degree burn wounds and dislocation was corrected by manual reduction. The burned limb was treated with exposure treatment. The wound area around the Kirschner pin was disinfected with 2% tincture of iodine at a fixed time every day. The eschar resolved without osteomyelitis. After 1 month, autografting was carried out at the bedside to cover the open wound and on the 56th postinjury day, roentgenograms taken at the bedside showed that the fracture had healed with good alignment and reposition. The limb was then fixed with plastic splinting instead of skeletal traction. The patient recovered fully on the 90th postinjury day.

Discussion

Burns associated with closed fracture of the femur can cause problems in management, rather than in diagnosis – which is not difficult by means of physical and roentgenographic examinations. Fracture healing, as we know, requires good immobilization, while the burn wound should be treated by frequent changes of dressing and operation; the result is contradiction in the management of these associated injuries. The skeletal traction adopted in the treatment of Case 3 had advantages in healing of both burn and fracture, as this therapy followed free checking of the fracture and management of the burn wound. With the topical use of 2% tincture of iodine on the wound around the Kirschner pin, osteomyelitis could be prevented. In addition, skin grafting could be carried out at the bedside without moving the patient.

Pruitt states[1] that skeletal traction has no major influence on various therapies including grafting, and the traction pin puncture through the burn wound will not cause infection in the burn tissue. Huang Jiasi stresses[2] that internal fixation of the bone should be performed with fairly high levels of technique and apparatus lest it should result in the bone failing to mend, wound infection, osteomyelitis, stiff joint and other severe consequences. Therefore, this operation cannot be regarded as a routine therapy for common fractures, especially in the case of splintered fractures. We consider that internal fixation of the bone should be avoided in cases of associated injuries for fear of complications, while skeletal traction may be a preferable therapy. Alternatively, internal fixation of the bone should be done as early as possible during the postinjury period; intensive measures must meanwhile be taken to prevent infection.

SEPTICEMIA

In the case of burns associated with mechanical injuries, the burn wound remains the main source responsible for the increased spread of septicemia.

In the management of these associated injuries, the surgeon tends to be engaged in treating the life threatening associated injuries and negligent in the reasonable management of the burn wound. According to the data presented by the PLA Third Medical College[3], the spread of septicemia accounts for merely 2.6% of the patients with a burn size of less than 29% of TBSA. Of the present five cases, three cases developed septicemia which was diagnosed on the basis of wound and blood cultures. This fact indicated that the spread of septicemia markedly increased in these associated injuries.

REFERENCES

1. Pruitt, B. A. Jr. (1970). Management of burns in the multiple injury patients. *Surg. Clin. N. Am.*, 1283
2. Huang Jia-si (1972). Fracture. In Huang Jia-si (ed.). *Surgery*. 2nd Edn., p. 926. (Beijing: The People's Medical Sciences and Health Pub.). (In Chinese)
3. Li Ao (ed.) (1977). *Symposium on Treatment and Research in Burns. The Third Military Medical College*. 1st edn., p. 161. (Beijing: The People's Medical Sciences and Health Pub.)

43 The Changes in Serum Ceruloplasmin and Copper in Burned Rats

GAO LANXING, XU ZHIQIN, WANG ZONGYIN and GU JINGFAN

Institute of Military Hygiene, Tianjin

Spurr[1] noted the anomalies of the ceruloplasmin zone in the electrophoresis of sera in severely burned patients. Of 16 cases of 20–26% BSA burns with such abnormal zones, only one survived. Sanchez-Agreda[2] showed that the trace elements such as copper, iron and zinc decreased in the sera of burned patients. A controversial result was reported by Sunderman *et al.*[3] who could not find any significant change in serum copper and zinc after thermal injury. With a view to further evaluating the effects of burns on serum ceruloplasmin and copper in well-controlled animals, experiments in rats with extensive third degree burns were designed, and are reported in this chapter.

METHODS

Male rats, body weight 290–320 g, were fed with a 10% casein ration (composition as shown in Table 43.1). The animals were divided at random into

Table 43.1 Composition of ration (percentages)

Constituents	Contents
Casein	10
Corn starch	50
Cane sugar	30
Vegetable oil	3
Cod-liver oil	2
Salt mixture*	4
Vitamin mixture†	1

*Calcium carbonate 300, calcium hydrophosphate 75, ferrous sulfate 20, potassium phosphate (dibasic) 420, magnesium sulfate 102, sodium chloride 170, manganese sulfate 5, potassium iodide 0.8, zinc chloride 0.41, copper sulfate 0.3 g
†Vitamin B_1 400, B_2 4000, nicotinic acid 2500, folic acid 200, vitamin B_{12} 15, *para*-aminobenzoic acid 5000, calcium pantothenate 1500, vitamin B_6 200, vitamin K 100, inositol 20000, biotin 50, choline 3000 mg, cane sugar added up to 1 kg

Table 43.2 Grouping of animals

Experiment	Group	Animal no.	Parameter
1	I (Burned)	10	Serum ceruloplasmin
	II (Control)	10	Serum ceruloplasmin
2	III (Burned)	10	Serum copper
	IV (Pair-fed)	10	Serum copper

four groups, each containing ten rats: Groups I (burned) and II (control) were used for determining ceruloplasmin; Groups III (burned) and IV (pair-fed, non-burned) for determining copper (Table 43.2).

The dorsum of each animal was shaved. Under ether anesthesia, a 20% BSA burn was inflicted by igniting 3% napalm in the amount of $0.6\,ml/cm^2$. The skin lesions thus produced were invariably third degree, which was proved by pathological sections. Blood samples were drawn for analysis before and 1, 3, 7 and 14 days after the injury. Ceruloplasmin was determined with Sunderman's method[3] and copper was determined with flameless atomic spectrophotometry (Sp 129 Atomic spectrophotometer).

The feed intakes and body weights were measured daily. The animals were fed ad lib, except group IV which was pair-fed to group III.

RESULTS AND DISCUSSION

Changes in serum ceruloplasmin

The contents of serum ceruloplasmin markedly increased on the first day postburn as compared to the control. It continued to increase and reached 810.9 activity units/100 ml per 30 min on the 14th postburn day (Table 43.3).

In the control group, the serum ceruloplasmin level did not change significantly throughout the experiment.

Ceruloplasmin is an acute-phase protein. Its main physiologic function is transportation of copper in the body. Through the activities of iron and amine oxidase, ceruloplasmin helps transform Fe^{2+} to Fe^{3+}, thus facilitating the transferring and coupling of transferrin and the oxidation of amines (such as

Table 43.3 Changes in serum ceruloplasmin in burned rats ($M \pm SD$ activity units/100 ml per 30 min)

Group	Before injury	After injury (days)			
		1	3	7	14
I (burned)	389.3 ± 34.8	424.6* ± 45.7	423.3* ± 70.4	499.7* ± 126.1	810.9† ± 239.5
II (control)	383.3 ± 28.2	365.8 ± 36.3	346.3 ± 37.3	359.2 ± 61.0	380.0 ± 36.7

Compared to the control: *$p < 0.05$; †$p < 0.01$

catecholamine). In this way, ceruloplasmin plays an important role in the maintenance of homeostasis of the body.

Some authors have suggested that immediately after the burns, the rapid increase in serum ceruloplasmin of the rats was probably due to the increased release of ceruloplasmin from the liver or decreased urinary excretion, secondary to the postburn rise in catecholamine, and decline in serum iron. The exact mechanism remains to be investigated.

Changes in serum copper

The serum copper of Group III animals decreased from $165.1 \mu g/100 ml$ before burns to $145.1 \mu g/ml$ on the first postburn day. In Group IV animals, the serum copper level also decreased from $166.5 \mu g/100 ml$ to $119.3 \mu g/100 ml$. As compared to the pair-fed animals, the burned rats showed significantly higher values of serum copper up to the 14th postburn day. At that time, the serum copper level increased to $318.5 \mu g/100 ml$, whereas the pair-fed animals recovered to their preburn level of $158.8 \mu g/100 ml$ (Table 43.4).

Table 43.4 Changes in serum copper in burned rats ($M \pm SD$ $\mu g/100 ml$)

Group	Before injury	After injury (days)			
		1	3	7	14
III (burned)	165.3 ± 38.1	145.1* ± 21.4	187.7 ± 40.0	202.4* ± 63.4	318.5† ± 84.1
IV (pair-fed)	166.5 ± 23.6	119.3 ± 4.1	153.3 ± 36.6	134.7‡ ± 18.5	158.8 ± 57.7

Compared to the pair-fed: *$p < 0.05$; †$p < 0.01$
Compared to the value before injury: ‡$p < 0.05$

The decrease in serum copper in the pair-fed animals was probably due to the sudden decrease in the feed intake. During the first postburn day, the daily feed intake of the burned rats decreased from $23.6 g$ to $5.2 g$; they then gradually recovered to $18.0 g$ 2 weeks later. Since the pair-fed animals were given a similar amount of feed as the intake of burned animals, their serum copper values showed a simultaneous decrease. However, it was shown that a third degree burn of 20% BSA would cause a marked increase in serum copper.

Ceruloplasmin is the carrier of copper. Each molecule of ceruloplasmin contains 8 atoms of copper. Copper absorbed from the intestine is first coupled with albumin or an amino acid, and then transferred to the liver. In the liver, copper is carried by ceruloplasmin probably in the form of a prosthetic group and transported to other sites in the body. The findings of the synchronous increase in both ceruloplasmin and copper, in the present study fit well with the above mechanism. Based on the values obtained from the control and pair-fed groups, the serum ceruloplasmin in the burned rats on the first, third, seventh and 14th postburn days increased by 16%, 22.2%, 39.1% and 113.4%, respectively, of that of the control animals, while the serum copper increased by

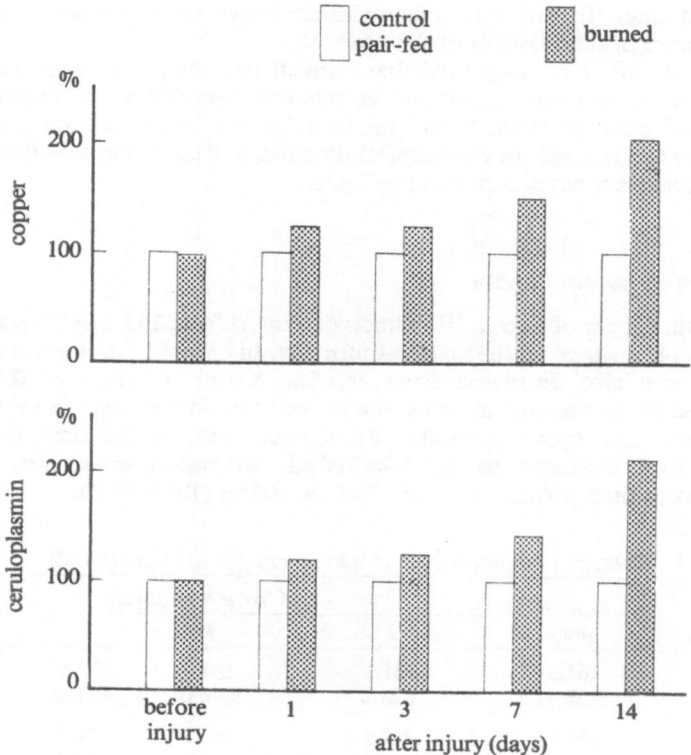

Figure 43.1 The relative contents of serum ceruloplasmin and copper in burned rats

21.6%, 22.4%, 50.2% and 100.5% of that of the pair-feds (Figure 43.1). The degrees of increase in ceruloplasmin and copper in different stages were quite similar.

To sum up, serum ceruloplasmin and copper in the rats with 20% third degree burns of the BSA markedly increased and did not recover in 2 weeks. The degrees of increase were basically similar.

REFERENCES

1. Spurr, E. D. *et al.* (1976). Some observations on ceruloplasmin in burned patients. *Burns,* **2**, 250
2. Sanchez-Agreda, N. *et al.* (1977). Trace elements in burned patients – studies of zinc, copper and iron in serum. *Burns,* **4**, 28
3. Sunderman, F. W. *et al.* (1970). Measurement of human serum ceruloplasmin by its P-phenylenediamine oxidase activity. *Clin. Chem.,* **16**, 903
4. Sinha, J. K. *et al.* (1980). Hormonal and associated metabolic alterations following burn injury. *Burns,* **7**, 16

44 Preliminary Experimental Observation on the Acute Rejection of Allotransplantation of the Kidney in Rabbits Treated by Traditional Chinese and Western Medicine

ZHU HONGYIN and WANG XUEPU
Research Laboratory of Plastic & Reconstructive Surgery. The Third Teaching Hospital, Beijing Medical College

Immunologic rejection is one of the problems of utmost concern to transplant teams. Up to now, it has not been solved satisfactorily. Recipients must take immunosuppressants for a long time. But most of the drugs used have severe side-effects. For example, they lower resistance against diseases, immunologic surveillance etc. So the recipients are very susceptible to infection and the rate of neoplasm formation increases. The principal side-effects of immuno-suppressants are listed in Table 44.1.

Table 44.1 The side-effects of immunosuppressants

Drug	Side-effects
Azathioprine	Bone marrow suppression, hepatic damage, gastroenteric reaction, infection
Cyclophosphamide	The same as azathioprine and hemorrhagic cystitis
Prednisone	Infection, peptic ulcer, bone necrosis
Antilymphocyte serum	Allergy, hemolytic anemia, thrombocytopenia, kidney damage, neoplasm
Cyclosporine A	Hepatic damage, delayed kidney damage

The immunosuppressants used at present act concentrically on the differentiation and proliferation of immunocompetent cells. But clinical practice shows that their effects are not satisfactory. The grafts are damaged by various factors released by immunologic reaction such as immunoadherence of the platelets, and erythrocytes impede the blood flow and active materials released by the platelets activate the mechanism of blood coagulation. The releasing of leukocyte chemotactic factors attracts leukocytes, the latter release lysosomes which damage the walls of blood vessels with their hydrolytic enzyme, causing

341

thrombosis and hemorrhage in the interstitium. The release of histamine leads to increased permeability of the vessel wall. Edema and cell accumulation in the interstitium finally further impede the blood flow, and the grafts die of ischemia. When investigating the acute rejection of kidney transplantation, special attention should be paid to the specific and nonspecific causes which lead to blood coagulation and vasospasm. The histologic manifestations of acute rejection are interstitium swelling, hemorrhage, monocyte infiltration and fibrinoid degeneration of blood vessel walls, blood stasis, thrombosis etc. As stated above, the immunosuppressants work at the early phase of immune reaction, but have no effect on the nonspecific damage at the later period.

We consider the changes caused by acute rejection are quite similar to those described in the 'stasis symptoms' of traditional Chinese medicine[1]. The report of Wuhan Medical College considered that the phenomena at the earlier stage of kidney graft are the same as those of 'blood stasis' in traditional Chinese medicine (TCM)[2]. There are two therapeutic principles in TCM: one is to strengthen the patient's resistance and the other to dispel the invading pathogenic factors[3]. Allergy falls into the category of invading pathogenic factors. Virtually, what expelling the invading pathogenic factors means in TCM is to suppress the immunologic function. 'Activating the blood flow and resolving blood stasis' is the TCM method that dispels the invading pathogenic factors[4].

The method of 'activating the blood flow and resolving blood stasis' includes the use of drugs to reinforce the vital energy in combination with drugs to remove 'heat' etc. By clinical and pharmacologic study, its mechanism has been made clearer. Its prime therapeutic action is to improve blood circulation and suppress immunoreaction[3,5-7] (Table 44.2).

The main purpose of the present chapter is to report the results of experimental observation using transplantations No. 3 (T No. 3) and No. 8 (T No. 8) in combination with Western immunosuppressants to treat acute rejection of allotransplantation of the kidney in rabbits.

MATERIALS AND METHODS

Animals

Hybrid male New Zealand rabbits, weighing 3 kg, were used. Donors and recipients were randomly chosen.

Table 44.2 The effect of TCM drugs 'for activating the blood flow and resolving stasis'

Therapeutic effect	Mechanism
Improving blood circulation	Adjusting permeability of the vessel wall, improving bloodstream, inhibiting agglutination platelets, promoting fibrinolysis, dilating vessel
Inhibiting immunity	Inhibiting antibody formation cell propagation, inhibiting blood coagulation antibody, strengthening the action of T-inhibitory cells

Table 44.3 Groups

Groups	Traditional Chinese medicine		Western medicine	
	T No. 3	T No. 8	Azathioprine	Prednisone
Control	—	—	—	—
Western medicine				
1.			20 mg, b.i.d.	20 mg, b.i.d
2.			20 mg, q.d.	20 mg, q.d.
3.			15 mg, b.i.d.	15 mg, b.i.d.
4.			10 mg, 6 days	20 mg, 6 days
			8 mg, 4 days	16 mg, 4 days
			5 mg, 4 days	10 mg, 4 days
			3 mg, 6 days	6 mg, 6 days
Combined TCM and Western				
T No. 3				
1.	20 g, b.i.d.		15 mg, 7–10 days	15 mg, 7–10 days
2.	20 ml, b.i.d.		15 mg, 2nd, 7th 14th, 21st, 28th days b.i.d.	15 mg, 2nd, 7th 14th, 21st, 28th days b.i.d.
3.	20 ml, b.i.d.		15 mg S.O.S.	15 mg S.O.S.
4.	20 ml, b.i.d.		20 mg, b.i.d. 3 weeks	20 mg, b.i.d. 3 weeks
T No. 8		20 mg b.i.d.	10 mg, 6 days 8 mg, 4 days 5 mg, 4 days 3 mg, 6 days b.i.d.	20 mg, 6 days 16 mg, 4 days 10 mg, 4 days 6 mg, 6 days b.i.d.

Table 44.4 Basis for gradation of rejection

Degree of rejection	Manifestation			
	Infiltration	Edema	Hemorrhage	Vessel damage
Nonrejection (0)	—	—	—	—
Minimal rejection (+)	Small patch	Mild	Mild	Intimal mild swelling
Moderate rejection (++)	Large patch	Moderate	Moderate	Fibrin deposit under intima
Marked rejection (+++)	Diffuse	Severe	Severe	Fibrinoid necrosis vessel obliteration

Table 44.5 Results

Groups	Rabbits (n)	Survival	Degree of rejection	Mean survival time (days)
Control	12	4–14	1–110	8.33
Western medicine				
1.	11	5–14	2711	8.55
2.	4	5–8	121–	7.22
3.	8	5–18	1331	10.85
4.	6	5–25	11–4	11
TCM combined with Western				
T No. 3				
1.	19	4–35	4951	7.2
2.	15	4–28	–942	11.8
3.	11	3–120	2711	20.18
4.	8	6–30	1331	14
T No. 8	9	4–61	135–	17.4

Kidney transplantation

A left orthotopic renal transplantation is performed using microsurgical techniques with end-to-end anastomosis of the renal artery and vein and ureter. The right kidney was removed 7–10 days after transplantation.

Drugs

Western drugs were azathioprine and prednisone. TCMs were T No. 3 and T No. 8 prepared by our laboratory. Both were made into decoction 20 cc per oz.

Groups

Animals were classified into unmodified control groups (I), Western drug group (II) and combined traditional Chinese and Western drugs group (III). Groups II and III are subdivided into four subgroups according to the different dosages used (Table 44.3).

Standard of diagnosis and basis for grading of acute rejection

In diagnosis of acute rejection no biopsy was done for experimental animals except for those which had survived for a markedly longer than average period of time. The diagnosis of rejection is based on renal swelling, proteinuria and decreased urine output. Autopsy was done and a specimen was taken for histopathologic examination on death of all animals. Classification of severity of rejection is based on the results of histopathologic findings, as shown in Table 44.4.

RESULTS

Unmodified control group

This comprised 22 rabbits. Minimal rejection was noted after 3–5 days, moderate rejection after 6–7 days and marked rejection after 9 days. Most of the experimental rabbits died about 12 days after transplantation. Only a few rabbits survived for about 2 weeks (Figure 44.1).

Experimental groups

The results are shown in Table 44.5.

Assessment of results

Using experimental animals as organ transplantation models to study the curative effects of immunosuppressive drugs has advantages which cannot be

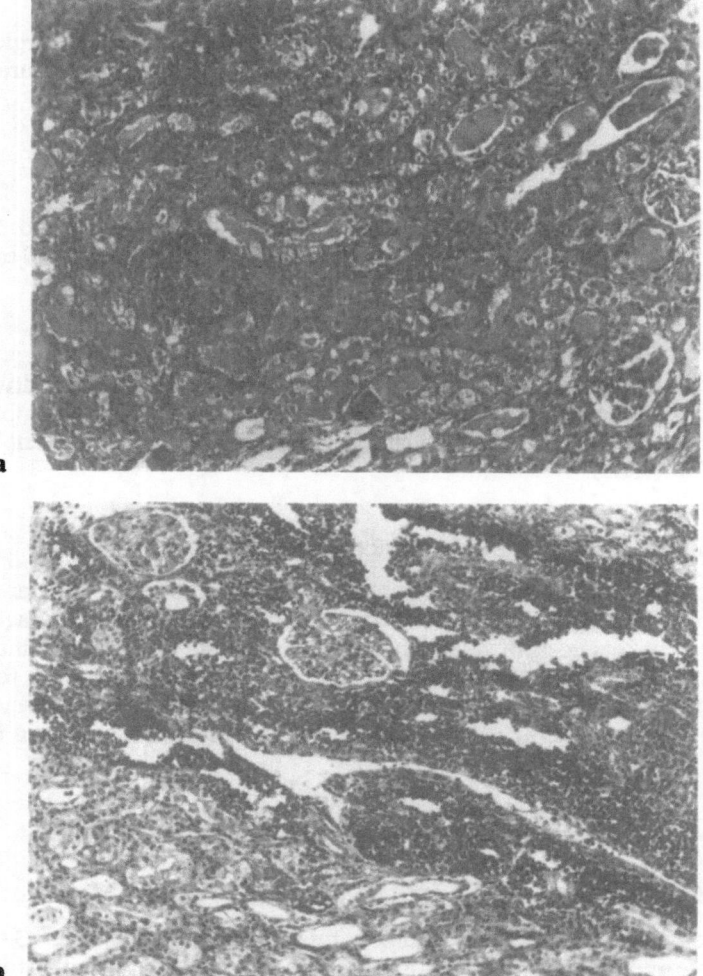

obtained by observation in vitro. Among its disadvantages are that the operative technique is more complicated, the consumption of manpower and material is greater, and many untoward factors intervene. The present raising and health conditions of animals at our laboratory cannot meet the desired requirements. So the rate of pneumonia and septicemia infection is high. These complications often cause the early death of animals operated on, thus preventing long term observation.

To meet these difficulties, we assessed the effect of drugs chiefly by post-mortem histopathologic examination of the grafted kidney and the side-effect of the drug in decreasing resistance as indicated by animal survival period.

The criteria for assessing the effect of the drug are as follows.

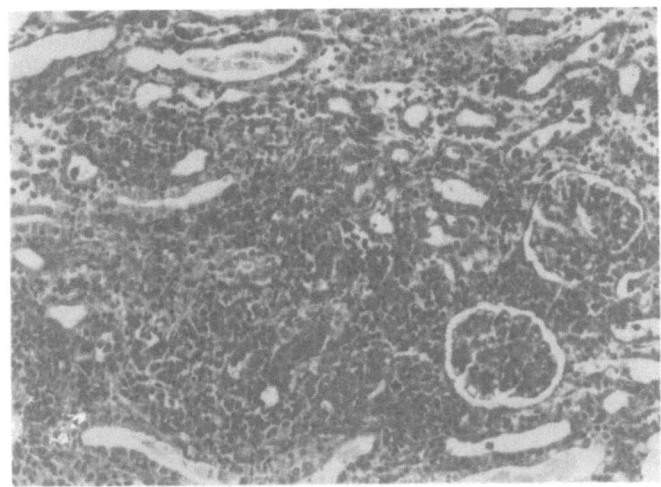

c

Figure 44.1 **a**. Rabbit No. 459. Four days after transplantation. Small patches of mononuclear cell infiltration in the interstitium, slight hemorrhage and widespread tubular necrosis.
b. Rabbit No. 458. Eight days after transplantation. Large patches of mononuclear cell infiltration in the interstitium, hemorrhage and fibrinoid change of the arteriolar wall
c. Rabbit No. 441. Eleven days after transplantation. Massive cellular infiltration and marked interstitial edema. Obliteration of lumen of the arterioles can be seen

(1) The assessment of effects on animals that died within 7 days. Some of the animals died of complications within 7 days. Under optical microscopy, the specimens in this category may be divided into two types. One type showed rejection in various degrees and the other showed no evidence of rejection. Cases of the first type, though the change might be slight (+), are counted as cases without effect. Cases of the second type, though no distinct effect was observed, as it occurred at the period when rejection barely takes place, could not serve as the basis to assess effects of the drug. So these cases are excluded from the statistics.

(2) Ineffective. Animals with any of the following findings are regarded as ineffective:

(a) rejection effect over (+), within 7 days after transplantation;
(b) rejection effect (+ +), within 15 days after transplantation;
(c) rejection effect (+ + +), 16–20 days after transplantation.

(3) Effective. The animals survived 8–15 days after transplantation.
     Urination appears nearly normal after removal of the right kidney. The cause of death is complication. Renal section only shows minimal rejection reaction (+). Generally at this period (8 days after transplantation) renal section of untreated animals would show moderate or massive rejection effect. So the effect of drugs in these cases could be defined.

(4)   Marked effect. Two types of animals fall into this category – animals that
survived for 15–19 days and whose sections showed rejection of moderate
level or below, and animals that survived for more than 20 days. Most
untreated animals died from rejection about 12 days after transplantation
and the sections showed severe rejection (Table 44.6).

Table 44.6   Standards for effect assessment

	Standards of assessment		
Effectiveness	Survival (days)	Rejection (autopsy)	Exception
No effect	1–7	over (+)	Animals that died
	7–15	(++)	within 7 days after
	16–19	(+++)	transplantation
Effect	8–15	(+) below	and showed no pathologic effect in
Marked effect	16–19	(++) below	the grafted kidney
	over 20		

The results of the experimental groups as classified by the above standards,
are shown in Table 44.8.

It should be pointed out that the grafted kidneys of all animals which have
survived for over 1 month after transplantation showed signs of chronic rejection. For example, animal No. 40, which received T No. 3 daily, survived for 120
days. During this period, azathioprine and prednisone were administered only
when signs of rejection – swelling and proteinuria etc – appeared, and when signs
of rejection disappeared administration of these two drugs was discontinued.
When the rejection reappeared the drugs were used again. This form of
administration was better than the others. But kidney biopsy done 40 days after
transplantation showed signs of chronic rejection (Figure 44.2; Table 44.7).

Table 44.7   Treatment of animal No. 40

Time of occurrence of rejection	Treatment (after transplantation)		Time of removing right kidney	Cause of death
1st 5 days after transplantation	Azathioprine Prednisone	15 mg b.i.d., 3 days		
2nd 14 days after transplantation	Azathioprine Prednisone	15 mg b.i.d., 3 days	9 days after transplantation	Chronic rejection
3rd 20 days after transplantation	Azathioprine Prednisone	15 mg b.i.d., 2 days		

Table 44.8 Evaluation of results

Group	Rabbits (n)	No effect	Effective	Marked effect	Exception
Control	12	11	—	—	1
Western medicine					
1.	11	5	6	—	—
2.	4	2	2	—	—
3.	8	4	2	2	1
4.	6	3	2	1	—
TCM combined with Western					
T No. 3					
1.	19	8	5	5	1
2.	15	9	4	2	—
3.	11	5	—	4	2
4.	8	3	3	2	—
T No. 8	9	4	1	3	1

DISCUSSION

Compared with the result of the untreated control group, both the immuno-suppressant group and the group treated with combined TCM and Western medicine show therapeutic effects.

Based on the data given in Table 44.8, the group treated with combined medicine show markedly better results than the group given immunosuppressant alone. According to statistical analysis (x^2 test), the ratio of animals having survived over 15 days is as follows:

$$x^2 = \frac{(22 \times 3 - 37 \times 2)^2 \times (22 + 37 + 2 + 13)}{59 \times 15 \times 24 \times 50} = 4.2181$$

$p < 0.05$.

TCM – T No. 8 group and immunosuppressant group:

$$x^2 = \frac{(26 \times 3 - 2 \times 5)^2 \times (26 + 5 + 2 + 3)}{31 \times 5 \times 8 \times 28} = 4.79447$$

$p < 0.05$.

So efficacy in the two groups treated with combined traditional Chinese and Western medicine is superior to that in the immunosuppressant group.

The immunosuppressant group is divided into four subgroups according to different dosages. Efficacy in the third and fourth subgroup with smaller dosage seemed better than that in the other two subgroups; statistical analysis $p < 0.05$. This shows the difference in efficacy.

Section of the autopsy specimens of the animals which have survived for over 1 month in the TCM group (Table 44.3) showed chronic rejection in the trans-planted kidney. This phenomenon demonstrated that the suppressive effect of this method on acute rejection is significant, but not so marked as it is on chronic rejection.

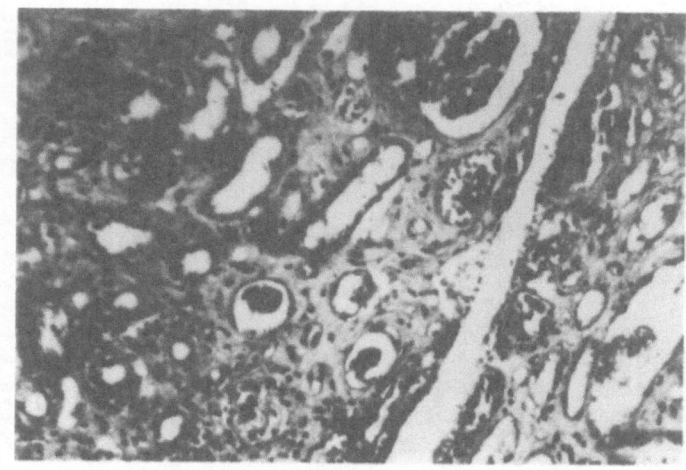

a

The study of suppressive effect on acute rejection of renal allotransplantation in rabbits, so far reported, showed that drugs such as azathioprine, prednisone, antilymphocyte serum and so on, except for cyclosporine A, failed to give satisfactory results. Though prednisone when administered continually is effective for acute rejection, its effective dose approximated an intoxicating dose.

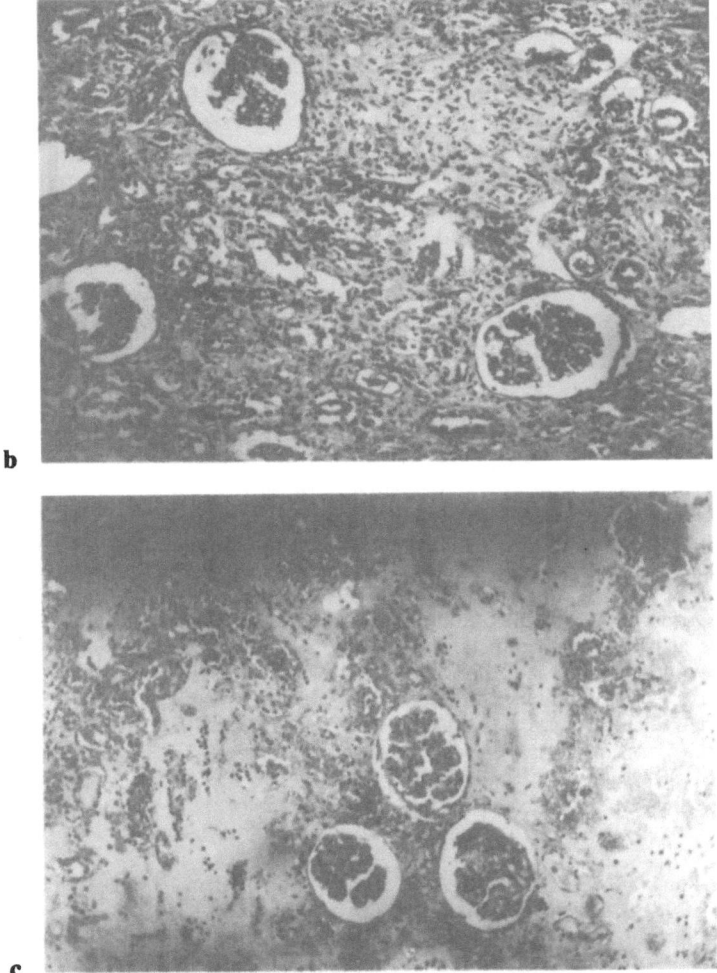

b

c

Figure 44.2 a. Rabbit No. 40. Fourth day. The section shows minimal cellular infiltration and interstitial collagen deposition.
b. Rabbit No. 40. Sixty-second day. Marked connective tissue proliferation and interstitial infiltration of rejection cells
c. Rabbit No. 40. 120 days. A greater part of the renal tissue lost its structure. Collapsed tubules and glomerular remnants can be seen

It is difficult for the animals to survive[8]. Use of TCM combined with Western drugs can reduce acute rejection of renal allotransplantation in rabbits and prolong their lives. So it is worthy of further study.

CONCLUSION

The search for a new immunosuppressant which can suppress the immunologic reaction and avoid severe side-effects is one of the urgent research topics in organ transplantation. Many investigators have been studying it from different angles and have achieved some progress. In the light of analyzing the patho-morphology caused by rejection and reviewing literature on 'activating the blood flow and resolving stasis', we tried to treat acute rejection with TCM combined with Western drugs. The experimental result suggested that this method could decrease the dosage of Western drugs and reduce their side-effects. There are 30–40 types of drug in daily use with the action of 'activating blood flow and resolving stasis'. In his *Correction of Medical Books*, Wang Zing-ren listed 22 varieties of prescriptions, from which we selected only a small number for our study. It would be a worthwhile piece of work to choose from them the most efficacious for this purpose.

REFERENCES

1. Qing Wan-zhang *et al.* (1977). Essentials of 'stasis symptoms' and the principles of activating the blood flow – a preliminary report. *J. Nature*, **2**, 115
2. Xia You-zhou *et al.* (1978). Use of combined traditional Chinese and Western medicine in the management of acute rejection of allotransplantation of kidney – a preliminary report. *J. Wuhan Med. Coll. (Transplant.)*, **4**, 66
3. Department of Combined Traditional Chinese and Western Medicine, Faculty of Basic Medical Sciences, Beijing Medical College (1978). Experimental studies on 'Huoxue Huayu' drugs. *Bull. Med. Technol. Beijing Med. Coll.*, **1**, 1
4. Department of Combined Traditional Chinese and Western Medicine, Faculty of Basic Medical Sciences, Beijing Medical College (1977). Studies on 'Huoxue Huayu' and its recent progress. *Bull. Med. Technol. Beijing Med. Coll.*, **2**, 117
5. Research Group of 'Huoxue Huayu', Shanghai First Medical College (1975). Scientific Research on Medicine (Special Collection of 'Huoxue Huayu'): Principles of 'Huoxue Huayu' and its application to clinical medicine. (Internal publication, 10)
6. Xu Li-na *et al.* (1976). Effects of 22 'Huoxue Huayu' drugs on the peripheral blood flow in dogs. *J. New Med.*, **5**, 38
7. Yan Lian-zuo *et al.* (1976). Effects of Chinese medicine 'Huoxue Huayu' herbs on the humoral immunologic responses in mouse. *J. Trad. Chinese Med.*, **9**, 61
8. Green, C. J. *et al.* (1978). Extensive prolongation of rabbit kidney allograft survival after short-term cyclosporin-A treatment. *Lancet*, **1**, 1182

Index